Current Perspectives on Nutrition and Health

Current Perspectives on Nutrition and Health

Edited by
Kenneth K. Carroll

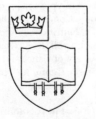

Published for The Royal Society of Canada by
McGill-Queen's University Press
Montreal & Kingston · London · Buffalo

© McGill-Queen's University Press 1998
ISBN 0-7735-1698-0 (cloth)
ISBN 0-7735-1724-3 (paper)

Legal deposit second quarter 1998
Bibliothèque nationale du Québec

Printed in Canada on acid-free paper

McGill-Queen's University Press acknowledges the
support of the Canada Council for the Arts for its
publishing program.

Canadian Cataloguing in Publication Data

Main entry under title:

Current perspectives on nutrition and health

These papers were prepared for a symposium held
at the University of Western Ontario, London,
Ontario, Canada, 16 to 19 June 1996, under the
sponsorship of the Royal Society of Canada, in
collaboration with the Centre for Human Nutrition,
the University of Western Ontario.

Includes bibliographical references and index.
ISBN 0-7735-1698-0 (bound)
ISBN 0-7735-1724-3 (pbk.)
1. Nutrition – Congress. 2. Diet in disease –
Congresses. 3. Nutritionally induced diseases –
Congresses. I. Carroll, K. K. (Kenneth Kitchener)
II. Royal Society of Canada. III. University of
Western Ontario. Centre for Human Nutrition.
RA784.C87 1998   613.2   C98-900200-4

Typeset in Palatino 10/12
by Caractéra inc., Quebec City

Contents

DIET AND CANCER

PRIORITIES FOR NUTRITION RESEARCH IN CANADA

KENNETH K. CARROLL

Foreword

The role of diet in maintenance of health and reduction of the risk of chronic disease is of continuing interest to health care professionals, to those concerned with the production and marketing of food, to governments coping with the escalating cost of health care, and to members of the general public. Research on the relationship between diet and chronic disorders such as cardiovascular disease, hypertension, kidney disease, diabetes, obesity, osteoporosis, and cancer has produced an abundance of data with vast implications for public health. Despite the overlap of interest in the role of diet in these various disorders, scientific meetings often focus on single diseases. Thus scientists and the public seldom have an opportunity to interact and consider the implications of this knowledge for overall health maintenance.

This symposium, like its predecessor in 1987, was designed to bring together leaders in this vast field to present to the scientific community and to the general public an update on different aspects of disease patterns, health maintenance, and dietary approaches to reducing the risk of chronic disease. It was sponsored by The Royal Society of Canada, in collaboration with the Centre for Human Nutrition at The University of Western Ontario.

This volume contains the proceedings of the symposium, which was held in the Richard Ivey School of Business Administration at The University of Western Ontario 16–19 June 1996. The format was similar to that of the 1987 symposium and included many of the same speakers. Like the earlier symposium it was focused on those diseases that have major implications for public health and are considered to be influenced by dietary patterns.

At the opening session on the evening of 16 June, participants were welcomed by Dr Paul Davenport, president of The University of Western Ontario, and Dr Robert H. Haynes, president of The Royal Society of Canada. There followed an introduction to the symposium by Dr Kenneth K. Carroll, director of the Centre for Human Nutrition, and the keynote address by Dr W. Phillip T. James.

As in the 1987 symposium, the program for the next two days consisted of four sessions of four speakers each, dealing with various aspects of the role of diet in health and disease. The first session was devoted to cardiovascular disease, and provided perspectives from various parts of the world, including Scandinavia, Eastern Europe, the South Pacific, and North America. Four diet-related health problems – hypertension, renal disease, diabetes, and obesity – were covered in the second session. The morning session on the second day dealt with diet and health maintenance and included presentations on osteoporosis, alcohol usage, the role of diet in the maintenance of health throughout life, and nutritional problems of the elderly. The afternoon session was devoted to presentations on various aspects of the role of diet in cancer.

The final session on the morning of Wednesday, 19 June, was entitled "Priorities for Nutrition Research in Canada." This featured a presentation on the development, consultation process, and highlights of a report from Health Canada on "Nutrition for Health: An Agenda for Action." This report originated from an International Conference on Nutrition convened by the World Health Organization (WHO) and the Food and Agriculture Organization (FAO) in Rome in 1993. At that conference Canada, along with other participating countries, endorsed a world declaration on nutrition and made a commitment to develop a national plan of action for nutrition. It is intended to reinforce healthy eating practices, to support nutritionally vulnerable populations, to enhance the availability of foods for healthy eating, and to support nutrition research. It is important that Canadians be aware of this plan and exert pressure on their elected representatives to ensure that it is implemented.

Several social events were planned in conjunction with the symposium. These included an all-day trip to Point Pelee on Sunday, 16 June. Point Pelee is Canada's smallest national park and, jutting as it does into Lake Erie, is the most southerly point on the Canadian mainland and is of particular interest to bird watchers, being part of the route followed by many migrating birds.

A banquet was held on Monday evening in the Great Hall of The University of Western Ontario. This was preceded by the Annual Shearer Public Lecture sponsored jointly by the Centre for Human Nutrition and the London-Region Interagency Nutrition Council (LINC). It was presented by Dr Helen Guthrie, Emerita Professor of the University of Pennsylvania, editor of *Nutrition Today*, and a graduate of Brescia College, The University of Western Ontario. The topic of her lecture was "Nutrition Today" and Dr Elizabeth Bright-See, chairman of the Department of Home Economics of Brescia College, acted as chairman. Following the banquet Dr David Kritchevsky entertained with a selection of his lyrics on themes relating to heart disease, set to well-known tunes. On Tuesday evening many of the participants travelled to the Shakespearean Theatre in the neighbouring town of Stratford for a performance of Meredith Willson's "The Music Man."

This compilation of presentations given at the symposium is primarily intended for dietitians, home economists, nutritionists, nurses, physicians, and other health care professionals concerned with the interpretation of research findings and their implementation for the general public. The educated lay person with an interest in the role of diet in health and disease may also find it a source of useful information.

Acknowledgments

The suggestion of holding a second symposium on diet, nutrition, and health came originally from Michael Dence, who at the time was executive director of The Royal Society of Canada. The idea was enthusiastically supported by Dr John Meisel, former president of the Society, and Dr Robert H. Haynes, its current president, and was approved by the Council of the Society.

We thank The University of Western Ontario and the Richard Ivey School of Business Administration for the use of facilities and for the excellent assistance of the staff with the physical arrangements, including audiovisual facilities, food services, and residence accommodation.

I particularly wish to thank my secretary, Charlotte Harman, for her invaluable assistance with correspondence, arrangements for the symposium, and the preparation of this volume, including the index. Thanks are also due to my wife, my colleagues, and students who assisted at the time of the symposium and helped to check the entries in the index.

We are most grateful to the organizations whose financial support made it possible to organize the symposium. In particular we wish to thank Dr John Meisel for arranging with Richard Van Loon, associate deputy minister, Health Canada, for major support by that ministry; Helen Bishop MacDonald, director of nutrition, Dairy Farmers of Canada, who responded promptly with a generous offer of support from that organization; and the Medical Research Council of Canada, who provided a substantial grant for the symposium. We also wish to express our appreciation to the other supporters and contributors to the symposium listed below.

Major Supporters
Health Canada
The Dairy Farmers of Canada
The Medical Research Council of Canada

Supporters
Canadian Atherosclerosis Society
Kellogg Canada Inc.
Heart and Stroke Foundation of Ontario
Merck Frosst Canada Inc.
Best Foods
International Olive Oil Council
Malaysian Palm Oil Promotion Council
State of Florida Department of Citrus

Contributors
Sandoz Nutrition
Serdary Research Laboratories Inc.
The Ontario Egg Producers' Marketing Board
Becel Heart Health Information Bureau
Eli Lilly Canada Inc./Boehringer Mannheim Canada
Tea Council of Canada
Uncle Ben's Rice
The Mutual Group

Finally we thank the individuals listed below, who chaired the scientific sessions and moderated the discussions that followed the presentations by each of the speakers.

Dr W. Robert Bruce, Department of Nutritional Sciences, University of Toronto
Dr Kenneth K. Carroll, Centre for Human Nutrition, The University of Western Ontario
Dr William F. Clark, Department of Medicine, The University of Western Ontario
Dr John Dupre, Department of Medicine, The University of Western Ontario
Dr M. Daria Haust, Department of Pathology, The University of Western Ontario
Dr Rudolf Poledne, Department of Preventive Cardiology, Institute for Clinical and Experimental Medicine, Prague
Dr Graham Pollett, Medical Officer of Health, Middlesex-London Health Unit, London, ON
Dr Bernard M. Wolfe, Department of Medicine, The University of Western Ontario
Dr Ernst L. Wynder, American Health Foundation, New York

Contributors

Dr Jonathan D. Adachi
Department of Medicine
St Joseph's Hospital
McMaster University
Suite 501, Charlton Avenue East
Hamilton, ON   L8N 1Y2

Dr Kenneth K. Carroll
Centre for Human Nutrition
Department of Biochemistry
The University of Western Ontario
London, ON   N6A 5C1

Dr S. George Carruthers
Department of Medicine
London Health Sciences Centre
University Campus
The University of Western Ontario
London, ON   N6A 5A5

Sonja L. Connor
Division of Endocrinology, Diabetes,
  and Clinical Nutrition
Department of Medicine, L465
Oregon Health Sciences University
3181 S.W. Sam Jackson Park Road
Portland, OR 97201-3098

Dr William E. Connor
Division of Endocrinology, Diabetes,
  and Clinical Nutrition
Department of Medicine, L465
Oregon Health Sciences University
3181 S.W. Sam Jackson Park Road
Portland, OR 97201-3098

M. Elisabeth Del Guidice
Department of Preventive Medicine
  and Biostatistics
Faculty of Medicine
University of Toronto
12 Queen's Park Crescent West
Toronto, ON   M5S 1A8

Dr Jean-Pierre Després
Lipid Research Centre
2705 Laurier Blvd, Bur. TR93
Ste-Foy, QC   G1V 4G2

Dr Guylaine Ferland
Centre de Recherche, Institut
  Universitaire de Gériatrie de
  Montréal
and Département de Nutrition
Université de Montréal
C.P. 6128, Succ. Centre-ville
Montréal, QC   H3C 3J7

George Ioannidis
Department of Medicine
St Joseph's Hospital
McMaster University
Suite 501, Charlton Avenue East
Hamilton, ON   L8N 1Y2

Dr W. Philip T. James
Rowett Research Institute
Greenburn Road
Bucksburn, Aberdeen
UK   AB21 9SB

Dr Jozef V. Joossens
Department of Epidemiology
Faculty of Medicine
University of Leuven
Capucijnenvoer 33
B-3000 Leuven, Belgium

Dr Harold Kalant
Addiction Research Foundation of
  Ontario, and Department of
  Pharmacology
Medical Sciences Building
University of Toronto
Toronto, ON   M5S 1A8

Dr Bertram L. Kasiske
Division of Nephrology
Department of Medicine
Hennepin County Medical Center
701 Park Avenue South
Minneapolis, MN 55415

Dr Hugo Kesteloot
Department of Epidemiology
Faculty of Medicine
University of Leuven
Capucijnenvoer 33
B-3000 Leuven, Belgium

Dr David Kritchevsky
The Wistar Institute
3601 Spruce Street
Philadelphia, PA 19104–4268

Dr J.I. Mann
Department of Human Nutrition
University of Otago
P.O. Box 56
Dunedin, New Zealand

Dr Gail McKeown-Eyssen
Department of Preventive Medicine
  and Biostatistics
Faculty of Medicine
University of Toronto
12 Queen's Park Crescent West
Toronto, ON   M5S 1A8

Joshua E. Muscat
American Health Foundation
320 East 43rd Street
New York, NY 10017

Mrs Heather Nielsen
Nutrition Programs Unit
Health Promotion and Programs
  Branch
Health Canada
Postal Locator 1917C
Tunney's Pasture
Ottawa, ON   K1A 1B4

Dr Sushma Palmer
Center for Communications, Health
  and the Environment (CECHE)
3333 K Street, N.W., Suite 110
Washington, DC   20007

Dr Alexandra Papaioannou
Department of Medicine
St Joseph's Hospital
McMaster University
Suite 501, Charlton Avenue East
Hamilton, ON   L8N 1Y2

Dr Pirjo Pietinen
National Public Health Institute
Department of Nutrition
Mannerheiminitie 166
Fin-00300 Helsinki, Finland

Dr Rudolf Poledne
Institute for Clinical and
  Experimental Medicine (IKEM)
Department of Preventive Cardiology
Prague, Czech Republic

Sylvie St-Pierre
Physical Activity Sciences Laboratory
PEPS, Laval University
Ste-Foy, QC   G1K 7P4

Dr Angelo Tremblay
Physical Activity Sciences Laboratory
PEPS, Laval University
Ste-Foy, QC   G1K 7P4

Dr Keiji Wakabayashi
Cancer Prevention Division
National Cancer Center Research
  Institute
1-1, Tsukiji 5-chome, Chuoku
Tokyo 104, Japan

Dr Thomas M.S. Wolever
Department of Nutritional Sciences
Faculty of Medicine
University of Toronto
Fitzgerald Building
150 College Street
Toronto, ON   M5S 3E2

Dr Ernst L. Wynder
American Health Foundation
320 East 43rd Street
New York, NY 10017

Keynote Address

W. PHILIP T. JAMES

The Evolution of Nutrition Research in Britain and Other European Countries

The evolution of nutrition research in Europe presents a fascinating picture because, however haphazard its development might seem to an individual scientist struggling to make an impact in his country, from a European perspective it is clear that we are now entering a new era. Nutrition is becoming an ever higher policy priority for most governments, for the European Union, and for other international bodies such as the United Nations. The same developments are evident, of course, in North America but the policy implications and responses are, for sociological reasons, very different. Nevertheless the reason for this renaissance in nutrition research seems to be the same on both sides of the Atlantic: the slowly emerging recognition that nutrition is the basis of many of the public health problems, currently so pressing, in ageing Western societies.

I would like to illustrate how two scientific endeavours have initiated change. First the agriculture research sector which, with its concern to produce appropriate food, has systematically funded new research opportunities in human nutrition. Second the epidemiological drive which, through the initiative of Keys and subsequent groups working in metabolic epidemiology, focused attention on diet as the basis of major health problems. Only later have the clinically orientated medical funding agencies responded and this response has usually been preceded by an academic-university recognition that students have become interested in nutrition because the media took up the issue of the importance of diet for personal health. In a previous lecture to a Royal Society Symposium here in London,

Ontario, I set out some of the battles that seem inevitably to develop in health policy making (1). Vested industrial interests often combine with naive government thinking on public health and diet to prevent coherent public health policies from being developed. These problems have re-emerged in Britain in the last few months as a dogma-driven government seems to near its electoral eclipse, but the detailed analysis of how scientific research in general, as well as nutritional research in particular, is supported must await another occasion.

Postwar Developments in European Nutrition Research

The European nutritional research field, postwar, was dominated by research in animal nutrition and studies on how manipulating the diet affected animal husbandry and production. Thus when I took over in 1982 the directorship of the Rowett Research Institute, I found it to be the largest nutrition research institute in the Western world and exclusively concerned with agricultural issues that were also the concern of 13 other British research institutes. This huge effort was seemingly justified by the priority assigned by the British government to self-sufficiency in food. There was a real determination that we would never again face the wartime crisis of growing less than a third of our food needs. This agricultural policy and research infrastructure was reproduced and promoted throughout Europe – and indeed throughout the world. Thus animal nutritionists dominated the nutritional journals, European nutrition societies, and European meetings, and often with a missionary zeal to improve the lot of small European farmers and their supporting industries. They were undertaking scientific research for the benefit of society by promoting the effectiveness of all the industries linked to farming.

U.K. Developments

I have described elsewhere how a reappraisal in Britain by the Neuberger Committee in 1973 set out a new agenda for nutritional research (2). Committee members were drawn from both agriculture and medicine and they recommended changes in both the relevant research councils. Thus the Dunn Nutrition Laboratory, where the hormonal nature of vitamin D had been discovered, was transformed in the early 1970s into an epidemiological and clinical centre, backed by the Medical Research Council. The Agricultural Research

Council also embarked on a completely new research program to reappraise the nutrient needs of humans. In 1982 I began the progressive addition of human studies to the animal research at the Rowett so that now our nutritional science applies to both animal and human nutrition throughout the institute. In addition to these institutional developments, a large number of personal university chairs in human nutrition have been established, initially by the Rank Prize Funds and subsequently by a large number of universities. Thus there are now 26 professors of human nutrition in our newly formed association for Britain and Eire.

Twenty years later the future of human nutrition research is again being reviewed by the U.K. government. Last year, as part of the Technology Foresight Programme, it was suggested that dietary aspects of ageing was, after biotechnology and bioengineering, the second highest priority, in terms of interest in the whole scientific spectrum of government activities, i.e., from defence through biological sciences to telecommunications, et cetera! Nutrition and the issue of interindividual variations in the response to diet were considered to have immense implications for both public welfare and for industry (3). This year, however, the U.K. government seemed to contradict these priorities by attempting to privatize, with about 50 other scientific centres, the 3 principal institutions now involved in food and nutritional research, viz., the Institute of Food Research, funded by the Biotechnology and Biological Research Council, the Medical Research Council's Dunn Nutrition Unit, and the Rowett, funded by the Scottish Office. This last development is a quirk of political fate in a government wedded, as a macho symbol of radicalism, to a break-up and privatization of all public sector operations and of any professional process. If its worst effects can be held at bay until the next election, then nutritional research may yet flourish. The current research themes in the 3 institutions are given in table 1.

The Agricultural Initiative in Human Nutrition

Note has already been made of the determination of the agricultural sector to promote the development of research in human nutrition, stimulated at least in part by the almost routine failure of the medical research community to accept its importance. With its postwar experiences of the value of substantial institutional effort to cope with complex problems, agriculture was much more willing than medical research workers to accept the value of promoting major programs

Table 1
The Principal Research Themes of the Nutrition Research Institutes in Britain

1 Dunn Nutrition Unit, Cambridge (Funded by the Medical Research Council)
  (a) Appetite control in humans: the role of macronutrients
  (b) Nutritional status and requirements of hospitalized, malnourished patients
  (c) Childhood growth and elderly osteoporosis
  (d) Colonic microbial metabolism and colonic carcinogenesis
  (e) Dietary carbohydrates: their measurement and intestinal effects
  (f) Epidemiological studies on diet and cancer
  (g) National nutritional surveillance of children and the elderly
  (h) Studies on protein-energy malnutrition in Gambian children
2 Institute of Food Research, Norwich and Reading (Funded by the Biotechnology and Biological Research Council)
  (a) Food metabolism and health: bioavailability of minerals and fat-soluble nutrients
  (b) Food choice and intake: choice and dietary change; mood and behavioural effects of food
3 Rowett Research Institute, Aberdeen (Funded by the Scottish Office)
  (a) The metabolic control of appetite and energy balance in humans and animals
  (b) The neurobiology of biorhythms
  (c) Maternal nutrition and fetal development
  (d) Intestinal processing and the systemic metabolism of peptides and amino acids
  (e) Intestinal development and health
  (f) The role of the intestinal microflora in health
  (g) The nutritional properties of plant foods and feeds
  (h) Free radicals and antioxidant processing
  (i) Trace elements and gene expression
  (j) Bone growth and turnover
  (k) International Feed Resource Unit

in human nutrition. Plant and animal genetic variations notwithstanding, the supply of an appropriate mix of nutrients for plant or animal growth was crucial and animal feed costs amounted to about 70% of all economic inputs in many enterprises.

The medical profession, by contrast, is dominated by the concept of the individual's unique and genetically determined metabolic propensity to disease, which has to be manipulated by drugs to produce dramatic changes evident to the physician and preferably to the patient also. Thus in Europe, and indeed in most of the rest of the Western world, it is the agricultural research organizations, e.g., Commonwealth Scientific and Industrial Research Organization (CSIRO) in Australia and the United States Department of Agriculture (USDA), who have taken up the challenge of research in human nutrition, and only later has the medical profession woken up to the substantial impact that dietary change can have.

Developments in Human Nutrition in the Netherlands

This has been well set out by Hautvast, who has made a great contribution in promoting an excellent undergraduate and PHD program in human nutrition research (4). The department itself began its activities in 1969 and has produced over 1000 students of nutrition and a large number of high-quality PHDs. Indeed the Netherlands, despite its small size, is one of the major forces in European nutritional research and many prominent investigators have developed, for example, major research programs in Bilthoven on obesity and cardiovascular disease, in Maastricht on sports nutrition and the role of dietary fatty acids in pregnancy, and in Zeist on nutritional epidemiology. Most of these endeavours owe their origins to the Wageningen School. More recently the nutritional impact of Wageningen has been further enhanced by the formation in 1994 of the graduate school, VLAG, for advanced studies in food technology, agrobiotechnology, nutrition, and health sciences. This graduate school aims to meld the interests of the Institute of Dairy Research in Ede with the TNO Nutritional Food Research Institute in Zeist, Utrecht University's Faculty of Veterinary Sciences, Nijmegen's Faculty of Medicine, and in Wageningen the Agrotechnological Research Institute, the Agricultural University, and the State Institute for Agriculture Quality Control.

Other European Initiatives

The diversion of agricultural funds into human nutrition also occurred in the early 1970s in Italy with its funding of Anna Ferro-Luzzi's Human Nutrition Unit in the National Institute of Nutrition. This centre was otherwise concerned with food technology and surveillance and some basic aspects of nutritional biochemistry. Elsewhere, however, there were more explicit initiatives.

Denmark, in 1986, decided to establish the Research Department of Human Nutrition within the Royal Veterinary and Agricultural University of Copenhagen. They wisely appointed Professor Isaksson, then retiring from the nutrition chair in Gothenberg, Sweden, to establish the centre, which rapidly flourished over its first three years. It is now led by Dr Astrup, who has expanded it rapidly, and in 1995 it took over a major new food sciences building. Its research areas are given in table 2.

France was not far behind with its Agricultural Research Service, INRA, establishing a division of human nutrition and building a

Table 2

The research themes of the Danish Nutrition Institute in Copenhagen
1 Nutrient effects on energy balance and obesity and related disorders
2 Diet and the prevention of cardiovascular disease and cancer
3 Minerals and trace element requirements
4 The determinants of dietary habits
5 Pediatric nutrition and subsequent health, especially bone growth
6 Nutrition in developing countries
7 Nutrition in prevention of osteoporosis

The research themes of the Human Nutrition Division of INRA, France
1 Energy and protein metabolism: their hormonal and nutritional regulation,
  particularly during ageing and stress
2 Role of complex carbohydrates and micronutrients (trace elements, vitamins,
  micro-components) in vegetables
3 Role of polyunsaturated fatty acid (PUFA): newborn requirements, trans-PUFA,
  cancerogenesis
4 Intestinal microflora: molecular characteristics, role in human health
5 Nutritional and hormonal regulation of digestion: exocrine and endocrine
  secretions, enterocyte and colonocyte metabolism of nutrients
6 Food safety: milk protein allergy, xenobiotics
7 Technology transfer in all these themes

The research themes of the German Nutrition Institute in Potsdam
1 Nutrition and cancer: the EPIC study and colonic responses to fibre
2 Nutrition and molecular genetics in hypertension; gene expression with stable
  isotopes; pathogenesis of obesity and amino acid requirements in adults
3 Study of intermediary and energy metabolism
4 Nutrition and the molecular control of carcinogenesis
5 Physiology of and immunological responsiveness to gut microflora
6 Oxidative stress and health: bioactive food components

The research themes of the Nutrition Research Institute in Oslo
1 Vitamin A: transport, metabolism, and function
2 Iron status, absorption and metabolism in deficiency and disease
3 Lipid metabolism and functional consequences
4 Food composition and surveys of food consumption nationally, in selected
  Norwegian areas and groups, and in the Third World
5 Development of new methods of dietary research and energy expenditure
6 Vitamin D deficiency as a health problem

---

specially designed unit for studies on energy and protein metabolism in 1990 in Theix linked up with the animal nutrition research in
the INRA centres in Clermont Ferrand. Its research themes are also
listed in table 2.

Germany then established its Potsdam Institute as a newly constituted Federal Centre for Studies on Human Nutrition with a

completely new research program under Barth's directorship. The centre is funded by both federal and local governments but, in this case, the funding relates – almost for the first time in Europe – to the medical research side. Table 2 includes its principal research fields.

Norwegian developments have also become very prominent with the opening of a major and beautifully designed centre at the medical school in Oslo to house the three original institutes for nutrition which included the Nordic School of Nutrition (table 2).

Other European University-Based Developments

The listing so far does not claim to be comprehensive and certainly does little justice to the renaissance in nutritional science in Europe. Spanish developments are now becoming much more prominent, with a new human nutrition unit in Reus Medical School in Tarragon, and a substantial interest in epidemiology and obesity research in Barcelona, to mention only a few Spanish initiatives. Sweden developed its facilities for human nutritional research in Uppsala and has supported a welter of world-class research in obesity and iron metabolism from Gothenberg and in molecular aspects of nutrition from Stockholm. In Ireland there has also been rapid progress to stimulate close interaction between centres of nutritional expertise in Dublin, Cork, Belfast, and Coleraine, with new chairs of nutrition established to promote a very effective research collaboration. Belgium's interest in nutrition has also always been strong since the early postwar epidemiological work on cardiovascular disease and more recent work on lipid metabolism and fetal development. The Leuven School, with the Maastricht Medical School, now runs the annual European Clinical Nutrition Course, with backing from the European Union and the European Diabetic Association.

Euragri

This is an informal group composed of the national directors of agricultural research within the European Union. They meet at regular intervals to discuss issues of concern to all or to a substantial portion of the EU. For the last three years they have been wondering how best to promote the development of human nutrition because they recognize that the whole of the agricultural food chain in Europe has been founded on a set of principles that no longer match modern concepts of human nutrition. They also recognize that a failure to anticipate or link the developments in plant selection and modification, animal production, food processing, or issues relating to food safety, with new concepts of human nutrition could cause them immense problems. After discussions with the EU and a wide range of scientists, they have now established a group, under the chairmanship of INRA's director general, Dr Chevassus, to assess and promote research in European priorities for human nutrition research. These will be linked to consumer interests and will be incorporated into the plant, animal, and food research programs. This ambitious program is now underway and symbolizes the commitment of those concerned with policy making in European agriculture to ensuring that the priority for both agriculture and food research should be human welfare and not the short-term profit of one sector of an industry involved in the food chain.

Nutritional Epidemiology

I consider that much of modern research into the nutritional basis of adult chronic diseases stems from the work of Keys and his colleagues. They combined, in a novel way, metabolic and nutritional epidemiology on coronary heart disease (CHD) with meticulous physiological studies on volunteers to monitor the effect of dietary fatty acids and cholesterol on serum lipids (5). Keys, having already conducted the classic Minnesota studies on semi-starvation (6), was therefore well able to take a physiological approach in his attempts to explain the extraordinary disparity in the rates of coronary heart disease in different parts of the world. I am emphasizing the physiological point because, with the explosion of epidemiological studies on cardiovascular disease and cancers on both sides of the Atlantic since the mid-1970s, the emphasis given to the process of surveys and their analyses has become extremely sophisticated but often seems to have diverted attention away from how best to explore the biological basis for so many of these diseases.

It seems reasonable to conclude that apart from the valuable follow-up studies on the Keys cohorts for CHD, the principal epidemiological effort in Europe has gone into surveillance systems, e.g., the MONICA surveys linked through WHO centres, and intervention studies, e.g., the WHO factory trial and Scandinavian lipid-lowering trials. These will doubtless be considered elsewhere in this volume. Britain was unusual in that the cardiovascular epidemiologists, e.g., Morris, Rose, Shaper, Mead, and Elwood, found it difficult to study diet in their modest cohort studies – indeed they were advised to give it up by Marr, the then expert on dietary surveys working with Morris. The Miller brothers' discovery of the importance of HDL-cholesterol levels (7), George Miller's identification of the role of fat in promoting pro-thrombotic changes (8), and his identifying the unusual propensity of Asian migrants to heart disease (9) led, however, to a more appropriate and integrated view of the complex processes leading to CHD. These, together with Renaud's meticulous metabolic epidemiological approach in France and elsewhere to the fatty acid effects on platelet function and clotting (10) and his recent secondary prevention trial on CHD (11), have all been singularly important in emphasizing the variety of dietary mechanisms that contribute to CHD.

These studies were underway as the U.K. battle for implementing national dietary guidelines raged, as set out in the symposium here six years ago (1). In Britain cardiological epidemiologists were divided. Thus Mead and Elwood seemed to consider diet to be of little importance compared with other risk factors, whereas Rose, Marmot, and Shaper accepted its role but dealt with other issues, such as the social class gradient or regional differences in CHD, with little emphasis on dietary methodology. Oliver was one of several cardiologists who were involved in drug trials and took the same jaundiced view of the potential hazards of diet as they did of drugs. Therefore the importance of diet as a major risk factor for cardiovascular disease depended, in Britain, on Rose, Shaper, and Marmot's constant efforts to highlight the value of a population approach to community dietary change. Their efforts were, however, constantly undermined.

Antioxidants and Cardiovascular Disease

Gey, then working for Hoffman-la-Roche on vitamin metabolism, played a major role in promoting epidemiological research on antioxidants by organizing a substantial cross-cultural case-control study of patients with myocardial infarction (12). The extension of these regional studies to encompass different areas with known rates of myocardial infarction revealed that the rates of smoking, hypertension and hypercholesterolemia could be good indices of individual risk within each community, but the community differences in cardiovascular disease were best explained by their strong association with the circulating α-tocopherol and vitamin C levels in the plasma (13,14). In smokers the best index of protection was the β-carotene concentration of adipose tissue (15) which probably served as a marker of vegetable intake. Other studies at the Rowett confirmed the lower plasma ascorbate concentration of smokers, their greater susceptibility to oxidative stress, and the remedial effects of α-tocopherol (16). Thus although much of the original biology on the cellular oxidative processes controlling LDL uptake by scavenger receptors in endothelium was North American (17), much of the clinical and epidemiological stimulus for this hypothesis came from Europe.

Fetal Nutrition and Adult Disease

This is very much a European development with Forsdahl (18) in the early days specifying a surprising link between the infant mortality rate in different regions of Norway and cardiovascular death rates 60 years later. Barker seemed to confirm this in Britain, despite concern for the confounding effect of persisting socio-economic differences. Barker has since undertaken a very large number of studies that have highlighted first the links between birth weight and subsequent hypertension, then between placental/birth-weight ratios and hypertension, and more recently between more subtle indices of disproportionate growth, e.g., the ponderal index or abdominal circumference at birth and the risk of glucose intolerance in 20-year-old adults, insulin resistance in middle age, and the risk of diabetes and coronary heart disease. These studies have been summarized in two books substantially written by Barker (19,20). Experimental support for fetal programming is extensive and long standing but more recently Hales and Barker (21) have suggested that a poor maternal diet – and a paucity of protein in particular – can lead to impaired pancreatic islet cell function. Perhaps more persuasively Jackson has induced hypertension in the offspring of rats fed a low-protein diet. This treatment seems to induce fetal hypercorticoidism by reducing the 11β-oxysterol dehydrogenase activity of the placenta, thereby allowing an excess of maternal cortisol to enter the fetal circulation (22).

Elsewhere (23) I have set out how maternal protein, iron, and essential fatty acid metabolism may affect fetal growth and placental function in different stages of pregnancy, but three other features may prove to be particularly important. First is the question of whether fetal malnutrition can lead to adult abdominal obesity as suggested by Law et al. (24). This can then be linked with Bjorntorp's demonstration of a hypothalamic-pituitary-adrenal (HPA) axis that is hyperresponsive to stress (25). This in turn invited the hypothesis that fetal hypercorticoidism induced, for example, by protein status changes in the mother may reset the HPA axis so that the hyper-responsiveness stimulates a Cushing-like syndrome thereby leading to abdominal obesity with all its complications, as in Syndrome X (23). If so this could explain the propensity to abdominal obesity, diabetes, and CHD in Asian migrants who initially have a low BMI and lean body mass and who eat a rice-based diet low in total protein and in a variety of essential amino acids.

Nutrient-Gene Interactions in Folate Metabolism

This may prove a particularly important explanation of part of the Barker hypothesis because it has long been known that folate deficiency can lead to small babies (26). This has been recently confirmed in the U.S. (27). Since, however, it has recently been shown that the folate requirements may be raised in 6% of individuals with a homozygous single base change in the gene controlling 5,10-methylene-tetrahydrofolate reductase (28) and that this astonishingly frequent abnormality is associated with neural tube defects (NTD) (29), it seems reasonable now to expect low birth weight (LBW) babies to show a higher prevalence of this reductase abnormality. They are also more likely to have hyperhomocysteinemia in their childhood and adult life if their folate intakes are "normal" for most Western societies. High levels of plasma homocysteine are now a recognized independent risk factor for CHD. Thus some of the Barker hypotheses may simply signify the outcome of modest maternal folate intakes on fetal growth and of adult folate intakes in those who have the gene defect. It is perhaps not coincidental that 400 mg folate is both the proposed preventive dose for NTD (30) and the intake needed to keep plasma homocysteine at their lowest level in an adult population (31).

Optimum Intakes of Nutrients and Dietary Bioactivity

One further emerging theme of European research concerns the issue of optimum nutrient intakes. With the recent proposals for EU-wide recommended dietary intakes (but in practice called reference nutrient intakes to highlight that these are a statistical reference point rather than true RDAs) comes the proposal by Gey (32) that there are optimum intakes of α-tocopherol and vitamin C that are higher than those needed to avoid deficiency disease. The folate findings, cited above, are another and the proposal by Fraga et al. (33) that 100 mg dietary ascorbate is needed to limit oxidative damage to DNA is a further example of shifting opinions. To these issues we now need to add a welter of European research into flavonoids (34) and other polyphenols and their effects on oxidative systems.

Progressive DNA Damage and Carcinogenesis

These studies on oxidative damage led to new work in the U.K. showing a progressive accumulation of DNA damage (35) and the options for manipulating oxidative changes by altering antioxidant intake (36). Smokers, with their increased ascorbate requirements, have 50–100% more damage than normal non-smoking British adults, but little is known as yet about these changes in people on higher antioxidant intakes, e.g., in the Mediterranean area.

Epidemiological research on cancer in Europe has not favoured the massive cohort studies that seem to be so readily funded in the U.S., but recently a large 50,000 individual cross-European (EPIC) study has been launched to assess diet in relation to cancer. The Cambridge group has, however, also been concentrating on metabolic studies, particularly in relation to colon cancer, with recent very sophisticated studies now suggesting that meat intakes can induce *de novo* N-nitroso compound formation within the colon, with an increase in ammonia formation (37). Red meat seems to be particularly conducive to promoting the formation of these N-nitroso compounds, perhaps because of the additional iron intake, but whether resistant starch and all the other non-starch polysaccharide components, often unmeasured for example in the AOAC method for fibre analysis, can counteract the effects of a high-meat diet as suggested by inter-country metabolic data (38–40) remains to be assessed.

These studies have another significance that may provide a European perspective on nutrition research and that relates to the approach to epidemiology. In North America especially, the cohort study is coming to be seen as the gold standard of epidemiological analyses whereas in Europe there is a clear recognition that such studies are fundamentally limited as analytical tools. Not only are there methodological errors in estimating food intake but these errors and the outcomes interact and multiply, as emphasized by the Cambridge statistical group (41,42). There is in addition a fundamentally important failure by some North American epidemiologists to recognize the role of interindividual variation in dietary responsiveness. Thus dietary cohort studies of CHD rarely link saturated fats to CHD disease rates because the genetically determined differences in basal LDL-cholesterol levels, and in their responsiveness to changes in saturated fatty acid intakes, are not taken into account. Thus, as in Keys' days, we need a combination of metabolic and epidemiological studies – preferably undertaken in the Swedish manner where subsets of a cohort may be asked to volunteer for detailed studies. The astonishing success rates of Scandinavian volunteer studies are not emulated elsewhere in Europe, but the Swedish approach does give a coherence to the metabolic-epidemiological perspective that is unprecedented. There is also great value in cross-country metabolic studies of defined and properly sampled population groups that allow the range of dietary intakes to be extended and thereby contribute to revealing the causal dietary factors. Intermediate indices of risk in the disease process are also invaluable in overcoming the problem of interindividual variations.

Analyses of Preventive Strategies in Public Health

In North America I suspect there is almost no understanding of public health in terms of policy making because it is usually assumed that the only basis for improving health is through individual education. This neglects the immense contribution of legislation and a huge variety of policy initiatives that extend well beyond taxation policies. In Europe, however, it has been well recognized for many decades that local and central governments have an important role to play in conditioning the environment so that individuals' habits are more conducive to health. Thus Norwegian policies have included agricultural initiatives, transport subsidies, and health service changes to promote the consumption of more appropriate foods and alert the population to the problems of CHD.

In Britain there was a remarkable acceptance by our right-wing government of the interplay of different sectors in determining dietary patterns, as set out in *Health of the Nation* (43). Now, however, we see a progressive backsliding in policy making as government seeks both to continue the promotion of individual rather than societal responsibilities and to respond to the lobbying efforts of vested industrial interests. Recently I was involved in producing a new analysis of the preventive measures for obesity based on both physiological and public health principles (44). Rose was the first to point out that the proportion of a population that is obese can be predicted confidently from the average BMI of the population (45). This implies that it is foolish to think of truncating a rising national or skewed distribution in body weights as a preventive measure. What is required is an examination of those factors that determine the secular increase in weight of the population, as explained elsewhere (46).

In essence two principal factors interact to induce a positive energy balance, viz., low physical activity and a high dietary energy density such as that found with a fat-enriched diet. This is clearly shown in physiological studies (47), but general epidemiological studies of dietary fat in relation to BMI are obscured by the seemingly enhanced sensitivity of those with familial obesity to weight gain (48). Women make considerable efforts to restrain consciously their eating in an attempt to remain thin and this also obscures the dietary fat–obesity relationship in cohort studies. Since the obesity report was produced Prentice has refined the analyses of physical activity and dietary fat and found in the U.K. that physical inactivity seems now to be particularly important (49).

Our analyses of physical activity lead to huge public health issues. If people need to remain physically active, e.g., with a physical activity level (PAL) of 1.7 to 1.8 times their basal metabolic rate, then our analyses show that this is very difficult to achieve by leisure activity alone. One needs 3–4 hours per day on one's feet, walking or cycling, to achieve these levels, but the whole of Western society's town planning is based on the motor car and on the idea of minimizing walking, climbing stairs, or cycling. In many North American cities it is difficult if not impossible to find the stairs in a hotel, cycle paths are relatively unknown, and walking is dangerous. Many supermarkets are out of reach of all those without a car and children are not encouraged to play in the street, to walk or cycle to school, or to limit their television viewing. Thus traffic and town-planning policies are fundamental to modulating spontaneous physical activity and since physically active children are the most responsive as adults to health promotion for taking exercise, we are clearly not recognizing the role of local and central government policies in modifying our lifestyles.

Management and Preventive Strategies for Obesity

New developments are underway in Scotland to change management strategies in obesity with newly defined criteria for the waist measurement as an index of risk. Management in primary health care centres is proposed with new approaches including the valid long-term use of obesity-slimming drugs to induce modest but sustained weight loss. A special centre is also proposed for the surgical management of severe obesity. This approach has been stimulated by the remarkable but still-not-fully published findings emerging from the national trial of gastroplasty in Sweden.

WHO is now considering the whole interplay of prevention and management strategies in view of the worldwide epidemic of obesity, so an international task force has been established to develop and promote more effective strategies for obesity prevention and management.

In Britain we followed the Health of the Nation initiative with a nutrition task force that aimed to cooperate with industry to reduce the fat content of normal foods by modest amounts. Unsurprisingly the food industry declared its satisfaction with the current composition of its foods and considered there was no room for reducing fat intakes further despite evidence from Scandinavia that this was possible. New food technology techniques also allow a remarkable reduction in the fat content of many processed foods without any deleterious organoleptic effects (50). Thus the health of the British continues to be sabotaged by those who simply declare that "education" is the answer. Yet all our analyses reveal that current food labelling and educational measures are not understood by the average child or adult. Given nutritionists' development of RDAs, based on ensuring, by the use of the 2 Standard Deviation limit, that everybody's needs are met, it could be argued that nutrition education should logically adopt a mean intelligence quotient minus 2 Standard Deviations as the limit above which everybody should be able to comprehend and indeed remember nutrition educational material. On these criteria I suggest that most, if not all, current nutritional educational techniques would fail but there seems to have been little research on this point.

These issues become important because our recent Scottish Diet Report (51) has been followed by an action plan to see how best to improve diet throughout life – from maternal feeding during pregnancy and breast-feeding through to old age. This is but one example of many recent national policy initiatives that highlight the new acceptance of diet as fundamental to health and the avoidance of a wide range of chronic diseases.

Conclusions

One can confidently predict that European nutrition research will expand and improve. The big challenge, however, is to see whether we can organize a pan-European approach to developing the resources, including facilities, that are appropriate for the newly recognized importance of nutrition in medical therapy and public health. With most nations trying to constrain their public spending, the pressure to arrest the escalating numbers of scientists will grow so nutrition research, seen as slow moving and difficult, will need to compete. This competition requires a recognition of the value of molecular biology to many nutritional studies and demands the promotion of high quality nutrition research so that it can be judged on the same basis as other scientific fields. We are now favoured, however, because of the widespread recognition in political and policy circles that nutrition is important.

Acknowledgments*

My understanding of the complex interrelationships between agriculture and health issues has been greatly enhanced by the support of my work by the Scottish Office Agriculture, Environment and Fisheries Department. Dr Ann Ralph has also helped me for many years in these endeavours; I am very grateful for this support.

REFERENCES

1 James WPT. Dietary guidelines and the development of a European policy. In: Carroll KK, ed. *Diet, nutrition, and health.* Montreal & Kingston: McGill-Queen's University Press, 1990:3–15.
2 Neuberger Committee. *Food and nutrition research. Report of Joint Agricultural Research Council and Medical Research Council Committee.* London: HMSO, 1973.

---

* This contribution was written during the last months of the Conservative government. Since May 1997 the Labour party has been in power and there has been a change in philosophy that may benefit attitudes to nutrition research in Britain.

3 Technology Foresight Steering Group. *Progress through partnership.* London: Office of Science and Technology, 1995.

4 Hautvast JG. The future of nutrition in Europe. *Eur J Clin Nutr* 1993;47(suppl 1):s96—s100.

5 Keys A. *Seven countries. A multivariate analysis of death and coronary heart disease.* Cambridge, MA, London: Harvard University Press, 1980.

6 Keys A, Brozek J, Henschel A, Mickelson O, Tayler HL. *The biology of human starvation.* Minneapolis: University of Minnesota Press, 1950.

7 Miller GJ, Miller NE. Plasma-high-density-lipoprotein concentration and development of ischaemic heart disease. *Lancet* 1975;1:16–19.

8 Miller GJ, Cruickshank JK, Ellis LJ. Fat consumption and factor VII coagulant activity in middleaged men. An association between a dietary and thrombogenic coronary risk factor. *Atherosclerosis* 1989;78:19.

9 Beckles GLA, Miller GJ, Kirkwood RR et al. High total and cardiovascular disease mortality in adults of Indian descent in Trinidad, unexplained by major coronary risk factors. *Lancet* 1986;2:1298–1300.

10 Renaud S, Godsey F, Dumont E, Thivenon C, Ortchanian E, Martin JL. Influence of long-term diet modification on platelet function and composition in Moselle farmers. *Am J Clin Nutr* 1986;43:136–150.

11 De Lorgeril M, Renaud S, Mamill N et al. Mediterranean α-linolenic acid-rich diet in secondary prevention of coronary heart disease. *Lancet* 1994;343:1454–1459.

12 Gey KF, Puska P. Plasma vitamins E and A inversely correlated to mortality from ischemic heart disease in cross-cultural epidemiology. *Annals New York Acad Sci* 1989;570:268–282.

13 Gey KF, Moser UK, Jordan P, Stahelin HB, Eicholzer M, Ludin E. Increased risk of cardiovascular disease at suboptimal plasma concentrations of essential antioxidants: an epidemiological update with special attention to carotene and vitamin C. *Am J Clin Nutr* 1993;57:787s–797s.

14 Gey KF, Puska P, Jordan P, Moser UK. Inverse correlation between plasma vitamin E and mortality from ischemic heart disease in cross-cultural epidemiology. *Am J Clin Nutr* 1991;43:326s–334s.

15 Kardinaal AFM, Kok FJ, Ringstad J et al. Antioxidants in adipose tissue and risk of myocardial infarction: the EURAMIC study. *Lancet* 1993;342:1379–1384.

16 Duthie GG, Arthur JR, James WPT. Effects of smoking and vitamin E on blood antioxidant status. *Am J Clin Nutr* 1991;53:1061s–1063s.

17 Steinberg D, Parthasarathy S, Carew TE, Khoo JC, Witzum JL. Beyond cholesterol: modifications of low-density lipoprotein that increase its atherogenicity. *N Engl J Med* 1989;320:915–924.

18 Forsdahl A. Are poor living conditions in childhood and adolescence an important risk factor for arteriosclerotic heart disease? *Br J Prev Med* 1977;31:91–95.

19 Barker DJP, ed. *Fetal and infant origins of adult disease.* London: BMJ Publishing Group, 1992.

20 Barker DJP. *Mothers, babies and disease in later life.* London: BMJ Publishing Group, 1994.

21 Hales CN, Barker DJP. Non insulin-dependent (type II) diabetes mellitus: thrifty genotype hypothesis. In: Barker DJP, ed. *Fetal and infant origins of adult disease.* London: BMJ Publishing Group, 1992:258–272.

22 Langley-Evans SC, Jackson AA. Increased systolic blood pressure in adult rats caused by fetal exposure to maternal low protein diets. *Clin Sci* 1994;86:217–222.

23 James WPT. Long-term fetal programming of body composition and longevity. *Nutr Rev* 1997;55:S31–S43.

24 Law CM, Barker DJP, Osmand C et al. Early growth and abdominal fatness in adult life. *J Epidemiol Community Health* 1992;46:184–186.

25 Bjorntorp P. Endocrine abnormalities of obesity. *Metabolism Clinical and Experimental* 1995;44(suppl 3):21–23.

26 Baumslag N, Edelstern T, Metz J. Reduction of incidence of prematurity by folic acid supplementation in pregnancy. *Br Med J* 1970;1:16–17.

27 Scholl TO, Hediger ML, Schall JI, Khoo C-S, Fischer RL. Dietary and serum folate: their influence on the outcome of pregnancy. *Am J Clin Nutr* 1996;63:520–525.

28 Whitehead AV, Gallagher P, Mills JL et al. A genetic defect in 5,10 methylenetetrahydrofolate reductase in neural tube defects. *Q J Med* 1995;88:763–766.

29 Steegers-Theunissen RPM, Boers GHJ, Trijbels FJM et al. Maternal hyperhomocysteinemia: a risk factor for neural-tube defects? *Metabolism* 1994;43:1475–1480.

30 Expert Advisory Group. *Folic acid and the prevention of neural tube defects – Report from an expert advisory group.* Department of Health, Scottish Office Home and Health Department, Welsh Office, Department of Health and Social Services, Northern Ireland, 1993.

31 Boushey CJ, Beresford SAA, Omenn GS, Motulsky AG. A quantitative assessment of plasma homocysteine as a risk factor for vascular disease. Probable benefits of increasing folic acid intakes. *JAMA* 1995;274:1049–1057.

32 Gey KF. Longterm adequacy of all major antioxidants, presumably in synergy with other vegetable-derived nutrients may help to prevent

early stages of cardiovascular disease and cancer respectively. *Internat J Vit Nutr Res* 1995;65:1–4.

33 Fraga CG, Motchink PA, Shigenaga MK, Helbock HJ, Jacob RA, Ames BN. Ascorbic acid protects against endogenous oxidative DNA damage in human sperm. *Proc Natl Acad Sci USA* 1991;88:11003–11006.

34 Knekt P, Jarvinen R, Reunanen A, Maatela J. Flavonoid intake and coronary mortality in Finland: a cohort study. *Br Med J* 1996;312:478–481.

35 Cole J, Waugh APW, Beare DM, Salat-Trepat M, Stephens G, Green MHL. HPRT mutant frequencies in circulating lymphocytes: population studies using normal donors, exposed groups and cancer-prone syndromes. *Prog Clin Biol Res* 1991;372:319–329.

36 Duthie SJ, Ma A-g, Ross MA, Collins AR. Antioxidant supplementation decreases oxidative DNA damage in human lymphocytes. *Cancer Res* 1996;56:1291–1295.

37 Bingham SA, Pignatelli B, Pollock JRA et al. Does increased endogenous formation of N-nitroso compounds in the human colon explain the association between red meat and colon cancer? *Carcinogenesis* 1996;17:515–523.

38 International Agency for Research on Cancer. International collaborative study on diet and large bowel cancer in Denmark and Finland. *Nutr Cancer* 1982;4:3–79.

39 Cummings JH, Bingham SA, Heaton KW, Eastwood MA. Fecal weight, colon cancer risk and dietary intake of non-starch polysaccharides (dietary fiber). *Gastroenterol* 1992;103:1783–1789 (abstract).

40 Cassidy A, Bingham SA, Cummings JH. Starch intake and colorectal cancer risk: an international comparison. *Br J Cancer* 1994;69:937–942.

41 Plummer M, Clayton D. Measurement error in dietary assessment: an investigation using covariance structure models. *Statistics in Medicine* 1993;12 part I:925–935: part II:937–948.

42 Plummer M, Clayton D, Kaaks R. Calibration in multi-centre cohort studies. *Int J Epidemiol* 1994;23:419–426.

43 Department of Health. *The health of the nation: A strategy for health in England.* London: HMSO, 1992.

44 Department of Health. *Obesity. Reversing the increasing problem of obesity in England. A report from the nutrition and physical activity task forces.* London: HMSO, 1994.

45 Rose G. Population distributions of risk of disease. *Nutr Metab Cardiovasc Dis* 1991;1:37–40.

46 James WPT. A public health approach to the problem of obesity. *Int J Obes* 1995;19(suppl 3):S37–S45.

47 Stubbs RJ. Macronutrient effects on appetite. *Int J Obes* 1995;19(suppl. 5):s11–s19.

48 Heitmann BL, Lissner L, Sorensen TIA, Bengtsson C. Dietary fat intake and weight gain in women genetically predisposed for obesity. *Am J Clin Nutr* 1995;61:1213–1217.

49 Prentice AM, Jebb SA. Obesity in Britain: gluttony or sloth? *Br Med J* 1995;311:437–439.

50 Brooker BE. Role of fat in bread doughs. *J Scanning Microscopes* Proc Found Adv Science and Medicine, USA, March 1995;17(5):v81/v82.

51 Scottish Office. *The Scottish diet. Report of a working party to the chief medical officer for Scotland*. Edinburgh: 1993.

Diet and
Cardiovascular Disease

SUSHMA PALMER and RUDOLF POLEDNE

Perspectives from Eastern Europe

From Poland to Bulgaria and across Ukraine and Russia, among the greatest threats to "life, liberty, and the pursuit of happiness," to productivity, social stability, and democracy is a further decline in an already bleak health picture in Central and Eastern Europe. Hungarians have among the highest cardiovascular disease (CVD) mortality rates in the world; Russian male life expectancy has fallen to 59 years in the last two decades and is dropping; lung cancer rates, already among the highest, are going up; once-stalled infectious diseases have re-emerged and spread.

A decisive breakthrough in reversing this trend can be made by targeted assistance to the professional community, raising public awareness of personal steps to improve health, and motivating policy makers to adopt progressive policies. In the United States, Australia, and elsewhere heart attack rates have fallen some 40% in the last three decades due to improved diagnosis and treatment but also in no small measure due to increased public awareness through television, newspapers, and other educational programs that have motivated people to improve their diets, reduce smoking, and take regular exercise. Most Russians, Poles, and others in the region are still struggling to accept the link between smoking and lung cancer, diet and heart disease.

The Center for Communications, Health and the Environment, formerly the Central European Center for Health and the Environment (CECHE), has been working throughout the region using various approaches to health promotion. The following provides some brief

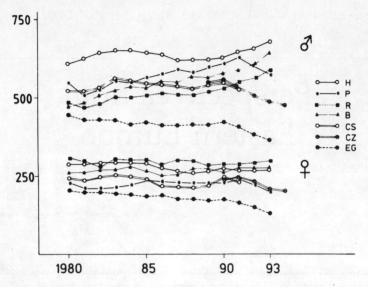

Figure 1. Total mortality. Number of deaths/100,000/year, under age 70. Data from World Health Statistics Annual (1)
H – Hungary; R – Romania; B – Bulgaria; CS – Czechoslovakia; CZ – Czech Republic; EG – East Germany.

glimpses of CECHE's programs, with special emphasis on a grass roots intervention program in two Czech communities – initiated by CECHE over the past four years, together with Stanford University and the University of California in San Francisco and three Czech institutions – using a combination of community-based and high risk intervention in an attempt to reduce risk factors for cardiovascular disease.

Total and CVD mortality have been rising since 1960 and this is apparent even in the 1980s in some of the countries of Central and Eastern Europe, as shown in figures 1 and 2. There is a general upward trend in mortality for men in Hungary, Poland, Bulgaria, and Romania between 1980 and 1990, with little change in Czechoslovakia and East Germany during that period. In women total and CVD mortality is relatively flat (figures 1 and 2). This contrasts with the sharp decline in CVD mortality in most Western nations during that time period. Within Central and Eastern Europe the picture is not uniform after 1990. In Hungary, Romania, and Bulgaria the rise in male mortality continues, whereas the Czech Republic and the former East Germany are showing a measurable decrease in the last few years.

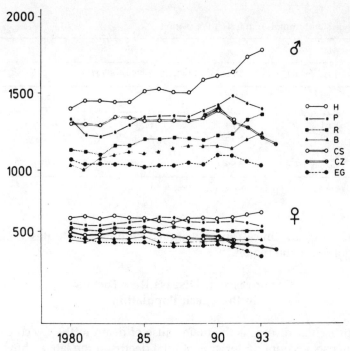

Figure 2. Cardiovascular disease mortality. Number of CVD deaths/100,000/year, under age 70. Data from World Health Statistics Annual (1). Country abbreviations as for figure 1.

What accounts for these adverse mortality trends in this region? Overall these countries show an extremely high prevalence of known risk factors, especially for cardiovascular diseases. Total serum cholesterol on average exceeds 6.0 mmol/l, hypertension exceeds 20% in the population, and obesity reaches the 40% mark in middle-aged women in many countries. Three WHO MONICA surveys conducted in several of these countries from 1981 to 1994 show the changes in blood pressure, serum cholesterol, smoking, and body mass index (BMI), and the cardiovascular and cerebrovascular diseases mortality trends are supported by changes in these risk factors (2).

The dietary picture is also bleak: fat intake in the region has nearly doubled in the last 50 years, as has the consumption of high-salt foods. Total fat intake ranges from 40–45% of calories, with 70–80% of the fat calories coming from saturated fat. This combination of

Table 1
Total Cholesterol (mmol/l) in Czech Population

	Male		Female	
Age	1988 (n = 1357)	1992 (n = 1142)	1988 (n = 1412)	1992 (n = 1211)
25–34	5.88	5.30	5.58	5.15
35–44	6.20	6.04	5.59	5.55
45–54	6.61	6.34	6.51	6.26
55–64	6.29	6.15	6.89	6.87
Σ	6.26 ± 1.15	5.99 ± 1.30	6.23 ± 1.25	5.95 ± 1.28

Source: Skodová Z et al. (3) and WHO MONICA Project (4).

epidemiological, clinical, and nutritional findings constitutes a high-risk profile for the region.

Cardiovascular Disease Risk Factors
in the Czech Population

Cardiovascular disease is the main cause of death in the Czech population also, accounting for 57% of total deaths in the late eighties. It is due to an unfavourable lifestyle, including a high frequency of smoking (almost 40% in men) and unhealthy diet. Total fat accounts for 40% of the energy intake, with a high proportion of animal fat (80% of total fat). These data were obtained from analysis of three-day dietary recall of a 1% sample of the population in six different districts of the Czech Republic, together with other biochemical data.

Total cholesterol concentration in men aged 25–64 years was 6.29 ± 1.15 mmol/l and 6.23 ± 1.25 mmol/l for women. Also triglyceride concentration was very high and 40% of Czech men displayed levels higher than 2.3 mmol/l (200 mg/dl) (table 1) (2–5). The frequency of obesity for both men and women is very high. The average BMI index for men in 1988 was 27.4 and for women 27.3.

Recent political and economic changes, entailing cessation of subsidies for meat, meat products, and dairy products, have led to dietary modifications and a consequent decrease in the frequency of risk factors, especially total serum cholesterol and BMI. In the Czech Republic cholesterol concentration dropped between 1988 and 1992 by 5% to 5.99 ± 1.3 mmol/l for men and 5.95 ± 1.28 for women (table 1). A significant decrease of BMI to 26.9 in men and 26.6 in

women was documented when data for 1988 and 1992 were compared. These changes have been followed by a decrease in CVD
mortality in each of the last four years.

The picture in certain other countries is just beginning to improve.
In the interim a combination of intensive professional training,
public education, policy changes, and reallocation of resources is
needed to combat this tragic public health profile.

In March 1992 CECHE formed a consortium of U.S. and Czech
partners and initiated a "Program for Reduction of Cardiovascular
Disease in the Czech Republic." The U.S. and Czech partners
included the Cardiovascular Research Institute at the University of
California in San Francisco, the Stanford University Center for Disease Prevention, CECHE, and in Prague, the Institute of Clinical and
Experimental Medicine, the National Institute of Public Health, and
the Second Medical Clinic of Charles University.

I. Partnerships in Health Program

The program – now in its fifth year – encompasses two distinct
though interlinked projects: a comprehensive Community-Based
Intervention Program to examine an entire community and undertake medical, educational, and other interventions to reduce CVD risk
factors in the community at large, and a High Risk Intervention Program to identify and treat individuals at high risk and those with
manifest coronary artery disease.

COMMUNITY-BASED INTERVENTION – DUBEC

The Community-Based Intervention Program targeted Dubec, a vil-
lage with 1800 inhabitants, east of Prague. It is modelled after the
Stanford 5 Cities Project and was carried out jointly by the Czech and
U.S. partners. It included a range of activities, beginning with an
analysis of the target community by Czech health professionals,
training of Czech physicians, nurses, dietitians, and other health professionals in the U.S., and on-site at Dubec, a baseline survey and
screening of the Dubec community, and implementation of medical
and community-wide interventions in Dubec for 18 months, beginning in January 1993. A repeat survey of risk factors in the population was also conducted. The final phase – now in progress – is the
evaluation of impact through compilation of the data on risk factors
and disease prevalence or incidence.

In the community program approximately 69% of the population, i.e., 881 adults and 235 children, participated in the baseline survey. The prevalence of high BMI and other risk factors, including coronary heart disease, cerebrovascular disease, and Type II diabetes, was high in Dubec. Overall, by U.S. criteria, nearly 50% of the Dubec population could have been designated as high risk.

However we set more practical goals, targeting approximately 26% of the Dubec adult population for primary prevention and 12% for secondary prevention. The remaining 62% constituted the community intervention group.

Community-based intervention included the following:

• Smoking cessation classes for adults.
• Stress control classes for adults.
• Nutrition intervention: A Healthy Dubec Fair in April 1993 spearheaded the nutrition intervention effort, especially in the school. Nutrition classes for adults and school cooks and a curriculum on healthy cooking in school was established.
• Physical exercise: A "Healthy Trail" was established for Dubec inhabitants to encourage participation in physical activity.
• Print materials: Several self-standing print materials as well as kits to support intervention efforts were used.

All major facets of the community – the mayor's office, school, kindergarten, and supermarket – were engaged in the intervention effort at Dubec. Preliminary analysis of data on knowledge and attitude overall indicated a strong positive response to intervention to change lifestyle. Further data analysis continues and some aspects of the community program have been extended to some 26 districts throughout the Czech Republic.

HIGH RISK INTERVENTION

The High Risk Intervention Program includes a diagnostic and treatment model, patterned after the University of California's Cardiovascular Research Institute, aimed at reducing risk factors in patients with established CVD. We established three new clinics: the High Risk Intervention Clinic (HRIC) established at Charles University for primary prevention for patients from Dubec who were identified at high risk as well as secondary intervention for those with CVD; a secondary prevention clinic at the Litomerice District Hospital (LDH) north of Prague for patients surviving myocardial infarction; and a secondary prevention clinic at the Institute for Clinical and Experimental Medicine (IKEM) for coronary artery bypass surgery patients.

High risk intervention took place at three clinics; HRIC has patients from Dubec whose low density lipoprotein (LDL) levels are between 130–160 mg/dl or who have other high CVD risk factors. They underwent individual evaluation and intensive interdisciplinary intervention, using dietary modification, weight control, and smoking cessation to reduce lipoprotein levels, blood pressure, and other risk factors to minimize the necessity of drug treatment.

Secondary prevention at LDH and IKEM, including a lipid-lowering diet, physical exercise, stress reduction, and prevention of smoking relapse, is sometimes accompanied by hypolidemic drugs when diet alone fails in reducing LDL levels.

The primary prevention group, monitored in an HRIC, showed the following prevalence of CVD risk factors:

- Non-high density lipoprotein (nHDL) Chol(%): over 50% of the clinic population had nHDL cholesterol exceeding 200 mg/dl.
- Diabetes: the prevalence of non-insulin-dependent diabetes mellitus (NIDDM) was exceedingly high, reaching the 15% mark in the primary prevention group.
- Smoking: the highest percentage of non-smokers was among the primary prevention group. The highest percentage of former smokers was in the post-bypass surgery clinic.
- Diastolic blood pressure: mean diastolic blood pressure exceeds 110 in the HRIC.
- Body mass index: the mean BMI is near the 30 mark.

Findings from high risk intervention have also been very encouraging. Smoking cessation has been remarkable in the Litomerice and IKEM groups, and there has been no relapse to date. At IKEM, within two months of dietary intervention, the percentage of patients with > 7.8 mmol/l (i.e., > 300 mg/dl) nHDL cholesterol has been reduced from 15.5 to 9, and those with 6.5 to 7.8 mmol/l (260–300 mg/dl) from 40.5 to 26.

POTENTIAL IMPACT

This is a brief summary of the salient points for the first three years. We have since extended the program to nearly 30 districts.

Overall we achieved average reductions of some 25% LDL cholesterol in the high risk groups, and this alone should reduce new or
recurrent coronary events by approximately 50%. Based upon the
experience at Stanford, a 15% overall reduction in mortality in the
community and in their coronary risk scores should be achieved in
the long run. The program experience to date shows that the techniques and approaches used could contribute significantly to reduction of CVD morbidity and mortality in the Czech Republic by the
end of this century, and in Central Europe as a whole since it has
disease patterns, a health care system, and a lifestyle similar to that
of the Czech Republic. The experience, the technology, and the training of manpower for these projects would simplify similar region-
wide implementation efforts that could substantially reduce CVD
morbidity and mortality in all of East-Central Europe.

II. Other CECHE Programs

CECHE is also carrying out several public educational and technical
assistance programs, many of which use mass media.

A FAMILY YEAR

A five-part television series, A Family Year, which has just been produced, gives another glimpse at challenges to human health faced by
Central and Eastern Europeans, and at traditional approaches and
personal attempts to overcome this historic legacy.

Slated to air in the winter of 1997 on national TV channels in Central Europe and possibly also the United States, A Family Year features ways in which families from the Czech Republic, Hungary,
Poland, and Russia are coping with environmental and health challenges. The series illustrates fundamental issues, self-help measures,
and targeted intervention successful in Western countries at cata-
lyzing individuals to change lifestyle and motivating decision
makers to adopt progressive policies. Each of five half-hour episodes
features one major topic – cigarette smoking and substance abuse,
diet and chronic disease prevention, maternal and child health,
health impact of environmental pollution, and others.

A Family Year is designed to motivate individuals and families to
take charge of their own health and environment. It is also meant to
reach decision makers and environmental health professionals to
help encourage policy changes and create positive lifestyle models.

Most of all with this series CECHE hopes to motivate Central and Eastern Europeans to use mass media creatively to stimulate, educate, and entertain the public.

III. Russian Non-Governmental Organization (NGO)-Assistance Program

Authoritarian rule and central government control have left behind a tragic public health legacy – rampant environmental pollution and a health care system distinguished by its lack of attention to disease prevention. The *Washington Post* states that "… the declining quality of health care, along with hazardous environmental conditions, poor occupational safety standards and sky-high smoking and alcohol-consumption rates are major factors in a perilous drop in the life expectancy of Russian men, which now stands at 57 years" (*Washington Post*, 13 September 1996). The 1994 UNICEF Regional Monitoring Study cautioned that the "health, nutrition and mortality crisis in Russia represents a clear threat to the political viability of the entire reform process."

Western assistance to date has tended to favour provision of supplies and aid to disaster victims, rather than alleviation of the root causes of increasing mortality and declining life expectancy. Health sector reform, while targeting new approaches to financing, has virtually ignored the need for a framework for disease prevention – the most fundamental, economically viable, long-term strategy for promoting health and increasing productivity.

This was the challenge facing CECHE – an American private voluntary organization operating in the region – in 1994, when it began a grass-roots program aimed at public health reform in Russia. At the hub of CECHE's Russian NGO project, funded by the U.S. Agency for International Development (USAID) through a subgrant from World Learning, Inc., were two Russian NGOs – the Health and Environment Foundation (HEF) in Moscow, started by Alexei Yablokov, President Yeltsin's former Minister of Ecology, and the Association of Physicians of the Don (ADP) in Azov, a progressive group of physicians pushing for health care reform. Over the next two years, with CECHE's financial assistance, technical support, and training in the rudiments of survival, HEF and ADP strengthened their organizations, launched health promotion programs, cultivated decision makers, developed media relations, and mobilized health care NGOs throughout Russia to form a cohesive network A direct outcome of this effort is the creation of the Russian Public Health Association (ROZA), an association spanning half of Russia's 89 oblasts and patterned after the World Federation of Public Health Associations (WFPHA). ROZA has assumed HEF's and ADP's agenda and leadership for public health education and policy reform – measures that potentially affect some 120 million people throughout Russia.

Other main outcomes of the Private Voluntary Organizations and Newly Independent States of the Former Soviet Union (PVO-NIS) Project are the following:

• Production and airing of public service announcements (PSAs) on the risks of cigarette smoke by national, regional, and local television channels.
• Launching and wide-scale distribution of two newsletters to health professionals and the health NGO community throughout Russia, and initiation of a third one for the general public.
• Commissioning and wide-scale dissemination of the first series of health policy reports "Health for All, All for Health" for policy makers in Russia, focusing on key public health issues such as increasing mortality and decreasing longevity, smoking, alcohol, and nutrition.
• Formation of a network of health-care NGOs encompassing over 50 NGOs – the first of its kind in Russia.
• Creation of a large database for the NGO network and the posting of a home page in English on the World Wide Web – which includes information on HEF's mission and current projects – thus enabling worldwide access to the latest information on health and environmental issues in Russia.
• Creation and implementation of an NGO-led regional grass-roots Alcohol Policy Program based on the WHO's model for Europe, which addresses the serious problem of alcohol abuse in Russia and incorporates education and policy measures.
• Development and successful local funding of a video education and information centre in Azov for teenagers, dedicated to substance abuse and sexual health.

Fundamental to the success of this program was the consultative and advisory role played by CECHE's long-standing and dynamic partners, including the American Institute of Cancer Research, Center for Science in the Public Interest, Georgetown University's

Child Development Center, and World Federation of Public Health Associations – all of Washington, DC – and the S.I. Newhouse School of Public Communications of Syracuse State University in Syracuse, NY.

Following in the footsteps of the Alcohol Policy Program is an emerging plan to attack the biggest killer in Russia today – cigarette smoking. Any grass-roots movement against cigarette smoking in Russia or Central and Eastern Europe and the Newly Independent States of the Former Soviet Union (CEE-NIS) must confront the Madison Avenue tactics of the Western tobacco giants that have invested over $1.5 billion in advertising in this region. In its continuing quest to promote health and prevent disease in the CEE-NIS, CECHE seeks support to equip ROZA and the NGO network as they attempt to remove this last iron curtain preventing Russians from achieving the quality of life so commonplace today in the West.

IV. Public Service Announcements (PSAs)

When Yul Brynner was dying of lung cancer he made an emotional appeal to fellow Americans to quit smoking. When CECHE developed its first crop of Russian anti-smoking PSAs in December 1993, it used humour and drama, played on the viewers' fear of being less attractive to the opposite sex, or stoked a nationalistic spirit in pointing to the lack of warnings on Russian cigarette packets when such warnings are mandatory in the West. Now CECHE has a new set of PSAs and a different approach – sound bites of ex-smokers seeking to persuade their fellow citizens to quit.

CECHE's Take Charge PSA program began in March 1993. These PSAs urge personal steps to avoid substance abuse, to minimize the impact of environmental pollution on health, and to consume a healthy diet, using limited resources. The program uses existing American PSAs as well as new ones designed and produced in collaboration with local partners. The first series, dubbed Your Fate Is In Your Hands, comprised five short programs developed jointly by CECHE, the National Centre for Health Promotion (NCHP) in Prague, Skyscraper Productions in London, and Syracuse University at Syracuse, NY. Audience scores for this series meant a resounding success. A second – Quit Smoking – series focused on substance abuse and encouraged Russians – particularly youth – to change their lifestyle and give up smoking.

V. Professional Training Programs

BIOCHEMICAL AND ENVIRONMENTAL EXCHANGES

In June 1996 the Trust for Mutual Understanding gave new direction to CECHE's Biomedical Sciences Fellowship Program – launched in 1990. The program provides up to three months of hands-on experience at North American institutions in biomedical and environmental health for CEE-NIS scientists. With support from anonymous philanthropic sources, grants from the Central European Development Corporation and Ronald Lauder, and in-kind support from participating North American and European host institutions, this program seeks to create a cadre of well-trained leaders in the region and to foster collaboration between them and their American counterparts. Since the program's inception over 60 professionals from Bulgaria, Croatia, the Czech Republic, Hungary, Poland, Russia, Yugoslavia, Romania, and Slovakia have received training at U.S., European, and Canadian institutions.

The 1996 fellows' fields of specialization ranged widely and generally reflected the priority of environmental health issues facing various CEE-NIS countries. Fellows were selected from over 70 applicants from eight countries.

CECHE's Trust-supported Environmental Sciences Exchange Program, which started in May 1996, permits exchanges between scientists from non-metropolitan areas of CEE-NIS and leading North American institutions. Up to 10 scholars per year – selected and screened by the Institute of Occupational Medicine and Environmental Health, Sosnowiec, Poland; Centre for Industrial Hygiene and Occupational Diseases, National Institute of Public Health, Prague, Czech Republic; and Health and Environment Foundation (HEF), Moscow, Russia – will participate in short-term collaborative research and study at American partner institutions. Environmental risk assessment and monitoring pertaining to the leading environmental health hazards, and morbidity and mortality in this region are among the high priority study topics.

CECHE's three American partners are the Environmental and Occupational Health Sciences Institute (EOHSI), of Piscataway, NJ; Northeast Regional Environmental Public Health Center, School of Public Health, University of Massachusetts, Amherst, MA; and Department of Environmental and Occupational Health (EOH), Graduate School of Public Health, University of Pittsburgh, PA.

MEDIA TRAINING

CECHE's mass media program seeks to enhance the programmatic, managerial, and organizational capacity and viability of media organizations in CEE-NIS through training and technical assistance; to use mass media for positive social impact, through demonstration programs that include training in CEE-NIS entities; to foster multimedia networking and collaboration among television, radio, and newspapers on sources, materials, and information; to disseminate the program and reach the general public through the broadcast media; and to promote excellence in and special focus on health and environmental programming for public education and policy reform.

In January 1996, as part of its effort to harness the power of the media to promote health and prevent disease, CECHE sponsored eight television producers and directors for training under the guidance of Karl Sabbagh, executive producer of Skyscraper Productions in London, U.K.

Representing major television broadcast outlets in Russia, Poland, Hungary, and the Czech Republic, the journalists received hands-on experience in fly-on-the-wall filming, whereby the camera "observes" the subjects going about their usual chores. CECHE's new television series, A Family Year, which served as a training laboratory, is slated for broadcast nationally in the region in late 1996. Participants critiqued the footage shot in each country and edited and presented it for discussion.

To further its goal of motivating journalists to participate in increasing health and environmental awareness through the media, trainees were introduced to award-winning editor Jane Stephenson at Diverse Productions for insight into Pulse, her weekly investigative health series broadcast in the U.K. Trainees explored the future of health and medical documentaries with Andrew Stevenson, the director and producer of the BBC series, Intensive Care, and visited Sindibad Films to study the latest non-linear editing equipment, Component Productions to view the latest in post-production facilities and wide screen framing, and the British Academy of Film and Television Arts to examine special techniques of documentary production. A second week of workshop and hands-on training in April 1996 concluded the two-week training program.

A pre- and post-evaluation conducted by Fiona Chew of Syracuse University's S.I. Newhouse School of Public Communications revealed a substantial increase in the participants' knowledge and awareness of effective and innovative production and communication techniques.

CECHE's Media Training Program was launched in 1994 to train promising young professionals in television, print, radio, and environmental health in the effective use of mass media for health-related issues. CECHE's ultimate goal is to create hubs of trained media professionals in each of its target countries and to institutionalize the use of mass media for effective use in health communications.

VI. Electronic Media

HEALTH PROMOTION BULLETIN

Last spring CECHE released the first issue of its new electronic publication, the NIS Health Promotion Bulletin. The bulletin contains short blurbs on current NIS programs striving to improve public health through public education to catalyze behavioural change. It targets key organizations, government bodies, academic institutes, and individuals in the health sector in the NIS. The bulletin is sent quarterly via e-mail. Its topics range from nutrition to substance abuse, environmental health, maternal and child health, and vulnerable groups. To date three issues have been produced in English, and plans are underway to distribute it also in Russian.

ENVIRONMENTAL COOPERATION BULLETIN (ECB)

The Environmental Cooperation Bulletin – re-launched on 1 October 1996 – is a monthly brief distributed electronically (by e-mail and fax) that covers a wide range of environmental projects, universities, and commercial entities operating in the former Soviet Union and Central and Eastern Europe. The ECB is circulated to over 1,000 groups and individuals in the NIS and North America, and lists timely publications available to professional environmentalists active in this region of unprecedented environmental decline. A major impact of the publication has been to stimulate cooperation among projects, including joint activities between government and non-government entities supported by international organizations, private donors, and commercial enterprises. The ECB is sponsored by the U.S. Environmental Protective Agency's Environment Committee of the Gore-Chernomyrdin Commission. Prior to May 1996 it was published by Kompass Resources International of Washington, DC.

VII. Future Agenda

The maturing of CECHE's region-wide community programs in CEE-NIS and relocation of its headquarters to Washington, DC, in May 1996 has brought a new awakening – the lessons learned to date have implications and applications far beyond the CEE-NIS region. The decentralization and economic transition taking place in Central Europe from an agricultural to an industrial base, from rural to urban society, is just as apparent in India and China, and it is posing new challenges to lifestyle and to health. CECHE has a unique opportunity to bring its special focus – application of media for positive social impact – to Asia and other parts of the world. This awakening will guide CECHE's direction as it considers the opportunity to address high priority issues such as improving child survival through community and public education programs in other parts of the world.

REFERENCES

1 *World health statistics annual*, 1994. Geneva: WHO, 1995.
2 Skodova Z, Pisa Z, Berka L, Cicha Z, Cerovska J, Emrova R, Hejl Z, Hrdlickoa K, Hoke M, Pikhartova J, Skalka P, Vojtisek P, Vorlicek P, Wiesner E. Myocardial infarction register in MONICA-Czechoslovakia Center. *Acta Med Scand* 1988;728(suppl):79–83.
3 Skodova Z, Pisa Z, Pikhartova J, Cicha Z, Vojtisek P, Emrova R, Berka L, Hoke M, Wiesner E, Valenta Z, Poledne R, Hronkova M. Development of the cardiovascular risk in the population of the Czech Republic. *Cor Vasa* 1993;35:178–182.
4 WHO MONICA Project. Myocardial infarction and coronary death in the WHO MONICA project. Registration procedures, event rates, and case fatality rates in 38 populations from 21 countries in four continents. *Circulation* 1994;90:583–612.
5 *Czech Health Statistics Year Book*, 1994. Prague, Czech Republic: UZIS 1995.

PIRJO PIETINEN

Diet and Cardiovascular Disease: The Nordic Experience

The Nordic countries (Finland, Sweden, Norway, Denmark, and Iceland) are a group of countries often referred to as Scandinavia. However Scandinavia is a geographical area covering only Sweden, Norway, and Denmark. The languages in these three countries are quite similar, but Finnish and Icelandic are totally different languages. The Nordic countries have strong ties, which have been strengthened by a political decision to maintain Nordic cooperation in many areas.

The aim of this paper is to describe what has happened in diet and cardiovascular diseases, especially coronary heart disease (CHD), in the Nordic countries during recent decades. Two of these countries, Norway and Finland, have had a food and nutrition policy for a long time and efforts to change the diet to prevent CHD have been exceptionally vigorous in both countries.

CHD mortality in the five Nordic countries is presented in figures 1 and 2. The graphs are based on WHO mortality statistics (ICD codes 410–414) and three-year moving averages. Finland had the highest CHD mortality in the early 1970s in both men and women, but by 1992 the differences have almost disappeared and all the countries have very similar rates, with Finnish men and Danish women having the highest mortality rates.

A comparison of Food Balance Sheet data from 1965 to 1990 shows that the diets in the Nordic countries have become similar in many ways (1). Some of the common trends have been increased consumption of low-fat dairy products, decreased consumption of edible fats,

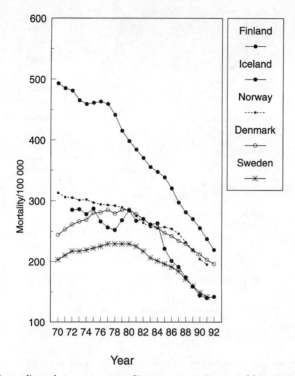

Year

Figure 1. Age-adjusted coronary mortality among 35–64-year-old men in the Nordic countries. Based on data from Statistics Finland.

and increased consumption of cheese, vegetables, and fruit, with the most dramatic changes taking place in Finland. The fat content of the diet has decreased towards the end of this period – in Finland and Norway it was only about 35% of energy in 1990, less so in Sweden, at about 37%, while there was no apparent change in Denmark where the fat content of the diet remained at about 43%.

Iceland

An analysis of trends in CHD death rates compared with expected rates computed from population surveys was recently carried out (2). CHD mortality decreased by 17–18% from 1970 to 1988. From 1981 to 1986 the myocardial infarction attack rate in men under 75 decreased by 23%. A decrease occurred in the level of all three major risk factors (smoking, total serum cholesterol concentration, and blood pressure)

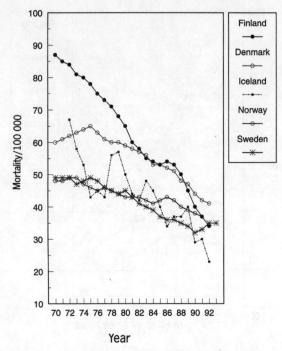

Year

Figure 2. Age-adjusted coronary mortality among 35–64-year-old women in the Nordic countries. Based on data from Statistics Finland.

after 1968. Altered food habits in Iceland coincided strongly with the observed decline in serum cholesterol concentrations. Decreased consumption of dairy fat and margarine alone would be expected to lower the serum cholesterol concentration by 0.3 mmol/l according to the Keys equation. In addition consumption of meat fat has decreased as more carcass fat is discarded during production and leaner meats have become available. Cholesterol values would accordingly be expected to have decreased more than 0.3 mmol/l as a result of changes in diet, as they indeed have (0.42 mmol/l among men and 0.75 mmol/l among women). The more dramatic fall in cholesterol concentrations among women was unexplained, but possibly women changed their diet to a greater extent. The calculated reduction in risk for the age group 45–64 was about 35%, which was closely similar to the observed decrease in mortality due to ischemic heart disease in that age group. In this study the changes in risk factors and ischemic heart disease incidence were coincident in women whereas in men there was a lag of several years.

Norway

The influence of dietary changes on serum cholesterol and CHD during the last century has recently been evaluated in Norway (3). Information about food consumption and nutrient intake is available from Food Balance Sheets as well as through household consumption surveys conducted since the beginning of the century. Data on mortality compiled from individual death certificates exist since 1928. During the last 20 years the National Health Screening Service has compiled information on serum cholesterol and other CHD risk factors of large samples of the population. To get a comparable series of the intake of energy, fat, saturated, monounsaturated, and polyunsaturated fatty acids, and cholesterol the authors made a food composition table covering the whole century. They also collected information on the consumption of coffee, fish, cod liver oil, vegetables, and fruit and the intake of vitamins A and C, selenium, iron, dietary fibre, salt, and alcohol.

From 1890 the energy percentage of fat in the Norwegian diet increased from 20 to 40 in the late 1970s and then decreased to 34 in the early 1990s. The dietary fatty acid pattern has changed considerably. Hydrogenation of oils for margarine production started in 1913. The intake of trans-fatty acids was highest, about 4% of energy, in 1958 and then decreased to 3% in 1990. The intake of cholesterol increased from below 80 mg/1000 kcal in the beginning of the century up to 180 mg/1000 kcal in 1950 and later decreased to about 150 mg/1000 kcal in 1990. Estimates made with the Keys equation on the basis of the Food Balance Sheets showed that the estimated serum cholesterol level increased from 1890, reached its peak during 1950s, and then decreased. Estimates based on the household consumption survey data showed a similar trend.

Norwegians are coffee drinkers and most of the coffee has traditionally been prepared by boiling. Filtered coffee has, however, taken an increasing share of the market, and the estimated effect on the decrease in serum cholesterol during the last 50 years is 0.13 mmol/l. Taken together the changes in dietary fats and coffee consumption have increased the estimated serum cholesterol level by 1 mmol/l from 1900 to 1959 and decreased it by 0.6 mmol/l from 1960 to 1991.

Based on population survey data the serum cholesterol level decreased by 0.43–0.81 mmol/l in men in three different areas and by 0.52–0.82 mmol/l in women from 1974 to 1991, which is a 7–12% decrease. The peak in CHD mortality was around 1970 and from 1971–1974 to 1991–1993 CHD mortality has decreased by 43% in men and 29% in women aged 50–59 years. The actual decrease in CHD mortality is thus greater than the estimated drop in risk. Other contributing factors could be increased intake of antioxidants and decreased salt intake. Daily salt intake is estimated to be about 10–12 g at present and it must have been higher in earlier times when salting was a food preservation method. However, reliable documentation is not available.

Sweden

CHD mortality in men was the lowest in Sweden among the Nordic countries in the early 1970s (figure 1). It increased slightly in the 1970s but has since about 1980 decreased again. Since Sweden has not carried out CHD risk factor surveys in representative population samples, no analysis on factors explaining the increase and the following decrease is available. Representative dietary surveys over time are also lacking and so only the Food Balance Sheets can show the changes in diet (1). The fat content of the Swedish diet was about 38% in 1965 and has since decreased to about 35%. The Swedish diet resembles the Norwegian diet except that fish consumption is lower.

Finland

Finland had the highest CHD mortality rate in the world in the late 1960s (4). From 1972 to 1992 CHD mortality declined by 55% in men and 68% in women. Changes in serum cholesterol, blood pressure, and smoking predicted a 44% decline in men and a 49% decline in women (5). Almost half of the decline was associated with the decrease in serum cholesterol concentration, which was 13% in men (from 6.8 mmol/l to 5.9 mmol/l) and 18% in women (from 6.7 mmol/l to 5.5 mmol/l) (6).

The Finnish diet has often been quoted as a peculiar diet, high in saturated fat and low in vegetables (7). However it has changed remarkably during the past 25 years and is now very similar to the diets in Sweden, Norway, and Iceland.

A recent analysis showed that the dietary changes account for the decrease in serum cholesterol (8). The total fat content of the Finnish diet changed from 38% of energy in the early 1970s to 34% in 1992, saturated fat content from 21% to 16%, and polyunsaturated fat content from 3% to 5%, and the intake of cholesterol decreased by 16%. Based on the Keys equation these changes could have decreased serum cholesterol level by 0.6 mmol/l in both genders. A shift from boiled to filtered coffee could have further decreased serum cholesterol by 0.3 mmol/l. Thus these changes together could explain a decrease of 0.9 mmol/l, and the average decrease has been 1.0 mmol/l. Several other changes in the diet have also been favourable. Fruit and vegetable consumption has increased two- to threefold during this time period. Supplementation of fertilizers with selenium has tripled the intake of selenium, which was very low (9).

Finland is the only Nordic country where sodium intake has been measured in population surveys since 1979 (8,10–12). There has been a decrease in daily sodium intake from about 13–15 g to 11–12 g sodium chloride among men and from 10–11 g to 8–9 g among women. Thus the salt content of the Finnish diet is now very similar to those of Denmark and Norway. There has been a decline in blood pressure during the period 1972–1992 (6). This can partly be attributed to better hypertension control by medication but supposedly the decrease in salt consumption has also contributed to this decline, since body mass index has increased in men (13) and alcohol consumption has increased in both genders (14).

Denmark

Denmark is in many ways different from the other Nordic countries. Evidently the geographical location close to central Europe has some influence on lifestyle. The smoking and drinking rates are highest in Denmark in both genders, and especially among women, and the diet still has a higher fat content than in the other countries, about 43% in 1990, based on the Food Balance Sheet data (1). A recent large dietary survey carried out in 1995 showed, however, that the fat content of the diet is now 37% (15). Saturated fatty acids represent 15%, cis-monounsaturated fatty acids 11%, polyunsaturated fatty acids 5%, and trans-fatty acids 1% of energy intake. The amount of sodium chloride in the diet is 8g/10MJ. Based on the dietary surveys conducted in 1985 and in 1995, adults consume less fats, milk and dairy products, cheese, sugar, and sweets. The consumption of meat, fruit, soft drinks, beer, and wine has increased.

Conclusions

The dietary changes in the Nordic countries have been quite favourable during recent decades and have contributed to the decline in

CHD mortality. The changes have been most dramatic in Finland. Compared to the other European countries and the U.S., there are still characteristics in the Nordic diet that should change even more. Vegetable and oil consumption are still relatively low. Efforts to increase the consumption especially of locally produced vegetables are, however, ongoing.

REFERENCES

1 Becker W, Enghardt H. Food consumption development in the Nordic countries 1965–1990 (in Swedish with an English summary). *Scand J Nutr* 1993;37:97–144.
2 Sigfusson N, Sigvaldason H, Steingrimsdottir et al. Decline in ischaemic heart disease in Iceland and change in risk factor levels. *Br Med J* 1991;302:1371–1375.
3 Johansson L, Drevon CA, Bjorneboe G-E Aa. The Norwegian diet during the last hundred years in relation to coronary heart disease. *Eur J Clin Nutr* 1996;50:277–283.
4 Keys A. Coronary heart disease in seven countries. *Am Heart Assoc Monograph* no 29, 1970.
5 Vartiainen E, Puska P, Pekkanen J, Tuomilehto J, Jousilahti P. Changes in risk factors explain changes in mortality from ischaemic heart disease in Finalnd. *Br Med J* 1994:309:23–27.
6 Vartiainen E, Puska P, Jousilahti P, Korhonen HJ, Tuomilehto J, Nissinen A. Twenty-year trends in coronary risk factors in North Karelia and in other areas of Finland. *Int J Epidemiol* 1994;23:495–504.
7 Artaud-Wild SM, Connor SL, Sexton G, Connor WE. Differences in coronary mortality can be explained by differences in cholesterol and saturated fat intakes in 40 countries but not in France and Finland. A paradox. *Circulation* 1993;88:2771–2779.
8 Pietinen P, Vartiainen E, Seppänen R, Aro A, Puska P. Changes in diet in Finland from 1972 to 1992: Impact on coronary heart disease risk. *Prev Med* 1996;25:243–250.
9 Varo P, Alfthan G, Huttunen JK, Aro A. Nationwide selenium supplementation in Finland – effects on diet, blood and tissue levels, and health. In: Burk RF, ed. *Selenium in biology and human health*. New York: Springer-Verlag, 1994:198–218.
10 Tuomilehto J, Puska P, Tanskanen A et al. A community-based intervention on the feasibility and effects of the reduction in salt intake in North Karelia. *Acta Cardiol J* 1981;36:83–104.

11 Pietinen P, Tanskanen A, Nissinen A, Tuomilehto J, Puska P. Changes in dietary habits concerning salt during a community-based prevention programme for hypertension. *Ann Clin Res* 1984;16(suppl 53):150–155.

12 Pietinen P, Vartiainen E, Korhonen HJ et al. Nutrition as a component in community control of cardiovascular disease (The North Karelia Project). *Am J Clin Nutr* 1989;49:1017–1024.

13 Pietinen P, Vartiainen E, Männistö S. Trends in body mass index and obesity among adults in Finland from 1972 to 1992. *Int J Obes* 1996;20:114–120.

14 Alcohol Statistical Yearbook 1994. The Finnish State Alcohol Company, 1995.

15 Andersen N, Fagt S, Groth MV, Hartkopp HB, Moller A, Ovesen L, Warming DL. Danskernes kostvaner 1995. *Levnedsmiddelstyrelsen, Sundhedsministeriet*, Publikation Nr 235, 1996 (in Danish with an English summary).

JIM MANN

Diet and Cardiovascular Disease: A South Pacific Perspective

Introduction

High rates of coronary heart disease (CHD) in the European populations of the South Pacific (predominantly residents of Australia and
New Zealand) and rapidly increasing rates in many of the indigenous populations, especially when exposed to rapid acculturation,
have resulted in a great deal of interest in the relationships between
diet and cardiovascular disease in this part of the world. This contribution deals with several nutrition issues relevant to preventive measures aimed at reducing CHD incidence in the South Pacific and in
particular to advice relating to the nature of dietary fat. Some of the
research findings presented here may also apply to certain other
population groups exposed over a short period of time to Western
culture and dietary habits. Reference will also be made to some other
relevant Australasian research relating to the effect of diet on various
cardiovascular risk factors – conducted principally on healthy individuals and patients of European descent – that may have more
widespread application to all populations with high CHD rates.

Coronary Heart Disease Trends amongst
People of European Descent in Australasia

Mortality rates for CHD, stroke, "all" cardiovascular disease, and
indeed for all causes have been decreasing in industrialized countries except for some in eastern and central Europe (1). In Australia

and New Zealand rates of both fatal and major non-fatal CHD have continued to fall steadily since the early 1970s (2,3). In New Zealand average percentage annual change (95% confidence intervals) during the years 1983 to 1992 are –5.5 (–7.4,–3.8) for European males and –4.8 (–7.0,–2.5) for European females (4). Attempts to explain these trends have been undertaken as part of participation in the World Health Organization MONICA project (5). Cross-sectional surveys measured CHD risk factors in Auckland, New Zealand, in 1982, 1986–8 and 1993–4. Over the 12-year period the prevalence of self-reported cigarette consumption declined significantly from 28.6% to 16.9% in men and from 24.5% to 14.8% in women. Mean blood pressure level fell by 4–6 mm Hg diastolic in men and women. Mean serum total cholesterol, fell from 6.18 mmol/l and 6.26 mmol/l in 1982 (in men and women respectively) to 5.73 and 5.60 in 1993–4. High density lipoprotein (HDL) cholesterol also fell from 1.19 and 1.42 mmol/l in men and women to 1.10 and 1.40 mmol/l. Mean body mass index (BMI) increased significantly from 25.6 to 26.4 in men and from 24.5 to 25.1 in women during this period.

Dietary data derived from other studies show that these changes occurred in parallel with a reduction in saturated and monounsaturated fatty acids, an increase in polyunsaturated fatty acids, and a small increase in dietary fibre (non-starch polysaccharide), in particular the insoluble form derived from cereal-based foods (Chisholm A, Mann J, unpublished data). These findings are comparable with those observed in other predominantly European populations. They suggest that a change in the nature of dietary fat (replacing a proportion of dietary saturated fatty acids with polyunsaturated fatty acids) leading to a reduction in low density lipoprotein (LDL), together with a reduction in cigarette smoking, can produce a reduction in CHD rates despite an increase in the frequency of obesity and a small but significant decrease in HDL. The reduction in HDL is not surprising, given the increase in at least two factors that are known to be associated with a decrease in levels of this lipoprotein – increasing adiposity and increased intake of polyunsaturated fatty acids. Given the strength of the total cholesterol:HDL-cholesterol ratio as a predictor of cardiovascular risk (6) it may at first glance seem surprising that an appreciable reduction in CHD could occur despite a deterioration in the ratio. However this observation serves to confirm other epidemiological data that suggest that HDL may be a less useful predictor in populations with low total and LDL cholesterol and for individuals in whom total and LDL cholesterol are decreasing

(Shepherd J, personal communication). Thus advice to reduce saturated fatty acids must remain the cornerstone of dietary advice aimed at reducing CHD, though it is conceivable that by preventing the decrease in HDL (e.g., by replacing saturated fatty acids with monounsaturated fatty acids of cis configuration rather than polyunsaturated fatty acids and by avoiding weight gain [7]) the decline in CHD might have been further accelerated. Furthermore the rapid increase in prevalence of obesity remains a major cause for concern because of the wide range of adverse health outcomes associated with adiposity, especially when the excess adipose tissue is centrally distributed.

Coronary Heart Disease Trends amongst People of Polynesian Descent in New Zealand

The recent (1990–2) mean CHD mortality rate for Maori men (232/100,000) in Auckland was almost double the rate for Pacific Island men (135/100,000) and more than double the rate for European men (103/100,000). Maori women had a threefold higher mean mortality rate (85/100,000) than European women (25/100,000). The mortality rate for Pacific Island women (42/100,000) was midway between those of the other ethnic groups (4). Rates amongst Maori men have changed little during the past 10 years (mean percentage annual change; 95% CI: −0.5; −3.0, 2.0). Mortality rates amongst Maori women and Pacific Islanders have shown fluctuations to the extent that it is impossible to discern trends with any degree of confidence.

Several research groups in New Zealand have attempted to explain the high CHD rates amongst the Maori who have inhabited New Zealand for about 1000 years and Pacific Islanders who have migrated relatively recently from Western Samoa, the Cook Islands, Nieue, Tonga, Tokelau, or Fiji. Cigarette smoking is common and rates of hypertension high amongst all people of Polynesian descent living in New Zealand, but particular interest has centred around lipoprotein-mediated risk of cardiovascular disease. Amongst Polynesian groups living in New Zealand, HDL cholesterol is lower and triglyceride levels higher than in European New Zealanders. Total and LDL-cholesterol levels are higher amongst Europeans (8). Ethnic-specific, age-adjusted mean lipid levels have been contrasted to determine which serum lipid is most consistent with the ethnic differences in coronary heart disease rates. High levels of triglyceride and low levels of HDL cholesterol appear to be important determinants of the ethnic differences in CHD mortality, whereas total and LDL cholesterol do not (8). It has been clearly shown that migrants from rural Tokelau to New Zealand tend rapidly to acquire higher levels of blood pressure, triglyceride, glucose, and uric acid and lower levels of HDL cholesterol than those observed in their islands of origin (9). BMI is a poor measure of adiposity in Polynesians (Swinburn B, personal communication), but it does seem as if these abnormalities occur with increasing obesity. It appears that the metabolic syndrome associated with insulin resistance, hyperinsulinemia, hypertension, hyperglycemia, hyperuricemia, and dyslipidemia (10), rather than raised levels of total and LDL cholesterol, explain the emerging epidemic of CHD. If this assumption is correct dietary advice to change the nature of dietary fat will probably on its own have little impact in reducing CHD in Polynesians and perhaps also other populations with similar predisposition to high CHD rates when exposed to relatively rapid acculturation. The various clinical and metabolic consequences of the metabolic syndrome are most likely to be reversed by weight loss and increased physical activity, and these aspects of health promotion, rather than reduction of saturated fatty acids, require greatest emphasis. However attention to the fatty acid profile of the diet to ensure optimum levels of HDL (as discussed below) is likely to confer additional benefits.

Dietary Fatty Acids and High-Density Lipoprotein

An enormous amount of research worldwide has been devoted to the study of the effects of the various dietary fatty acids on lipids and lipoproteins and other cardiovascular risk indicators (11). A summary of the effects on lipids and lipoproteins is shown in figure 1. In summary it would seem that myristic, palmitic, and elaidic (C18:1, n-9 trans) acids have the most marked adverse effect in elevating total and LDL cholesterol, when compared with carbohydrate or oleic acid. Elaidic acid (derived especially from hydrogenated vegetable oils) may also be associated with elevated lipoprotein (a) and reduced levels of HDL and in epidemiological studies has been associated with an increased risk of CHD (13). Thus it is regarded as a particularly undesirable fatty acid. Linoleic acid has a powerful effect in lowering total and LDL cholesterol, but in large amounts tends to reduce HDL levels. n-3 polyunsaturated fatty acids, and in particular eicosapentaenoic acid, reduce triglycerides and very low density lipoproteins but have a variable effect on LDL, sometimes

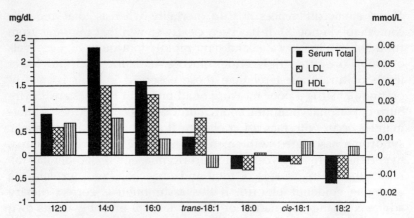

Figure 1. Effects of individual dietary fatty acids on serum total, LDL and HDL cholesterol when 1% of energy from carbohydrates in the diet is replaced by 1% of energy
from the fatty acid in question. Reprinted by permission from Katan et al. (12)

even producing elevations (14). Stearic acid is regarded as neutral
with regard to effect on lipids and lipoproteins, but may have an
adverse effect on thrombogenesis. Of all the common dietary fatty
acids cis oleic acid appears to be associated with the most favourable
lipoprotein profile in terms of both HDL and LDL.

Relatively little information is available regarding coconut oil, a
preferred fat source amongst Polynesian people. It is rich in lauric
and myristic acids and restriction is usually recommended in dietary
guidelines aimed at reducing saturated fatty acids. Because in the
South Pacific the alternative to coconut oil is hydrogenated vegetable
oil or dairy fats and because limited experimental data suggested that
at least in part the hypercholesterolaemic effect of coconut oil might
be due to an increase in HDL cholesterol, we have carried out a series
of controlled experimental studies to quantify the effects of lauric
acid and coconut oil on lipids and lipoproteins (15, 16). Twenty-eight
European New Zealanders (13 men, 15 women) participated in a randomized crossover study that aimed to compare butter, coconut oil,
and safflower oil as predominant fat sources in diets with a percentage of total fat that was comparable with that usually eaten in New
Zealand. The participants followed each experimental diet while continuing their usual daily activities, but a range of measures was
adopted to ensure compliance. Changes in serum triglyceride fatty
acids mirrored the component fatty acids of the test fats, suggesting

Table 1
Plasma Lipids and Lipoproteins During Coconut Oil, Butter, and Safflower Oil Diets

Diet	*TC	LDL-C	HDL-C	VLDL-C	Tag	HDL/LDL
Butter (B)	‡5.61 ± 0.93	4.10 ± 0.90	1.14 ± 0.20	0.33 ± 0.18	1.97 ± 1.01	0.30 ± 0.09
Coconut (C)	5.51 ± 0.86	3.87 ± 0.85	1.21 ± 0.20	0.40 ± 0.35	1.66 ± 0.97	0.33 ± 0.10
Safflower (S)	5.04 ± 0.91	3.51 ± 0.85	1.11 ± 0.20	0.44 ± 0.43	1.75 ± 0.97	0.32 ± 0.08
B v C†	n/s	p < 0.05	p < 0.01	n/s	n/s	p < 0.05
B v S	p < 0.0001	p < 0.001	n/s	n/s	n/s	n/s
C v S	p < 0.0001	p < 0.01	p < 0.001	n/s	n/s	n/s

* All variables expressed in mmol/l, except for HDL-C/LDL-C
† Statistics by paired student's t-tests
‡ All variables expressed as mean ± SD

along with carefully kept diet records a high level of compliance with the experimental diets. Diets were planned so that each included similar amounts of the predominant fatty acid of each test fat. Thus it was possible to compare the effects of lauric, palmitic, and linoleic acids as well as coconut oil, butter, and margarine respectively. Total and LDL cholesterol were significantly higher on the diet containing butter than on the coconut oil diet when levels were higher than on the safflower oil diet. Apolipoprotein A1 was significantly higher on the coconut oil diet than on the other two diets and HDL cholesterol showed a similar trend, which did not achieve statistical significance. Thus the ratios of HDL and apolipoprotein A1 to LDL cholesterol and total cholesterol were similar on the coconut oil and safflower oil diets, and on both diets the ratio was more favourable (i.e., higher) than that observed on the butter diet.

A comparable study was undertaken in 41 healthy Pacific Islanders living in New Zealand. The results were broadly comparable, but perhaps even more striking is that the HDL-cholesterol levels on the coconut oil diet were significantly higher than on both the butter and safflower oil diets. Thus despite consisting predominantly of saturated fatty acids, a diet high in coconut oil was associated with ratios of HDL-C/LDL-C and ApoA1/ApoB similar to that seen with safflower oil. The least favourable lipoprotein profiles were seen on the butter diet (tables 1 and 2). There was no significant difference in the HDL-C/(ApoA1 + ApoA2) molar ratio between the three diets and no significant difference in cholesterol ester transfer activity between the butter and coconut diets. Increased formation of HDL may explain the

54   Diet and Cardiovascular Disease

Table 2
Plasma Apolipoprotein Concentrations During Coconut Oil, Butter, and Safflower
Oil Diets

Diet	Apo A1 (g/l)	Apo AII (g/l)	Apo B (g/l)	Apo A1/Apo B
Butter (B)	†1.23 ± 0.18	0.34 ± 0.08	1.00 ± 0.22	1.30 ± 0.40
Coconut (C)	1.33 ± 0.28	0.35 ± 0.08	0.87 ± 0.38	1.68 ± 0.53
Safflower (S)	1.16 ± 0.14	0.35 ± 0.08	0.76 ± 0.18	1.60 ± 0.38
B v C‡	n/s	n/s	p < 0.01	p < 0.0001
B v S	n/s	n/s	p < 0.001	p < 0.0001
C v S	p < 0.001	n/s	p < 0.05	n/s

† All variables expressed as mean ± SD
‡ Statistics by paired student's t-tests

higher levels of HDL-C on a coconut-rich diet. These results may help
to understand the low CHD rates observed in Polynesian people who
consume a diet relatively high in saturated fatty acids and why lipoprotein-mediated atherosclerosis risk and CHD rates increase with
dietary change on migration to New Zealand. However, more importantly, they suggest that especially for Polynesian people, for whom
low levels of HDL may be a particularly important risk factor, coconut
oil should not be included with other sources of saturated fatty acids
to be avoided. Polynesian people are unlikely to use olive oil or safflower oil as a substitute for coconut oil, but are more likely to change
to dairy fats rich in palmitic and myristic acids or hydrogenated vegetable fats high in trans unsaturated fatty acids. While a reduction in
total fat may help to facilitate weight loss in those who are overweight and obese, the use of moderate amounts of coconut oil as part
of a fat-reduced diet seems acceptable. The results may also have
wider application. While coconut oil might still be regarded as a less
desirable oil than for example olive oil, it may be more appropriate
for use in manufactured food than hydrogenated vegetable oils.

Variation in Plasma Cholesterol Response to Dietary Lipid

Two research groups in Australasia have had a longstanding interest
in the variation in plasma cholesterol response to dietary lipid. Nestel's group in Adelaide has made several helpful observations. They
have confirmed earlier findings that some individuals are more sensitive than others to changes in the nature of dietary fat and furthermore

that those individuals who respond to changes in saturated fatty acids are also more likely to respond to changes in the amount of dietary cholesterol (17). More recently they have shown that gender, body mass index, and age have an important influence on response of plasma lipid to changes in dietary fat plus cholesterol (18). Women, younger people, those with a lower body mass index, and those with lower plasma cholesterol appear to respond by preferentially using HDL$_2$ cholesterol for any rise in plasma cholesterol. On the other hand men, especially older men with higher cholesterols and raised body mass index, respond in a presumably less favourable manner by transporting excess plasma cholesterol in LDL cholesterol. The difference of 0.09 mmol/l in HDL cholesterol and 0.06 mmol/l in HDL$_2$ cholesterol between men and women in their response to a high-fat, high-cholesterol diet translates into a potential increase in the risk of myocardial infarction in men of 7–13% compared with women on the same diet. Thus the benefits of a low-fat, low-cholesterol diet would appear to be slightly greater for men than women despite the same change in total cholesterol, as there is a greater fall in LDL cholesterol and a smaller fall in HDL cholesterol.

Our own research group has clearly demonstrated individual consistency in response to changes in dietary lipid, utilizing the double crossover experimental design. Sixty-seven free-living volunteers were repeatedly challenged with diets high in saturated fat or polyunsaturated fat for six-week periods (19). Similar average changes in cholesterol, virtually identical with those predicted from the Keys equation, masked a wide range of individual responses. Response was not related to compliance. In all participants the change in cholesterol observed when the nature of the dietary fat was changed on the two occasions was correlated ($r = 0.31$, $p = 0.01$) but the degree of correlation between the two sets of responses was greater in the 46 consistent responders than in the 21 variable responders ($r = 0.71$ vs $r = 0.21$). Mean difference in cholesterol between the diets rich in saturated and polyunsaturated fats during the two crossovers were 1.16 and 0.95 mmol/l for the consistent hyper-responders and 0.18 and 0.18 mmol/l for the consistent minimal responders. In consistent responders changes in total cholesterol in response to increasing saturated fats correlated with baseline cholesteryl ester transfer activity, total cholesterol, triglycerides, and apolipoprotein B. A more recent study (20) has identified three genes where common variation may determine an individual's response to dietary change. Genotype was determined at the apolipoprotein (apo)B locus (signal peptide), apoCIII (c1100-T) and lipoprotein lipase (LPL) gene loci (HindIII). In those individuals classified as consistent responders the frequency of the apoB signal peptide-24 allele was significantly higher than amongst those with a variable response. None of the other polymorphisms showed a significant frequency difference between groups. Both apoB and apoCIII genotypes were associated with the correlation between response during the first and second crossovers, while those with one or more apoB SP24 alleles and those with the apoCIII genotype CC had a significantly higher correlation than those with other genotypes (0.46 [p = 0.05] vs 0.12 [NS] and 0.31 [p = 0.05] vs 0.02 [NS] respectively). Neither apoB nor apoCIII genotypes were associated with effects on the magnitude of the response to dietary change. However individuals with the LPL HindIII genotype H+H+ had a significantly smaller change in mean TC in response to diet than those with one or more H-alleles (9.3% vs 14.4%, p = 0.03). Thus variation at the apoB and apoCIII locus affects the consistency of response to change in dietary fat content, while variation at the LPL gene locus affects magnitude of response. Our studies also provide some confirmation that individuals with the genotype apoE4E4 have the highest initial cholesterol levels as well as the most marked changes when altering the nature of dietary fat.

These findings in no way alter the need for a population strategy to reduce CHD risk in populations with high rates of the disease (21). However they do raise the possibility that when dealing with high risk individuals it may soon be possible to identify those who are likely to benefit most from dietary modification and to target advice towards them.

REFERENCES

1 Thom TJ. International mortality from heart disease: rates and trends. *Int J Epidemiol* 1989;18(suppl 1):520–528.
2 Public Health Commission. *Our health, our future.* Wellington: Public Health Commission, 1994.
3 Russell MA, Dobson AJ. Age specific patterns of mortality from cardiovascular disease and other major causes, 1969 to 1990. *Aust J Public Health* 1994;18:160–164.
4 Bell C, Swinburn B, Stewart A, Jackson R, Tukuitonga C, Tipene-Leach D. Ethnic differences and recent trends in coronary heart disease incidence in New Zealand. *NZ Med J* 1996;109:66–68.

5 Jackson R, Yee RL, Priest P, Shaw L, Beaglehole R. Trends in coronary heart disease risk factors in Auckland 1982–94. *NZ Med J* 1995;108:451–454.

6 Grover S, Coupal L, Hu X-P. Identifying adults at increased risk of coronary disease. How well do the current guidelines work? *JAMA* 1995;274(10):801–806.

7 Rivellese AA, Auletta P, Marrota G et al. Long term metabolic effects of two dietary methods of treating hyperlipidaemia. *Br Med J* 1994;308: 227–231.

8 Scragg R, Baker J, Metcalf P, Dryson E. Serum lipid levels in a New Zealand multicultural workforce. *NZ Med J* 1993;106:96–99.

9 Stanhope JM, Sampson VM, Prior IA. The Tokelau Island migrant study: serum lipid concentrations in two environments. *J Chron Dis* 1980;34:45–55.

10 Frayn KN, Coppack SW. Insulin resistance, adipose tissue and coronary heart disease. *Clin Sci* 1992;82:1–8.

11 Mensink RP, Katan MB. Effect of dietary fatty acids on serum lipids and lipoproteins. *Arterioscler Thromb* 1992; 12:911–919.

12 Katan MB, Zock PL, Mensink RP. Effects of fats and fatty acids on blood lipids in humans: an overview. *Am J Clin Nutr* 1994;60(suppl): 986s–990s.

13 Nestel P, Noakes M, Belling B et al. Plasma lipoprotein lipid and Lp(a) changes with substitution of elaidic for oleic acid in the diet. *J Lipid Res* 1992;33:1029–1036.

14 Sullivan DR, Sanders TAB, Trayner IM, Thompson GR. Paradoxical elevation of LDL apoprotein B levels in hypertriglyceridaemic patients and normal subjects ingesting fish oil. *Atherosclerosis* 1986;61:120–134.

15 Cox C, Mann J, Sutherland W, Chisholm A, Skeaff M. Effects of coconut oil, butter, and safflower oil on lipids and lipoproteins in persons with moderately elevated cholesterol levels. *J Lipid Res* 1995;36:1787–1795.

16 Cox C, Mann J, Sutherland W, Chisholm A, Skeaff M. Effects of coconut oil, butter and safflower oil on lipids and lipoproteins in persons with moderately elevated cholesterol levels. *J Lipid Res* 1995;36:1787–1795.

17 Clifton PM, Kestin M, Abbey M, Drysdale M, Nestel PJ. Relationship between sensitivity to dietary fat and dietary cholesterol. *Arteriosclerosis* 1990;10:394–410.

18 Clifton PM, Nestel PJ. Influence of gender, body mass index, and age on response of plasma lipids to dietary fat plus cholesterol. *Arteriosclerosis* 1992;12:955–962.

19 Cox C, Mann J, Sutherland W, Ball M. Individual variation in plasma cholesterol response to dietary saturated fat. *Br Med J* 1995;311:1260–1264.
20 Humphries SE, Talmud PJ, Cox C, Sutherland W, Mann J. Genetic factors affecting the consistency and magnitude of changes in plasma cholesterol in response to dietary challenge. *Q J Med* 1996;89:671–680.
21 Lewis B, Mann J, Mancini M. Reducing the risks of coronary heart disease in individuals and in the population. *Lancet* 1986;1:956–959.

SONJA L. CONNOR AND WILLIAM E. CONNOR

Pathogenic and Protective Nutritional Factors in Coronary Heart Disease

Historically and to the present time a vast amount of evidence in both humans and animals has pointed to certain dietary factors that produce atherosclerosis and coronary heart disease. The evidence for the crucial role of nutritional factors in the causation of atherosclerosis and its chief clinical consequence, coronary heart disease, goes back to the early years of this century. Ignatovski and Anitschkow in Russia demonstrated that feeding rabbits animal foods, cholesterol, and fat caused hypercholesterolemia and atherosclerosis (1,2). At about the same time de Langen demonstrated that the Dutch diet, rich in animal foodstuffs, would elevate the cholesterol level in Javanese seamen who were accustomed to a diet of rice, fish, fruits, and vegetables and who had little atherosclerosis in contrast to the Dutch (3). The link between nutrition and atherosclerosis was the dietary causation of hyperlipidemia which, when sustained, caused atherosclerosis. However it was not until the 1950s that a precise definition was delineated of which dietary factors caused and which prevented hyperlipidemia and atherosclerosis. This research continues to the present. Dietary therapy should be regarded as the mainstay for the prevention and treatment of hyperlipidemia and coronary heart disease. This is true regardless of the cause, genetic or nutritional. The advantages of dietary therapy are listed in table 1.

Permission has been granted by McGill-Queen's University Press to use segments, tables, and figures from (83).

Table 1
The Advantages of the Dietary Therapy of Hyperlipidemia and Atherosclerosis

1 Inexpensive
2 Can become habitual and can be used by the entire family
3 Safe over the lifetime
4 Will achieve therapeutic goals without drugs in many patients
5 Will augment the action of all lipid-lowering drugs
6 Is antithrombotic as well

Table 2
The Effect of Major Dietary Factors upon Plasma Lipids, Lipoproteins and
Coronary Heart Disease

Pathogenic dietary factors
   Dietary cholesterol
   Saturated fat
   Trans fatty acids
   Total fat
   Total calories with adiposity
   Alcohol (in some individuals)
Protective dietary factors
   Polyunsaturated fat: omega-6-rich vegetable oils and omega-3-rich fish and
      fish oils
   Monounsaturated fat*
   Soluble fibres (pectin, beta glucans, guar gum)
   Antioxidants, especially vitamin E
   Saponins
   Folic acid
   Vegetable protein
   Other substances from vegetables not yet identified

* Very high amounts of polyunsaturated and monounsaturated vegetable fat, while resulting in
a hypocholesterolemic effect overall, would produce postprandial hypertriglyceridemia and
increased remnant formation, except for the fish oils.

From the perspective of the prevention and treatment of coronary
heart disease, the major clinical catastrophe of atherosclerosis, it is
useful to divide nutritional factors into two groups, as is illustrated
in table 2. There are protective nutritional factors and pathogenic
nutritional factors. Cholesterol, saturated and total fat, and excess
calories in the current Western diet are especially pathogenic and
cause hyperlipidemia in susceptible individuals by affecting both
the synthesis and secretion of lipids into the plasma and the removal

Table 3
Causes of Hyperlipidemia

---

1 Overproduction of apo B, VLDL and LDL cholesterol and triglycerides, and
   subsequent secretion into the plasma
2 Defective removal by the liver of: the remnants of chylomicrons and VLDL by the
   apo E receptor, LDL by the apo B-100 receptor

---

of lipids from the plasma (table 3). In addition saturated fat is thrombogenic.

Some dietary factors have a hypolipidemic action and are protective against coronary disease. This is most clearly illustrated in a comparison of France and Finland in 1977, with France having a coronary mortality one-fourth that of Finland. While both countries had similar intakes of saturated fat and cholesterol, France had a much higher intake of protective factors from vegetables and olive and peanut oils and a much lower intake of milk and the thrombosis-producing fatty acids that come from its butterfat content (4). It must also be appreciated that certain dietary factors, such as fatty acids, can affect thrombosis, an event that adds greatly to the organ ischemia produced by atherosclerotic blockage of blood flow.

These important nutritional factors will be discussed in detail to provide the theoretical and practical basis for the dietary treatment of hyperlipidemia and prevention of coronary disease. This article will conclude with a perspective about plasma lipid/lipoprotein changes expected as a result of making dietary changes, the dietary treatment of patients with specific lipid/lipoprotein abnormalities, the use of diet in diabetes and hypertension, and the interrelationships of dietary and pharmaceutical therapy.

Dietary Cholesterol

After absorption dietary cholesterol enters the body via the chylomicron pathway and is removed from the plasma by the liver as a component of chylomicron remnants. After dietary cholesterol is removed by the liver, it enters the hepatic pool of cholesterol. The quantity of cholesterol in the liver profoundly affects the catabolism of LDL. This effect is mediated through the LDL receptor (5–7). Conversely a drastic decrease in dietary cholesterol will increase the LDL receptor activity in the liver, enhance LDL removal, and hence will lower plasma LDL-cholesterol levels.

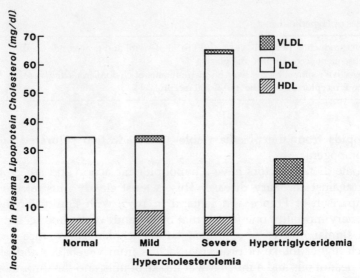

Figure 1. The effects of a 1000 mg cholesterol diet upon the plasma lipoproteins in 25 subjects who comprised a heterogeneous group (normals, moderate and severe hypercholesterolemics and hypertriglyceridemics). The preceding control diet was cholesterol free. Both dietary periods were four weeks in length.

Twenty-six separate metabolic experiments over the past 30 years, involving 196 human subjects and patients, have shown profound effects of dietary cholesterol upon plasma total and LDL-cholesterol levels (8–10). These data document the importance of dietary factors in hyperlipidemia associated with any phenotype or genotype. At one extreme are the Tarahumara Indians, who have an average plasma cholesterol level of 120 mg/dl. They consume a low-cholesterol, low-fat diet and respond to an increase in dietary cholesterol with a 23% increase in plasma cholesterol and a 31% increase in LDL-cholesterol concentrations (11). This is similar to an increase of 17% in the mean plasma cholesterol that occurred when 1000 mg of dietary cholesterol was added to a cholesterol-free diet in 32 subjects (11 normal and 7 with type II-a mild, 5 with II-a severe, and 9 with type IV hyperlipidemia) (figure 1). LDL cholesterol increased significantly in all groups, indirectly showing the effects of dietary cholesterol on the LDL receptor.

Patients with familial hypercholesterolemia respond to reduction of dietary cholesterol. The plasma cholesterol level decreased 18 and 21% in two homozygote hypercholesterolemic patients in response to a cholesterol-free diet (12).

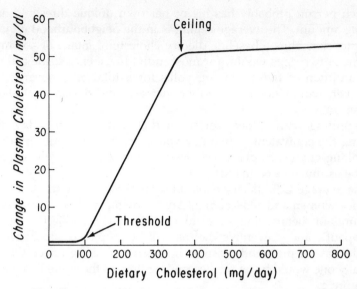

Figure 2. The effects upon the plasma cholesterol level of gradually increasing the amount of dietary cholesterol in human subjects whose background diet is very low in cholesterol content. See the text for discussion of the threshold and ceiling concepts.

Adding more cholesterol to an already substantial cholesterol intake (e.g., from 475 to 950 mg/day) will not necessarily increase the plasma cholesterol level. This phenomenon has been reported from time to time and mistakenly interpreted as showing that dietary cholesterol has no effect on plasma total and LDL-cholesterol levels. These dietary cholesterol feeding studies have been extensively reviewed for those who wish to explore the subject more fully (9,13).

The effect on the plasma cholesterol level of gradually increasing amounts of dietary cholesterol is shown in figure 2. These findings are supported by both animal and human experiments. In the context of a cholesterol-free diet the amount of dietary cholesterol necessary to produce a measurable increase in plasma cholesterol is termed "the threshold amount" (about 100 mg/day). As the dietary cholesterol is increased, the plasma cholesterol level increases and then ultimately plateaus. The amount of dietary cholesterol at this inflection point is termed "the ceiling amount" (about 300–400 mg/day). Increasing the dietary cholesterol further does not lead to higher levels of plasma cholesterol, even though phenomenally large amounts may be fed.

Each person probably has his or her own unique threshold and ceiling amount. The average ceiling is in the neighbourhood of 300–400 mg/day. Thus a baseline dietary cholesterol intake of 500 mg/day from two eggs would, for most individuals, exceed the ceiling. The addition of two more egg yolks for a total of 1,000 mg/day, however, would not then further increase the plasma cholesterol concentration.

Beginning with a low-cholesterol diet under 100 mg/day and adding the equivalent of two egg yolks, or 500 mg, would produce a striking change in plasma cholesterol concentration. This change can be as much as 60 mg/dl (14).

The average U.S. dietary cholesterol intake is about 300–400 mg/day for women and 400–500 mg/day for men (15). Decreasing these amounts of dietary cholesterol to 100 mg/day, the objective of the therapeutic and preventive diet as will be amplified subsequently, would have a profound plasma cholesterol lowering effect. Operationally one would be on the descending limb of the curve illustrated in figure 2.

Effects of Dietary Fats upon the Plasma Lipids and Lipoproteins

Both the amount and kind of fat in the diet affect plasma lipid concentrations. The total amount of dietary fat is important because the formation of chylomicrons in the intestinal mucosa and their subsequent circulation in the blood are directly proportional to the amount of fat that has been consumed. A fatty meal will result in large numbers of chylomicrons and will impart the characteristic lactescent appearance to postprandial plasma three to five hours after eating. "Remnant" production from chylomicrons is proportional to the number of chylomicrons synthesized. Chylomicron remnants resulting from the action of lipoprotein lipase are cholesterol rich and are atherogenic particles (16). Postprandial lipemia is, of course, intense after the usual Western diet and may be present for many hours before being cleared. A typical Western diet with 110 g of fat produces 110 g of chylomicron triglyceride per day. Not only is this lipemia (the composite of chylomicrons and remnants) atherogenic but it may also promote thrombosis (16). Postprandial lipemia is lessened by physical activity and by a diet low in fat and/or a diet containing omega-3 fatty acids from fish (17,18). Postprandial lipemia is intensified and is prolonged in patients with fasting hypertriglyceridemia whose clearance mechanisms are already impaired, i.e., especially patients with type IV and type V hypertrig-lyceridemia. There is even impaired chylomicron clearance in patients with familial combined hyperlipidemia, whose fasting trig-lyceride values are elevated (19).

Saturated Fatty Acids

Fats with different chemical structures have different effects on the plasma cholesterol levels. Fats may be divided into three major classes based on the degree of saturation of their fatty acids. Long-chain, saturated fatty acids have no double bonds, are not essential nutrients, and are readily synthesized in the body from acetate. However, saturated fatty acids in the diet have a powerful hyper-cholesterolemic effect, increase the plasma concentrations of LDL, and are thrombogenic as well. Animal fats tend to be highly satu-rated (30% or more of the fat is saturated) and contain little polyun-saturated fatty acid except for the fats of fish and shellfish, which are, contrastingly, highly polyunsaturated.

The molecular basis for the effects of dietary saturated fat on the plasma cholesterol level is now well understood. It rests upon its influence on the LDL-receptor activity of liver cells as described by Brown and Goldstein (5,20). Dietary saturated fat suppresses mes-senger RNA synthesis for the LDL receptor, which decreases hepatic LDL receptor activity, decreases the removal of LDL from the blood, and thus increases the concentration of LDL cholesterol in the blood (7,21). Dietary cholesterol augments the effect of saturated fat by further suppressing hepatic LDL-receptor activity and raising the plasma LDL-cholesterol level. Conversely a decrease in dietary cho-lesterol and saturated fat increases the LDL-receptor activity of the liver cells, enhances the hepatic pickup of LDL cholesterol, and lowers the concentration of LDL cholesterol in the blood (21).

Some saturated fats, such as coconut oil, also increase the synthesis of cholesterol and LDL in the liver (22). Metabolic studies suggest that one can expect an average plasma cholesterol decrease of 20% by maximally decreasing dietary cholesterol and saturated fat (14).

Besides natural sources of saturated fats, the hydrogenation of liquid vegetable oils can saturate some of the unsaturated fatty acids. Large quantities of highly hydrogenated fat should be avoided to keep the total saturated fat low. Monounsaturated "trans" fatty acids, isomers of the cis oleic acid, are important by-products of the hydrogenation process. It must be appreciated that trans fatty acids are also present in butterfat and in beef, for example. The hydrogenation process occurs through bacterial action in the rumen of the cow. Trans fatty acids are oxidized for energy as are other fatty acids.

In a study in which large amounts of trans fatty acids were consumed (10% kcal), the plasma LDL-cholesterol level was significantly increased (23). However the average trans fatty acid intake in the United States is 2–4% of energy intake and is much lower than the saturated fat intake of 13–14% of energy intake (24).

A study in 56 subjects showed that lightly hydrogenated margarine was clearly preferable to butter when the overall diet was low in fat and high in complex carbohydrate and fibre (25). A dietary coronary trial from England showed that foods containing saturated and trans fatty acids enhanced coronary occlusion (26,27). Men who ate more foods containing myristic, palmitic, and stearic acids (milk, cheese, butter, lamb, and other red meats) had progression of coronary artery disease, whereas men who restricted foods containing these fatty acids stabilized their coronary lesions. The trans fatty acids from those foods also correlated positively with progression of coronary lesions. Conversely vegetable fats, including the trans fatty acids from margarine, were not associated with progression of coronary lesions in this study.

The trans fatty acid intake would be cut in half if a patient reduced the total fat intake from 37–40% to 20% kcal. Further if the patient used small amounts of liquid vegetable oil and select margarines that have been only lightly hydrogenated (those in which a liquid vegetable oil is listed as the first fat ingredient), the trans fatty acid intake would be less than 1% kcal. The softer a margarine is at room temperature the less hydrogenated it is. Peanut butter is so lightly hydrogenated that its fatty acid composition is little affected by this process. The daily use of small quantities of the lightly hydrogenated soft margarines does not constitute a problem in the treatment of hyperlipidemia.

Attention has been called to the fact that some saturated fats do *not* seem to cause hypercholesterolemia (see table 4). Medium chain triglycerides (c8 and c10 saturated fatty acids) are water soluble and are handled metabolically more like carbohydrate than fat. They are transported to the liver via the portal vein blood rather than as chylomicrons. These fatty acids do not elevate the plasma cholesterol concentration.

Dietary stearic acid, an 18-carbon, saturated fatty acid, also has a limited effect upon the plasma cholesterol concentration. Excessive

Table 4
Effects of Different Saturated Fatty Acids on Plasma Cholesterol Levels

Fattty Acid	Action
c8:0, c10:0 medium chain	Neutral
c12:0 lauric	Increase
c14:0, c16:0 myristic, palmitic	Increase
c18:0 stearic	Neutral

stearic acid from the diet is converted into oleic acid, a monounsaturated fatty acid, by the desaturase enzyme in the liver. Feeding
animals large quantities of stearic acid, such as cocoa butter, which
contains a considerable percentage of its total fatty acids as stearic
acid (33%), results in the deposition of oleic acid rather than stearic
acid in the adipose tissue, as would occur with mono- and polyunsaturated fat feeding (28). Another consideration is the potential
for stearic acid to promote thrombosis (26,29). In the study from
England that was discussed earlier, stearic acid was associated with
progression of coronary lesions (26). The authors suggested that
stearic acid is thrombogenic through both platelet actions and the
activation of clotting. The development of a thrombus in a coronary
artery severely obstructed from atherosclerosis, of course, leads to
myocardial infarction or sudden death in coronary patients (27).

The practical importance of these observations about stearic acid
is limited because it is present in foods that also contain appreciable
amounts of the other saturated fatty acids (palmitic, myristic, and
lauric) that cause hypercholesterolemia. One of these, palmitic acid,
is the most common saturated fat found in our food supply. Palmitic
acid has 16 carbons and is intensely hypercholesterolemic in humans
(30). Myristic acid and lauric acid with 14 and 12 carbons, respectively, are also very hypercholesterolemic in humans (30). It is these
fatty acids present in saturated dietary fats that cause their untoward
effects. Amounts of stearic acid in the American diet are not great
compared with palmitic acid (table 5). Also the equations developed
for the prediction of plasma cholesterol change have been based
upon the changes produced by a given fat including its concentration of stearic acid. Thus all of the information that has accumulated
about the hypercholesterolemic and atherogenic properties of beef
fat, butterfat, lard, palm oil, cocoa butter, and coconut oil remains
completely valid.

Table 5
Sources of Specific Saturated Fatty Acids in Foods and Fats

Food	Fatty Acids
MCT oil*	c8:0, c10:0
Coconut oil	c12:0, c14:0
Butter	c14:0, c16:0, c18:0
Beef tallow, lard	c16:0, c18:0
Palm oil	c16:0
Cocoa butter (chocolate)	c16:0, c18:0

* MCT oil = medium chain triglyceride oil

The Cholesterol–Saturated Fat Index of Foods

As already indicated the major plasma cholesterol–elevating effects of a given food reside in its cholesterol and saturated fat content. To help understand the contribution of these two factors in a single food item and to compare one food with another, we have computed a cholesterol–saturated fat index (CSI) for selected foods (31) (see figure 3). The formula for the CSI is: CSI = (1.01 × g saturated fat) + (0.05 × mg cholesterol), where the amounts of saturated fat and cholesterol in a given amount of a food item are entered into this equation. The higher the CSI of a food the greater the hypercholesterolemic and atherogenic effect. This cholesterol–saturated fat index is a representation of how much a given food will decrease the activity of the LDL receptor and, hence, will raise the level of LDL cholesterol in plasma. Worldwide the CSI of a country's diet is highly correlated with the mortality from coronary heart disease (4).

In this context it is particularly instructive to compare the CSI of fish versus that of moderately fat beef. An 85 g portion of cooked fish contains 58 mg of cholesterol and 0.31 g of saturated fat. This contrasts to 72 mg of cholesterol and 10.3 g of saturated fat in 85 g of 30% fat beef. The CSI for the fish is 3, and for the beef 14, almost five times greater. The caloric value of these two portions also differs greatly (100 kcals for fish and 310 kcals for beef). The CSI of cooked chicken and turkey (without the skin) is also lower than that of beef and other red meats and the total fat content is considerably lower. The saturated fat in an 85 g serving of poultry is 1.5 g, the cholesterol is 71 mg, and the CSI is 5. Table 6 lists the CSI for various foods. Shellfish have low CSIS because their saturated fat content is extremely low despite the fact that their cholesterol or total sterol content is 2.5 to 3 times higher than fish, poultry, or red meat. Shellfish have an average CSI

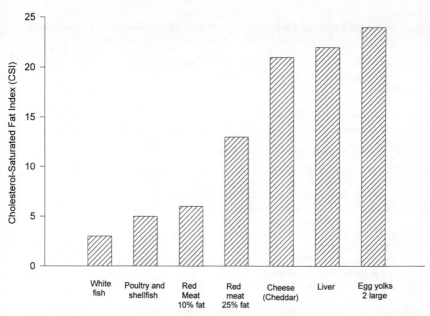

Figure 3. The cholesterol–saturated fat index (CSI) of 85 g of fish, poultry, shellfish, meat, cheese, egg yolk, and liver. The CSI for poultry is the average CSI for cooked light and dark chicken without skin. The CSI for shellfish is the average CSI of cooked crab, lobster, shrimp, clams, oysters, and scallops. The CSI for cheese is the average CSI of cheddar, Swiss, and processed cheese.

of 4 per 85 g. This means that when considering both cholesterol and saturated fat, shellfish, like poultry, is a better choice than even the leanest red meats. Even though salmon is a higher-fat fish, it has a low CSI and is preferred to meat. We have now calculated the CSI for 1000 foods and incorporated this concept in a book along with low-fat, low-cholesterol recipes (32,33).

Monounsaturated Fatty Acids

The second class of dietary fats consists of the characteristic mono-unsaturated fatty acids present in all animal and vegetable fats. For practical purposes oleic acid, having one double bond at the omega-9 position, is the only significant dietary monounsaturated fatty acid (figure 4). In general the effects of dietary monounsaturated fatty acids have been "neutral" in terms of their effects on plasma choles-terol concentrations, neither raising nor lowering them, as a recent review indicated (34). They are, however, cholesterol lowering when

Table 6
The Cholesterol–Saturated Fat Index (CSI) and Kilocalorie Content of Selected Foods

	CSI*	kcalories*
Fish, poultry, red meat (3 oz or 85 g cooked)		
Shellfish (oysters, scallops, clams)	3	114
Whitefish (snapper, perch, sole, cod, halibut, etc.)	3	100
Shellfish (shrimp, crab, lobster)	5	85
Poultry, no skin	5	154
Salmon, chinook	6	173
Beef, pork, and lamb:		
10% fat (ground sirloin, flank steak)	6	176
15% fat (ground extra lean, pork chop)	8	211
25% fat (ground lean, stew meat, rump roasts)	13	286
30% fat (typical ground beef, ground lamb, steaks, ribs, lamb chops, pork sausage, roasts)	14	310
Cheese (1 oz or 28 g) – cheeses in italics are used frequently by staff and patients		
Fat-free cheeses (Cheddar, Jack, ricotta, cream, Healthy Choice, Alpine Lace, Kraft Free Singles)	< 1	41
Lite part-skim mozzarella, low-fat ricotta, *Light Laughing Cow*, Weight Watchers, Lite-Line	2	62
Jarlsberg Lite, low-cholesterol "filled" cheese (Scandic Mini Chol, Hickory Farms Lyte)**	4	65
Part-skim mozzarella, light cream cheese/Neufchatel, Lappi, light Cheddar, light jack (*Kraft Light Naturals*, Alpine Lace, Velveeta Light or other part-skim cheeses)	4	65
Cheddar, Swiss, Jack, Brie, Feta, Montrachet, American, cream cheese, processed cheese (cheese slices, cheese spreads, Velveeta, American)	7	95
Eggs		
Whites (2)	0	33
Egg substitute (equivalent to 2 eggs)	0	51
Whole (2)	24	149
Fats (1/4 cup or 4 tablespoons)		
Reduced-fat peanut butter	4	375
Peanut butter	6	382
Mayonnaise, fat free	trace	47
Mayonnaise, *Best Foods Low Fat*	1	100
Mayonnaise, Light	4	197
Mayonnaise	8	396
Canola oil	4	482
Olive oil	7	477
Most vegetable oils – average of 7 oils	8	481
Canola oil margarine	6	407
Other soft vegetable margarines	9	401
Margarine-butter blends	23	462
Soft shortenings	13	453
Butter	35	407
Coconut oil, palm oil	37	476

Table 6
(continued)

	CSI*	kcalories*
Frozen desserts (1 cup)		
Fruit ices, sorbets	0	258
Nonfat frozen yogurt	1	200
Sherbet or frozen yogurt (low-fat)	2	234
Ice milk	4	234
Ice cream, 10% fat	11	285
Rich ice cream, 16% fat	19	357
Specialty ice cream, 19% fat	26	588
Milk products (1 cup)		
Skim milk or powdered nonfat	1	86
1% milk, buttermilk	2	102
2% milk	4	121
Whole milk (3.5% fat)	7	150
Cottage cheese, nonfat	< 1	141
Cottage cheese (1% fat)	2	164
Cottage cheese, low-fat (2%)	4	203
Cottage cheese (4% fat)	8	217
Light liquid non-dairy creamers: soybean oil	1	140
Liquid non-dairy creamers: soybean oil	4	306
Sour cream, nonfat	1	166
Sour cream, low-fat	14	320
Sour cream, typical	36	449
Imitation sour cream (IMO)	41	479

* Averages
** Cheeses made with skim milk and vegetable oils.

compared to saturated fat. Reports that Mediterranean basin populations that consume olive oil in large quantities have fewer heart
attacks than people in the United States, however, have led to further
investigations of the atherogenic properties of the monounsaturates.
Studies have shown that large amounts of monounsaturated fat, like
polyunsaturated oils, lower plasma total and LDL-cholesterol levels
when compared with saturated fat (35). Furthermore unlike polyunsaturated oils, monounsaturated fat did not lower the plasma HDL-
cholesterol level. However, distinct from omega-3 fatty acids from
fish oil, monounsaturated fat does not decrease the plasma triglyceride
concentrations. Furthermore monounsaturated fat has no known
effect upon prostaglandin metabolism or upon platelet function. As
will be indicated later, omega-3 fatty acids are antithrombotic; monounsaturated fat has no such action.

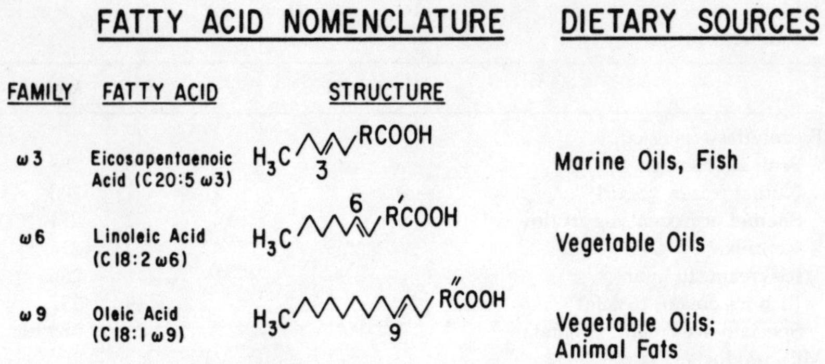

FATTY ACID NOMENCLATURE   DIETARY SOURCES

FAMILY	FATTY ACID	STRUCTURE	
ω3	Eicosapentaenoic Acid (C20:5 ω3)	H_3C ⋀⋀⋀RCOOH 3	Marine Oils, Fish
ω6	Linoleic Acid (C18:2 ω6)	H_3C ⋀⋀⋀⋀RCOOH 6	Vegetable Oils
ω9	Oleic Acid (C18:1 ω9)	H_3C ⋀⋀⋀⋀⋀RCOOH 9	Vegetable Oils; Animal Fats

Figure 4. Nomenclature for fatty acids. Fatty acids can be organized into families according to the position of the first double bond from the terminal methyl group. Typical fatty acids from three common families are shown in this figure. Omega-3 fatty acids all have three carbons between the methyl end and the first double bond. Besides eicosapentaenoic acid (C20:5) shown here, other common omega-3 fatty acids are linolenic acid (C18:3) and docosahexaenoic acid (C22:6). Linoleic acid (C18:2) and arachidonic acid (20:4) are the most important omega-6 fatty acids. Oleic acid (C18:1) is the most common fatty acid in the omega-9 family.

There are several additional points to be made in regards to these studies: 1. The "Mediterranean diet" is also rich in fish, beans, fruit, and vegetables, and is low in both saturated fat and cholesterol. These could be the decisive factors that influence the lessened incidence of coronary disease and the lower plasma cholesterol levels. 2. Olive oil is low in saturated fatty acids (which raise plasma cholesterol levels); this is why the recent metabolic experiments have shown some cholesterol lowering from large amounts of monounsaturated fat in the diet. 3. Large amounts of any kind of fat should be avoided to lower the risk of other diseases such as obesity and colon or breast cancer. In addition all fats, after absorption as chylomicrons, are acted upon by lipoprotein lipase to form remnant particles that circulate in the blood. These remnant particles are atherogenic. Our translation of the latest research on monounsaturated fats is to recommend that patients include them in small amounts as part of a general lower-fat eating style, but not to consider them as especially protective.

Polyunsaturated Fatty Acids

The third class of fatty acids are vital constituents of cellular membranes and serve as prostaglandin precursors. Because they cannot be synthesized by the body and are only obtainable from dietary sources, they are "essential" fatty acids (36). The two classes of polyunsaturated fatty acids are the omega-6 and omega-3 fatty acids (figure 4). Omega-6 and omega-3 fatty acids are not interconvertible. The most common examples of omega-6 fatty acids are arachidonic acid, 20 carbons in length with four double bonds (20:4), and its dietary precursor, linoleic acid (18:2). Linoleic acid is found in many foods and especially in the vegetable seed oils, whereas there is little arachidonic acid in the diet. Linoleic acid is converted to arachidonic acid in the liver. Since the basic structure of omega-6 fatty acids cannot be synthesized by the body, 2–3% of the total energy in the diet must consist of linoleic acid to meet the metabolic requirements of the body for the omega-6 structure.

Omega-3 fatty acids differ from omega-6 fatty acids in the position of the first double bond. Counting from the methyl end of the molecule, this double bond is at the third rather than the sixth carbon as for the omega-6 fatty acids. Omega-3 fatty acids are also "essential." They are important membrane components of all organs, especially the brain, retina, and sperm. The dietary sources of omega-3 fatty acids are plant foods, some but not all vegetable oils, and leafy vegetables. Fish and shellfish are especially rich in omega-3 fatty acids. Linolenic acid (c18:3) is obtained from the vegetable products. Eicosapentaenoic acid (EPA, c20:5) and docosahexaenoic acid (DHA, c22:6) are derived from fish, shellfish, and phytoplankton (the plants of the ocean). These fatty acids are highly concentrated in fish oils. Once either the omega-3 or omega-6 structure comes into the body as the 18-carbon linoleic or linolenic acid, the body can synthesize the longer chain and more highly-polyunsaturated omega-6 or omega-3 fatty acids (20 and 22 carbons), but the synthesis is rate limited. A safe intake of omega-3 fatty acids would be 0.4 to 0.6% of total calories and is especially important in infant nutrition and during pregnancy (37).

EPA and DHA are present in the diet in two forms: as triglyceride in the adipose tissue of fish, usually present between muscle fibres, and as membrane phospholipids of the muscle of fish. These highly polyunsaturated fatty acids occupy the middle position of the glycerol skeleton for both triglycerides and phospholipids. In either of these dietary forms EPA and DHA are efficiently absorbed from the intestinal tract (38). After absorption EPA and DHA readily associate with membranes and are found in the four plasma lipid classes: triglycerides, free fatty acids, cholesterol esters, and phospholipids.

Ultimately they are stored in the adipose tissue. We have found they even reach the brain and the retina.

There are distinctly different functions in the body for omega-3 and omega-6 fatty acids (39). Both serve as substrates for the formation of different prostaglandins and leukotrienes and are abundant in phospholipid membranes. Both omega-3 and omega-6 fatty acids are concentrated in nervous tissue. Omega-3 fatty acids are rich in the retina, brain, spermatozoa, gonads, and many other organs. Omega-6 fatty acids are concentrated in the different plasma lipid classes (cholesterol esters, phospholipids, etc.) and in addition play a role in lipid transport.

Polyunsaturated fatty acids in large amounts, either the omega-6 or omega-3 structure, reduce plasma total and LDL-cholesterol concentrations in normal and hypercholesterolemic individuals (8). The situation is somewhat different in hypertriglyceridemic individuals or in those with combined hyperlipidemia. Only the omega-3 fatty acids from fish and fish oil have a decided hypotriglyceridemic effect. VLDL, in particular, is decreased by the omega-3 fatty acids (40). Isotopic studies have shown that the hypotriglyceridemic effect of omega-3 fatty acids occurs as a result of the depression of triglyceride, VLDL and apoprotein B synthesis in the liver, and also accelerated catabolism of VLDL from the plasma (41). In some patients with type IV hypertriglyceridemia and in some patients with combined hyperlipidemia, there have been reports of an increase in LDL as the plasma triglyceride falls after fish oil administration. This increase in LDL also occurs when gemfibrozil is given to these patients. In the severely hypertriglyceridemic type V patients, however, large doses of fish oil (10–15 g/day) produce a dramatic clearing of chylomicronemia and lower both triglyceride and cholesterol concentrations. Fish oil also promotes the clearing of chylomicrons after the administration of a fatty meal. This would be of particular benefit in the type V patient in whom there is great difficulty in clearing chylomicrons. Most experiments have not shown plasma triglyceride lowering from the omega-6 vegetable oils.

In the early days of dietary therapy for hyperlipidemia, it was suggested that large amounts of a vegetable oil such as corn oil could be used to treat hypercholesterolemia. However, its high content of the omega-6 fatty acid linoleic acid was probably not beneficial. It promoted obesity and gallstone formation and, more importantly, may have been carcinogenic, as suggested by animal studies. In current diets for the treatment of hyperlipidemia, omega-6 polyunsaturated fatty acids are not increased from the current amount in the Western diet, which averages about 6–8% of total calories. When saturated and monounsaturated fatty acids are decreased, they should not be replaced in total by equivalent amounts of polyunsaturated fatty acids from liquid vegetable oil, margarines, or shortenings.

Omega-3 fatty acids from fish have important effects whether or not the diet is high in saturated fat. In either instance omega-3 fatty acids produced a lowering of plasma cholesterol, triglyceride, and especially VLDL (about 50%) (42). With the low–saturated fat diet there was an additional action; further plasma cholesterol lowering occurred as LDL declined 25%. Thus an ideal diet would be low in saturated fat and high in omega-3 fatty acids.

It is not known exactly how much the intake of omega-3 fatty acids should be increased to achieve optimum effect. One study from the Netherlands indicated that men who included fish in their diet twice a week had fewer deaths from heart disease (43). A similar protective effect from eating fish occurred in the Seattle study. Men who ate a weekly meal of salmon had a 50% reduction in cardiac arrest, a most compelling statistic (44). In a prospective trial in Wales the prescription of two fish meals per week led to both a reduction in total mortality and in coronary events (45). Even very low-fat seafood contains an appreciable amount of omega-3 fatty acids, up to 40% or more of total fatty acids. Eating a total of 12 oz of a variety of fish and shellfish each week would provide 3 to 5 grams of omega-3 fatty acids as well as protein, vitamins, and minerals. The fish could be fresh, frozen, or canned without affecting the quantity of omega-3 fatty acids. The patient with hyperlipidemia can only expect to have beneficial effects from following this dietary advice, especially if the fish replaced meat in the diet, meat being a major source of saturated fat. Also to be considered are the antithrombotic actions of fish oil mediated through inhibition of the thromboxane A2 in platelets (39) and the enhanced clearance of chylomicrons (17,46). Other effects of fish oil include inhibition of platelet-derived growth factor, alteration of certain functions of leukocytes, reduction of blood viscosity, greater fibrinolysis, inhibition of intimal hyperplasia in vein grafts used for arterial bypass (47), and, most recently, reduced risk of primary cardiac arrest (44). Fish oil serves as a therapeutic agent in certain hyperlipidemic states, especially the chylomicronemia of type V hyperlipidemia. Thus fish oils have discrete effects not only upon the plasma lipids and lipoproteins but also upon the atherosclerotic and thrombotic process.

Carbohydrate

If the total fat content of a hypolipidemic diet is reduced from the current Western fat intake of 35–40% of the total calories to only 20%, and if the protein of the diet is kept constant, then the difference in caloric intake between a high-fat diet and a low-fat diet would ideally be made up by increasing the complex carbohydrate content of the diet. Epidemiological evidence buttresses this basic concept since populations ingesting a high-carbohydrate diet from complex carbohydrates have low plasma cholesterol levels and a low incidence of coronary disease.

Are there harmful effects from a high-carbohydrate diet? It was demonstrated more than 25 years ago that a sudden increase in the amount of dietary carbohydrate in Americans accustomed to a high-fat diet would dramatically increase the plasma triglyceride concentration. After many weeks of the new diet, however, adaptation occurs and the hypertriglyceridemia subsides. If the dietary carbohydrate is gradually increased as fat is reduced, the hypertriglyceridemia does not occur. Thus high dietary carbohydrate should not be regarded as a problem, but rather as a caloric replacement for the saturated fat removed from the diet. For example we increased the dietary carbohydrate intake gradually from 45% kcal to 65% kcal over a 28-day period in eight mildly hypertriglyceridemic subjects. There was a significant fall in the mean plasma cholesterol level, from 232 to 198 mg/dl. The mean plasma triglyceride level remained constant, 213–230 mg/dl (48).

In a low-fat, high-carbohydrate diet the majority of the carbohydrate is in the form of cereals and legumes and not as sucrose or other simple sugars. Americans commonly consume about 20% of the total calories as sucrose or other simple sugars, about half of their carbohydrate intake. In the dietary changes being suggested, sugar intake would fall to about 10% of the total calories. Sucrose, in large quantities, is mildly hypertriglyceridemic. The primary point is that all simple sugars, including sucrose, are potent promoters of obesity; they are extremely low in bulk and have a high caloric density.

Fibre, Saponins, and Antioxidants

Dietary fibre is a broad, nondescript term that includes several carbohydrates thought to be indigestible by the human gut. These include cellulose, hemicellulose, lignin, pectin, and beta glucans. In humans dietary fibre promotes satiety through its bulk and produces larger stools and a more rapid intestinal transit, factors that may prevent certain diseases of the colon (i.e., diverticulitis, colon cancer). Interest in the hypolipidemic effects of fibre dates back at least 30 years. Fibre added to semi-synthetic diets fed to rats has usually had a plasma cholesterol–lowering effect. Ingesting fibre, predominantly in an insoluble form such as wheat bran, has probably not had a hypocholesterolemic effect in humans. Soluble fibre may be different. Large amounts of soluble fibre (17 g/2000 kcal), such as that contained in oat bran or beans, produced a 20% reduction of plasma total and LDL-cholesterol levels (49). These decreases were at least in part the result of concurrent weight loss. In a recent study a more modest effect was achieved. Very high intakes of food rich in soluble fibre lowered plasma cholesterol levels 5% more than was achieved by a Step Two diet that was high only in insoluble fibre. LDL and HDL were also reduced (50). One way that soluble fibre acts to lower cholesterol levels is to bind bile acids in the gut and prevent their reabsorption. This is the same mechanism as the bile acid–binding resins like cholestyramine. Rich sources of soluble fibre include fruits, oats and some other cereals, legumes, and vegetables.

A high-fibre diet is certainly integral to the dietary concepts for the treatment of hyperlipidemia. The consumption of more foods from vegetable sources will automatically mean a higher consumption of both total and soluble fibre. Such foods are bulky and have a low caloric density which is helpful for the overweight patient. A feeling of satiety occurs from the consumption of high-fibre foods that also are low in calories. It is likely that foods high in fibre have a mild hypolipidemic effect. If oat bran is consumed in place of bacon and eggs for breakfast, this high-fibre food would also have a beneficial effect indirectly, since it is replacing foods high in cholesterol and saturated fat. Finally plant foods rich in fibre may also contain other hypocholesterolemic substances. One of these is a group of compounds called saponins, which, in monkeys, had a hypocholesterolemic action (51). Saponins bind cholesterol present in the gut lumen and prevent its absorption.

Other dietary factors that may be important in prevention of the atherogenic process are contained in fruits, vegetables, grains, and beans. Besides soluble fibre and saponins, as already mentioned, we should also consider the role of the antioxidants contained in these foods in preventing the oxidation of LDL, since oxidized LDL is believed to be particularly pathogenic in the atherosclerotic process

(52–55). A study in 80 subjects who consumed a 10% fat diet and exercised daily resulted in increased resistance of LDL to oxidation (56). The antioxidant factors in plant foods include beta carotene, ascorbic acid (vitamin C), and alpha tocopherol (vitamin E) (54,57). Of these antioxidant vitamins, only vitamin E in a dose of 400 units per day has been shown to lower the incidence of coronary heart disease in survivors of myocardial infarction and at the same time to be safe (58). In regard to taking supplemental vitamins to prevent coronary heart disease, an editorial concluded that while the evidence is suggestive, we need other trials before supplements of other antioxidant vitamins should be administered. Possible harmful effects have not been studied either (59). The important point is that when dietary fat is reduced the consumption of fruits, vegetables, and beans is enhanced, which would increase the intakes of the desirable antioxidants in a more natural and physiological form.

Protein

The dietary treatment of hyperlipidemia involves, in general, a shift from the consumption of protein derived from animal sources, such as meat and dairy products, to the consumption of more protein from plants. The nutritional adequacy of such protein shifts is assured because mixtures of vegetable proteins, plus the provision of ample low-fat animal protein sources, provide for essential amino acid requirements. Ranges of protein intake from 25 to 150 g/day have been tested for effects on blood lipids and have been found to have no effect within amounts commonly consumed by Americans. Experiments in animals, however, suggest that an animal protein such as casein is definitely hypercholesterolemic and a vegetable protein such as soy protein is hypocholesterolemic (60). There are suggestions, moreover, that the consumption of vegetable protein may have some hypocholesterolemic action in humans. There has been a shift in the sources of protein in the U.S. from the early 1900s (52% vegetable, 48% animal) to 1980 (68% animal, 32% vegetable), suggesting there has been an increase in the methionine intake (61). A higher intake of methionine, coupled with a lower intake of folic acid if there is a low consumption of vegetables and fruits, could theoretically result in a higher plasma homocysteine level, which has been associated with increased risk of atherosclerosis (62,63). Also it may be postulated that a shift in protein intake to include more vegetable protein carries no risk and may confer some benefit to the hyperlipidemic individual. Milk protein consumption, in a world-wide epidemiological survey, correlated directly with the incidence of coronary heart disease (4).

Calories

Excessive caloric intake and adiposity can contribute to both hyper-triglyceridemia and hypercholesterolemia by stimulating the liver to overproduce triglyceride and VLDL (64). This is especially true for abdominal or visceral obesity in which mobilized free fatty acids from the adipose tissue are carried directly to the liver via the portal circulation and stimulate VLDL synthesis. The plasma triglyceride and VLDL concentrations of hypertriglyceridemic patients are greatly reduced by weight reduction and are increased by weight gain (64). There is little direct evidence, however, that the LDL receptor and plasma cholesterol and LDL concentrations are directly affected by caloric excess. Nonetheless it is known that obese individuals have a total body cholesterol production higher than that of normal weight individuals. Weight reduction and fasting, which involve a decrease in the consumption of cholesterol and saturated fat, would be expected to increase LDL receptor activity and improve LDL levels in hyperlipidemic patients. It is therefore reasonable to advise caloric control and the avoidance of obesity in the dietary management of hyperlipidemia. The role of increased physical activity is most impor-tant in weight control. The consumption of a self-selected research diet that is low in fat and high in complex carbohydrate and fibre has resulted in weight loss and, if the subjects also exercised, there was an improvement in plasma lipids and lipoproteins (65).

When excessive dietary cholesterol and fat are combined with excessive calories, a particularly potent hyperlipidemic effect occurs. Such a "holiday" diet occurs particularly in the United States between Thanksgiving and New Year's. The effects of such dietary excesses were actually studied in the Tarahumara Indians of Mexico, a people habitually accustomed to a very low-fat diet (66). After a suitable baseline period in which they consumed their typical diet, Tarahu-mara Indians of both sexes were given a diet high in cholesterol, fat, and calories. Within two weeks their plasma lipids had increased tre-mendously: total cholesterol 31%, LDL 39%, HDL 31%, and plasma triglyceride 18%. Body weight gain averaged 7–8 pounds for each individual. The composite action of all of these potent dietary hyper-lipidemic factors was certainly greater than any one of them alone.

Alcohol

In the past few years there has been confusion over the relationship of alcohol consumption and factors related to coronary heart disease. Alcohol consumption correlates well with higher values of HDL in the blood and reduced mortality from coronary heart disease (67–70). Since HDL plays a role in "reverse" cholesterol transport, this finding has encouraged some to drink more with the idea that alcohol is "good for the heart." These findings related to alcohol, HDL, and coronary disease, however, are too scant, contradictory, and complex to lend themselves to any definite conclusions. From a clinical point of view the typical patient attending a lipid clinic who is overweight and consuming two or more drinks per day could have some problems that are directly related to alcohol consumption itself. Usually such patients are overweight and hypertriglyceridemic, and have low HDL concentrations (71,72). One aspect of the treatment for hypertriglyceridemia is to reduce alcohol consumption or even stop it completely, since alcohol ingestion can increase plasma triglyceride levels. Alcohol also has a high caloric content of 140 kcals per drink. Two to three drinks a day can contribute 300–400 kcals to an already hypercaloric state, thus stimulating further the synthesis of triglyceride and VLDL by the liver (73). Even more importantly alcohol has so many adverse social, psychological, and physical effects that the astute physician would not recommend alcohol even if it would increase HDL levels. On the contrary the best evidence indicates that those who drink are least likely to enjoy good health. In our Lipid Disorders Clinic we suggest that people restrict alcohol consumption to no more than 2–4 drinks per week in order to avoid adverse effects upon the plasma lipids and lipoproteins.

Coffee and Tea

Because of the enjoyment people derive from coffee, almost a national pastime, there is great interest in the ever-conflicting reports on the relationship between coffee and coronary heart disease. One study from Europe does make some sense in that boiled coffee, which would extract most of the ingredients that might have any effect upon health, is positively associated with a higher incidence of coronary heart disease (74). The methods of coffee preparation in North America are generally different (instant, percolated, and drip coffee). In a recent U.S. study the consumption of 720 ml of filtered coffee raised the plasma cholesterol slightly (both LDL and HDL alike) in contrast to no effect from the same amount of decaffeinated coffee (75). A theoretical reason why large quantities of coffee might be harmful relates to its caffeine content. Caffeine stimulates the release of epinephrine, which increases free fatty acid concentrations. The production of VLDL and triglyceride would be expected to increase as a consequence. No one has defined precisely what an excessive coffee intake is. When patients ask us we generally suggest no more than four cups per day. Tea, on the other hand, has not been associated with any disease. In fact tea drinkers, if anything, seem to have less coronary heart disease. Whether a patient chooses to drink decaffeinated, regular, or no coffee or strong tea at all really becomes a matter of personal choice.

Minerals and Vitamins

Under the assumption that daily requirements have been met in the diet, there is no information to indicate that additional vitamins and minerals above and beyond the content of a nutritionally adequate diet will have any effect upon the plasma lipid concentrations. This comment applies equally to vitamin C (76), vitamin E (77), and beta-carotene, all enthusiastically consumed by the public without there being some conclusive proof of benefit in hyperlipidemia. However these vitamins do serve as antioxidants and, as discussed earlier, oxidized LDL enhances atherosclerosis (78). Theoretically antioxidants would prevent the oxidation of LDL and would inhibit atherosclerosis. Long term, possibly harmful effects of large doses of these antioxidant vitamins are also not known. A low consumption of vegetables and fruits would result in a low intake of folic acid, possibly raise the plasma homocysteine level, and increase risk of atherosclerosis (62,63). We favour the view that all people should usually obtain the desired amounts of minerals and vitamins from food. Several million years of human evolution occurred without the use of nutritional supplements. The prescribed low-fat diet has ample quantities of vitamins and minerals and this would be an additional protective characteristic.

The Dietary Design to Achieve Optimal
Plasma Lipid–Lipoprotein Levels

In view of the evidence about the role of dietary factors in the causation of hyperlipidemia and subsequent coronary heart disease, it

        Diet and Cardiovascular Disease

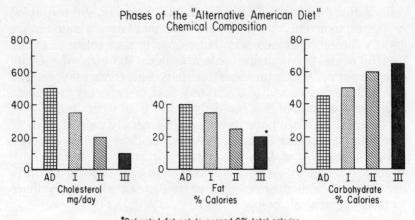

Figure 5. The cholesterol, fat, and carbohydrate contents of the typical U.S. diet (AD) and the three phases of the low-fat, high–complex carbohydrate diet (I, II, and III).

should be possible to indicate the features of the most effective diet to prevent and treat hyperlipidemia (14). The major features of this "maximal" diet are that it is low in cholesterol, low in fat and saturated fat, and, reciprocally, high in complex carbohydrate and fibre (figure 5). The first objective is to reduce cholesterol consumption from 500 to less than 100 mg/day (note that only foods of animal origin contain cholesterol). This requires keeping egg yolk consumption to a minimum, since much of the dietary cholesterol comes from egg yolk. Half of this is from visible eggs and half from eggs incorporated into processed foods. Meat, poultry, and fish also are limited. Non-fat dairy products are recommended.

The second objective is to reduce fat intake by one-half from 40 to 20% of calories. This can be done by avoiding fried foods, reducing the fat used in baked goods by one-third, and using low-fat dairy products. A good guide to use in selecting foods is to choose main dishes with no more than 10 g of fat per serving. For other dishes choose those with no more than 5 g of fat per serving. Added fat should be limited to two teaspoons per day for women and children and four teaspoons per day for teenagers and men. Peanut butter should be eaten no more than twice a week as part of a meal and not as a snack; nuts, olives, and avocados used sparingly as condiments. The daily fat allowance in calories and grams for a 20% fat diet is given in table 7.

Table 7
The 20% Fat Diet: Daily Fat Allowance in Calories and Grams for Different Caloric
Levels

| Calorie levels | Daily Fat Allowance | | Appropriate for |
	Calories	Grams	
1200	240	27	Weight loss
1600	320	36	Weight loss
2000	400	44	Women/children
2400	480	53	Women
2800	560	62	Men/teens
3200	640	71	Men/teens/exercisers
3600	720	80	Exercisers

The third objective is to decrease the current saturated fat intake by two-thirds, from 14 to 5% of calories. This requires eating limited amounts of red meat or cheese no more than twice a week, using lower-fat cheeses (20% fat or less), limiting ice-cream and chocolate to once a month, using soft margarines and oils sparingly, and avoiding products containing coconut and palm oil.

When people are advised to decrease the amount of fat in their diets, they usually think only of visible fat and are surprised to learn that fat added at the table represents only 22% of their total fat intake. Decreasing dietary fat would be very difficult without knowing that 78% is invisible, with the majority coming from red meat, cheese, ice cream and other dairy products, baked products, and fat used in food preparation.

The fourth major dietary objective is to increase the carbohydrate content. If dietary fat is reduced from 40 to 20% of calories and protein kept constant at 15% of calories, then carbohydrate intake must be increased from 45 to 65% of total calories. In practical terms this means that at least two complex carbohydrate–containing foods should be eaten at each meal. For example eating toast and cereal for breakfast, a sandwich (2 slices of bread) or bean soup and non-fat crackers at lunch, and 1–2 cups of rice, pasta, potatoes, corn, etc., with bread at dinner. Snacks should be of a complex carbohydrate type, such as baked chips, popcorn, or low-fat crackers and low-fat cookies. This is a significant change as most Americans currently limit carbohydrate foods to no more than one per meal. To reach the increased carbohydrate objective the patient must also eat 3–5 cups of legumes per week and 2–4 cups of vegetables per day. While research increasingly supports the value of a high-carbohydrate diet, many people are reluctant to adopt it because "starchy" foods are associated with weight gain because they are typically combined with foods high in fat and calories (oil, cheese, sour cream, etc.). Patients need recipes and convenience foods that combine complex carbohydrates with low-fat ingredients to provide tasty dishes. The carbohydrate objective, however, is essential if the fat intake is reduced and body weight is to be maintained. Another objective is to eat 3–5 pieces of fruit per day with a concomitant decrease in refined sugar intake from 20% of calories to 10%. This means that sweets (pop, candy, or baked desserts) are limited to no more than two servings per week.

A Phased Approach to the Dietary Treatment of Hyperlipidemia

A realistic view is that even well-motivated patients have difficulty making abrupt changes in their dietary habits. It may take many months and even years to change patterns of food consumption. Therefore the changes recommended from the current Western diet of most hyperlipidemic patients should be approached in a gradual manner, with each of three phases introducing more changes toward the eating pattern ultimately required for maximal therapy.

We call this changing from Phase I (making substitutions) to Phase II (eating meatless, cheeseless lunches and trying new recipes) to Phase III (doing every day what used to be done once a week). People need to change slowly and gradually by trying new recipes (33,79) and new food products one at a time and incorporating those they like into their lifestyles. How far and how fast one progresses through the phases depends on the energy and interest for trying new recipes and new products. There needs to be continual exposure to new foods and recipes if change is to become permanent and the eating style is to keep up with current tastes. For example fajitas (stir-fried vegetables and chicken in a flour tortilla) are a fairly recent addition to the U.S. cuisine. Now there are many recipes for fajitas and many restaurants serve them. Eating styles are continually being remodelled so people need continual inspiration for trying low-fat recipes and food products.

The goal of Phase I is to modify the customary consumption of foods very high in cholesterol and saturated fat (table 8). This can be accomplished by deleting egg yolk, butterfat, lard, and organ meats (liver, heart, brain, kidney, gizzards) from the diet and by

Table 8
Summary of the Suggested Dietary Changes in the Different Phases of the Low-Fat,
High–Complex Carbohydrate Diet

Phase I	Avoid foods very high in cholesterol and saturated fat: delete egg yolk, butterfat, lard, and organ meats
	Substitute soft margarine for butter, vegetable oils and shortening for lard, skim milk for whole milk, egg whites for whole eggs
Phase II	Eat meatless, cheeseless lunches
	Gradually use less meat and more fish, chicken, and turkey: no more than 6–8 oz once a day
	Use less fat and cheese
	Acquire new recipes
	Make low-csi, low-fat choices when eating out
Phase III	Eat mainly cereals, legumes, fruit, and vegetables
	Use meat as a condiment; eat fish twice a week
	Use low-csi, low-fat cheeses
	Save these foods for use only on special occasions: extra meats, regular cheese, chocolate, candy, and coconut

using substitute products when possible: soft margarine for butter, vegetable oils and shortenings for lard, skim milk and skim milk products for whole milk and whole milk products, and egg whites and/or egg substitutes for whole eggs. Patients are also encouraged to trim fat from meat and remove skin from chicken, choose commercial food products lower in fat and csi such as for cheeses and frozen yogurt, modify favourite recipes by using less fat and sugar, and decrease the use of table salt (use a lower sodium salt such as Lite Salt).

In Phase II a reduction in meat consumption is the goal, with a gradual transition from the presumed American ideal of up to a pound of a meat a day to no more than 6–8 oz per day (table 8). Meat can no longer be the centre of the meal, particularly for two or three meals a day. The goal is to eat meatless, cheeseless lunches. Some ideas for lunch with and without sandwiches have been detailed in sample menus and recipes (33,79). In addition in Phase II we propose the use of less fat and cheese and fewer products containing salt. For example encouragement is given to cut down on fats used as spreads, on/in salads, and in cooking and baking. When eating out patients are encouraged to make low-csi, low-fat choices.

Substitute recipes have been developed to replace recipes that are centred on meat or high-fat dairy products (cream cheese, butter, sour cream, cheese) as the principal ingredients. Since these foods are to be eaten in smaller amounts or even omitted (butterfat), the patient needs to find recipes that use larger amounts of grains, legumes, vegetables, and fruits. Examples of such recipes are included in (33) and (79).

In Phase III the maximal diet for the treatment of hyperlipidemia is attained (table 8). The cholesterol content of the diet is reduced to 100 mg per day, and saturated fat is lowered to 5–6% of total calories. Since cholesterol is contained only in foods of animal origin, these changes mean that meat consumption in particular must be further reduced. Meat, fish, and poultry should be used as "condiments" rather than "aliments." With this philosophy the meat dish will no longer occupy the centre of the table. Instead meat in smaller quantities will spice up dishes based on vegetables, rice, cereal, and legumes much as Asian, Indian, and Mediterranean cookery has been doing for eons. The total of meat and poultry should average 3–4 oz per day, but the use of poultry should be stressed because of its lower content of saturated fat. The recommendation is to eat fish twice a week. Note the low cholesterol–saturated fat index (CSI) of fish (table 6), shared also by shellfish. Because of a low CSI up to 6 oz of fish can be used in place of meat in Phase III of the diet. Also all fish contain omega-3 fatty acids that are antithrombotic.

Shellfish are divided into two groups: higher-CSI shellfish (shrimp, crab, and lobster) and lower-CSI shellfish (oysters, clams, and scallops). Both contain omega-3 fatty acids and have a low fat content. Because of differences in CSI content, higher-CSI shellfish are more restricted in the daily diet than are the lower-CSI shellfish, i.e., 3 oz vs 6 oz per day. The lower-CSI shellfish contain other sterols (e.g., brassicasterol) that are more analogous to plant sterols. These are poorly absorbed by humans.

The use of special lower-CSI, low-fat cheeses is an important component of Phase III (see table 6). Other goals include using no more than 4–7 teaspoons of fat per day as spreads and salad dressings, in cooking and baking, and from commercially prepared foods; decreasing the amount of salt used in cooking; drinking 4–6 glasses of water per day; and enjoying a wide variety of new foods and a repertoire of new and savoury recipes. The sample menus in references (79) and (33) give some idea about the eating pattern in Phase III.

An eating habit questionnaire, The Diet Habit Survey, can be used to classify the diet as the typical Western diet (40% fat) and as Phase I (30%), II (25%), and III (20%) of the low-fat, high–complex carbohydrate diet (80). The Diet Habit Survey is related to plasma cholesterol change, measures eating habits directly, reflects nutrient composition indirectly, is quick to administer, and is inexpensive to analyze. Thus it is useful as a research questionnaire and helpful in the dietary management of patients with hyperlipidemia and coronary heart disease.

Predicted Plasma Cholesterol Lowering from the Three Phases of the Low-Fat, High–Complex Carbohydrate Diet

As has been emphasized both dietary cholesterol and saturated fat elevate plasma cholesterol levels, whereas monounsaturated fat is neutral and polyunsaturated fats have a mild depressing effect. In stepwise fashion the cholesterol and saturated fat of each phase of the diet are successively reduced, with Phase III providing for the lowest intakes. According to calculations derived from Hegsted and co-workers (81), changing from the current American diet to Phase III of the low-fat, high–complex carbohydrate diet would provide for maximal plasma cholesterol lowering, an estimated average decrease of 20%. Phase II would produce a 14% lowering and Phase I, 7%. These plasma cholesterol changes for all phases offer the possibility of improved plasma levels, depending on the amount of dietary modification, with Phase III as the ultimate goal. Figure 6 illustrates the theoretical plasma cholesterol lowering for three people who have very different initial plasma cholesterol levels based on genetic differences, while consuming the current American diet. Regardless of the initial plasma cholesterol level, everyone's level decreases as dietary changes are made, approximately 5–7% per phase.

The Applicability of the Low-Cholesterol, Low-Fat, High-Carbohydrate Diet in the Treatment of the Various Phenotypes and Genotypes of Hyperlipidemia

We emphasize a single dietary approach for the treatment of all forms of hyperlipidemia (8,82–84). There need not be a different diet for each phenotype of this clinical problem. Instead, as indicated and further illustrated in table 9, this dietary approach deals effectively with the disturbed pathophysiology in all of these phenotypes, regardless of the lipoprotein disturbance (chylomicrons, VLDL, IDL, and/or LDL). (For a thorough discussion of the phenotypes and genotypes of hyperlipidemia, please see references [82] and [84].) The reduction in dietary cholesterol and saturated fat will increase LDL receptor activity. The plasma cholesterol and LDL will then decrease. Lower dietary fat

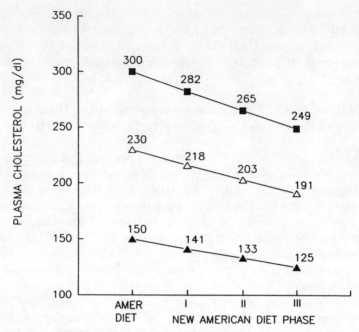

Figure 6. Theoretical plasma cholesterol changes for three people changing from the American diet to a low-fat, high–complex carbohydrate diet. *The New American Diet* Phases I, II, and III.

intake means that fewer chylomicrons would be synthesized. A reduction in fat intake with an increase in high-fibre foods from vegetables and grains usually leads to a slightly reduced caloric intake with some weight loss and a reduction in VLDL synthesis.

In types I and V hyperlipidemia it may be necessary to restrict the fat below the suggested 20% of total calories. In these conditions the amount of dietary fat is a trial-and-error proposition. Fat may need to be restricted to less than 10% of calories, with the diet composed primarily of fruits, vegetables, grains, beans, and fish, with a little chicken. In chylomicronemia the cholesterol intake is of lesser importance, so shellfish can be consumed safely. Fish and shellfish also contain omega-3 fatty acids, which would tend to depress the synthesis of VLDL by the liver. Should caloric restriction be necessary in order to attain ideal body weight, the use of the very low-fat diet plus increased physical activity would be the approach to follow. Even in familial hypercholesterolemia we have found the influence

Table 9
How the Low-Fat, Low-Cholesterol Diet Will Affect the Plasma Lipids and Lipoproteins

Dietary Factor Affected	Plasma Lipids-Lipoproteins					Phenotype Affected
	Cholesterol	LDL	Trigly-ceride	VLDL	Chylomicrons & remnants	
Cholesterol 100 mg/da	↓↓↓	↓↓↓				II-a, II-b
Saturated fat 5% of calories	↓↓↓	↓↓↓				II-a, II-b
Total fat to 20% of calories	↓	↓	↓		↓↓↓	All phenotypes esp. I and V
Complex CHO, fibre and plant foods	↓	↓	↓			All phenotypes
Protein, more vegetable less animal	↓	↓				No information
Caloric reduction for the overweight	↓	↓	↓↓	↓↓	↓↓	II-b, III, IV, V

of diet to be crucial in attaining the lowest possible LDL concentrations. In fact we suspect that the LDL receptor of these patients is even more susceptible to the effects of dietary cholesterol and saturated fat, since the number of LDL receptors is already reduced about 50%.

It is important to be aware that the HDL-cholesterol level will increase with a high-fat, high-cholesterol diet (85). A low-fat diet will decrease HDL. It has been suggested that the increase in HDL cholesterol in response to a high-cholesterol, high–saturated fat diet is a defensive mechanism to counteract the concomitant increase in LDL cholesterol (86). However populations such as the Tarahumara Indians, whose diets are very low in fat and very high in complex carbohydrates, are known to have HDL-cholesterol levels that are pathologically low by U.S. standards (87). Both Tarahumara men and women have average HDL-cholesterol levels of 28–29 mg/dl. Other populations that eat low-fat diets have also been observed to have low HDL-cholesterol levels (88,89). Since these populations have low LDL-cholesterol levels and little coronary heart disease, the low HDL-cholesterol level is not a risk factor. The physiological response to a low-fat diet is a 10–20% decrease in the HDL-cholesterol level (48). Since LDL-cholesterol lowering is even greater, the LDL-to-HDL ratio is little changed or even improved. Also a recent study indicated that a lower HDL-cholesterol level resulting from a low-fat, high–complex carbohydrate diet is different from a genetically low HDL-cholesterol level and that the coronary risk is not enhanced (90).

The Use of the Low-Fat, High–Complex Carbohydrate Diet in Diabetic Patients, Pregnant Patients, Children, and Hypertensive Patients

The approach to diabetic patients who are also hyperlipidemic involves the same dietary considerations as for the treatment of hyperlipidemia generally. Phase III of the diet has been used successfully in both juvenile-onset and maturity-onset diabetic patients, insulin-dependent and non-insulin-dependent. Clearly involved in this treatment is the appropriate control of carbohydrate as well as lipid metabolism by means of adequate amounts of insulin, increased physical activity, and weight reduction when the patient is overweight. The great propensity of diabetic patients to atherosclerotic vascular disease makes control of their hyperlipidemia of particular importance. The principles we have outlined can be utilized fully with benefit to these patients.

Pregnancy constitutes a particularly difficult situation because in most pregnant women there will be a 40–50% increase in plasma lipids and lipoproteins (chiefly LDL) in physiological circumstances. A hyperlipidemic patient who becomes pregnant should continue on the same diet advised previously for the treatment of her hyperlipidemia, supplemented by vitamins and minerals, as is usual in pregnancy. In pregnant patients with familial hypercholesterolemia, the Phase III diet is utilized as before, with some increase in calories to allow for the desired weight gain. In the type I or V hypertriglyceridemic pregnant patient there is apt to be a profound augmentation of the usual hyperchylomicronemia, and strict adherence to the 5–10% fat diet is often necessary to avoid acute pancreatitis.

The single-diet concept for the treatment of hyperlipidemic children can be applied as for adults. For those above age four years, no more than 3 oz of meat per day is the goal. The amount of meat should be adjusted to caloric intake for children younger than four years of age. Egg yolk, organ meat, and butterfat are eliminated from the diet, even for infants. In fact formula-fed infants already consume a cholesterol-free, low–saturated fat diet. Dietary iron is obtained from fortified cereals, whole grains, and beans. Human breast milk, commercial infant formula, or whole cow's milk is recommended before weaning or until the infant eats sufficient table food to provide adequate calories for growth. This usually occurs sometime between one and two years of age. The child can then be switched to skim milk and other non-fat dairy products. Throughout childhood the greatest thing parents can do is be a nutritional role model. By serving low-fat, high–complex carbohydrate foods at home, the fat and cholesterol children consume away from home will have less effect. What children see happening at home in food preparation and consumption will ultimately help them develop food habits useful for their lifetime.

For the rare infant with type I hyperlipidemia the fat content of human milk or infant formulas is much too high. A basic skim milk formula will have to be used to avoid the abdominal pain and episodes of pancreatitis to which these patients are so prone. However, sufficient amounts of essential fatty acids must be provided. These can be prescribed separately as canola or soybean oil, to yield at least 2–4% of total calories. Such oils will provide both omega-6 and omega-3 essential fatty acids. In this way much of the fat intake will be from linoleic and linolenic acids and very little total fat will be taken in. Success in several infants with the type I disorder has been achieved using this dietary approach and has resulted in the abolition of episodes of abdominal pain.

Special attention must be given to hypertensive, hyperlipidemic patients for several reasons. First, coronary heart disease and atherosclerotic brain disease are common causes of death in hypertensive patients. Second, some diuretic agents (thiazides) and beta blockers are hyperlipidemic in themselves, so that the usual hypertensive patient will have an increase in plasma lipids from the use of these agents alone. Thus hypertensive individuals given thiazides should have additional dietary therapy in the form of the single-diet approach. Furthermore the genetic syndrome of both hypertension and hypertriglyceridemia (hypertensive dyslipidemia) requires simultaneous treatment of both conditions. Finally a salt-restriction program can readily be incorporated to provide for the additional treatment of the essential hypertension as this is desired by the physician. The correction of obesity and lessening of alcohol intake may also have blood pressure–lowering effects. In order to combine the dietary treatment of hypertension and that of hyperlipidemia in a single diet, a stepwise reduction in salt use is also advocated and incorporated into the different phases (79).

Interrelationships between Dietary and Pharmaceutical Therapy of Hyperlipidemic States

The use of hypolipidemic drugs, which may be necessary in some patients, should not be regarded as an alternative form of therapy but as an additive therapy. Dietary factors can assist or interfere with the actions of all hypolipidemic drugs. The mechanisms by which dietary factors and drugs affect the plasma lipoproteins are reasonably well known, and their interactions can be deduced. A good example is the interaction between the HMG Co-A reductase inhibitor, lovastatin, and dietary cholesterol and saturated fat. Lovastatin increases hepatic LDL-receptor activity, promoting the removal of LDL from the plasma and the lowering of plasma cholesterol levels (20). Dietary cholesterol and saturated fat do the opposite; they decrease the hepatic LDL-receptor activity and, ultimately, raise the plasma total and LDL-cholesterol levels (21). The full benefit of lovastatin will not be achieved unless the diet also contains low amounts of cholesterol and saturated fat. When hyperlipidemia persists after the correction of metabolic errors (e.g., diabetes mellitus) or endocrine abnormalities (e.g., hypothyroidism), diet will then play a more dominant role in the correction of the hyperlipidemia.

Although dietary therapy remains the cornerstone in the treatment of hyperlipidemia, many patients will require additional pharmaceutical treatment in order to obtain the therapeutic objectives. In this connection some patients may believe that once they are started on drug therapy they no longer need to pay as much attention to their diet as when they were not receiving drug treatment. Nothing could be further from the truth. The two modes of therapy are not mutually exclusive but are instead complementary. Dietary treatment may obtain a lowering of the plasma LDL and total cholesterol of at least 10% but which may be as much as 15–20%. This will continue to be the case when pharmaceutical treatment is added. Then the patient will receive plasma lipid lowering from diet plus the additional lowering from medication.

The complementary nature of diet and drugs together is easily noted during the holiday period from Thanksgiving to New Year's when weight gain and additional intakes of cholesterol and saturated fat from holiday foods occur. Patients who are well controlled on diet and drug therapy continue their medication but their levels of plasma cholesterol and LDL, as well as VLDL and triglyceride, often increase during this holiday period. This particular premise was put to the test in a metabolic feeding study in patients with familial hypercholesterolemia who were well controlled on diet and then were given 40 mg of lovastatin per day. When they were given a diet high in cholesterol and saturated fat, while still maintaining the same dose of lovastatin, the plasma cholesterol level increased from 246 to 289 mg/dl, a 17.5% increase. LDL cholesterol increased even more, 20%. When it is considered that the dietary factors of cholesterol and saturated fat have a primary effect in decreasing LDL-receptor activity (21) and that lovastatin has a primary action in increasing LDL-receptor activity (20), it then becomes apparent that a diet high in cholesterol and saturated fat may nullify some of the beneficial effects of lovastatin.

Similar responses may occur in patients with types IV or V hyper-lipidemia. Weight gain and a high-fat diet can nullify the effects of gemfibrozil in maintaining lower plasma triglyceride concentrations. When a patient whose lipid values have previously been under good control with good adherence to diet and medication has a deterioration in lipid values, it is reasonable to question whether the previous dietary lifestyle changes have been disregarded. In diabetic hyper-triglyceridemic patients the dietary deviations will upset glycemic control as well. Many times when this matter is explained to the patient, he/she is then able to return to their previous excellent dietary lifestyle with a concomitant decrease in the plasma triglyceride and cholesterol levels and, if diabetic, better glucose control.

Summary

The principal goal of dietary prevention of atherosclerotic coronary heart disease is the achievement of physiological levels of the plasma total and low density lipoprotein (LDL) cholesterol, triglyceride and very low density lipoprotein (VLDL) cholesterol, and chylomicrons. These goals have been well delineated by the National Cholesterol Education Program of the U.S. National Heart, Lung and Blood Institute (91). Dietary treatment is first accomplished by enhancing LDL-receptor activity and at the same time depressing liver synthesis of cholesterol and triglyceride. Both dietary cholesterol and saturated fat decrease LDL-receptor activity and inhibit the removal of LDL from the plasma by the liver. Saturated fat decreases LDL-receptor activity, especially when cholesterol is concurrently present in the diet. The total amount of dietary fat is also of importance. The greater the flux of chylomicron remnants into the liver, the greater is the influx of cholesterol. In addition factors that affect VLDL and LDL synthesis could be important. Of most importance is obesity. Excessive calories enhance triglyceride and VLDL synthesis and thereby LDL synthesis. Weight loss and omega-3 fatty acids from fish oil inhibit synthesis of both VLDL and triglyceride by the liver.

The optimal diet for the treatment of children and adults is similar and has the following characteristics: cholesterol (100 mg/day or less), total fat (20% of kcals, 5% of kcals as saturated fat with the balance from omega-3 and omega-6 polyunsaturated and monounsaturated fat), carbohydrate (65% kcals, at least two-thirds from starch, including 11–15 g of soluble fibre), and protein (15% kcals). This low-fat, high-carbohydrate diet can lower the plasma cholesterol 18–21%. This diet is also an antithrombotic diet, thrombosis being another major consideration in preventing coronary heart disease. Dietary therapy is the mainstay of the prevention and treatment of coronary heart disease through the control of plasma lipid and lipoprotein levels.

REFERENCES

1 Anitschkow N. Experimental arteriosclerosis in animals. In: Cowdry EV, ed. *Arteriosclerosis*. New York: MacMillan, 1933:271–322.

2 Ignatovski A. Influence of animal food on the organism of rabbits. *Izv Imp Voyenno-Med Akad Peter* 1908;16:154–176.

3 de Langen C. Het cholesteringegehalte van het bloed in Indie. *Geneeskd Tijdschr Ned Indie* 1922;62:1–4.

4 Artaud-Wild SM, Connor SL, Sexton GJ, Connor WE. Differences in coronary mortality can be explained by differences in cholesterol and saturated fat intakes in forty countries but not in France and Finland. *Circulation* 1993;88:2771–2779.

5 Brown MS, Goldstein JL. Lipoprotein receptors in the liver: control signals of plasma cholesterol traffic. *J Clin Invest* 1983;72:743–747.

6 Sorci-Thomas M, Wilson MD, Johnson FL, Williams DL, Rudel LL. Studies on the expression of genes encoding apolipoproteins B100 and B48 and the low density lipoprotein receptor in nonhuman primates. *J Biol Chem* 1989;264:9039.

7 Fox JC, McGill HC, Jr, Carey KD, Getz GS. *In vivo* regulation of hepatic LDL receptor mRNA in the baboon – differential effects of saturated and unsaturated fat. *J Biol Chem* 1987;262:7014.

8 Connor WE, Connor SL. Diet, atherosclerosis and fish oil. In: Stollerman H, Siperstein M, eds. *Advances in internal medicine*, 35th ed. Chicago: Year Book Publishers, 1989:139–172.

9 Hopkins PN. Effects of dietary cholesterol on serum cholesterol: a meta-analysis and review. *Am J Clin Nutr* 1992;55:1060–1070.

10 Fielding C, Havel R, Todd K, Yeo K, Schoetter M, Weinberg V et al. Effects of dietary cholesterol and fat saturation on plasma lipoproteins in an ethnically diverse population of healthy young men. *J Clin Invest* 1995;95:611–618.

11 McMurry MP, Connor WE, Cerqueira MT. Dietary cholesterol and the plasma lipids and lipoproteins in the Tarahumara indians: a people habituated to a low-cholesterol diet after weaning. *Am J Clin Nutr* 1982;35:741–744.

12 Carter GA, Connor WE, Bhattacharyya AK, Lin DS. The cholesterol turnover, synthesis and absorption in two sisters with familial hypercholesterolemia (Type IIA). *J Lipid Res* 1979;20:66–77.

13 Roberts SL, McMurry MP, Connor WE. Does egg feeding (i.e. dietary cholesterol) affect plasma cholesterol levels in humans? The results of a double-blind study. *Am J Clin Nutr* 1981;34:2092–2099.

14 Connor WE, Connor SL. The dietary prevention and treatment of coronary heart disease. In: Connor WE, Bristow JD, eds. *Coronary heart disease: prevention, complications, and treatment.* Philadelphia: Lippincott, 1985:43–64.

15 Gordon T, Fisher M, Ernst M et al. Relation of diet to LDL cholesterol, VLDL cholesterol and plasma total cholesterol and triglycerides in white adults. *Atherosclerosis* 1982;2:502.

16 Zilversmit DB. Atherogenesis: a postprandial phenomenon. *Circulation* 1979;60:473–479.

17 Harris WS, Connor WE, Alam N, Illingworth DR. The reduction of postprandial trigylceridemia in humans by dietary n-3 fatty acids. *J Lipid Res* 1988;29:1451–1460.

18 Weintraub M, Rosen Y, Otto R, Eisenberg S, Breslow JL. Physical exercise conditioning in the absence of weight loss reduces fasting and postprandial triglyceride-rich lipoprotein levels. *Circulation* 1989;79:1007–1014.

19 Cabezas M, de Bruin TWA, Jansen H, Kock LAW, Kortlandt W, Erkelens DW. Impaired chylomicron remnant clearance in familial combined hyperlipidemia. *Arterioscler Thromb* 1993;13:804–814.

20 Brown MS, Goldstein JL. A receptor-mediated pathway for cholesterol homeostasis. *Science* 1986;232:34–47.

21 Spady DK, Dietschy JM. Interaction of dietary cholesterol and triglycerides in the regulation of hepatic low density lipoprotein transport in the hamster. *J Clin Invest* 1988;81:302–309.

22 Spady DK, Dietschy JM. Dietary saturated triacylglycerols suppress hepatic low density lipoprotein receptor activity in the hamster. *Proc Natl Acad Sci USA* 1985;82:4526–4530.

23 Mensink RP, Katan MB. Effect of dietary trans fatty acids on high-density and low-density lipoprotein cholesterol levels in healthy subjects. *N Engl J Med* 1990;323:439–445.

24 ASCN/AIN Task Force on Trans Fatty Acids. Position paper in trans fatty acids. *Am J Clin Nutr* 1996;63:663–670.

25 Chisholm A, Mann J, Sutherland W, Duncan A, Skeaff M, Frampton C. Effect on lipoprotein profile of replacing butter with margarine in a low fat diet: randomised crossover study with hypercholesterolaemic subjects. *Br Med J* 1996;312:931–934.

26 Watts GF, Jackson P, Burke V, Lewis B. Dietary fatty acids and progression of coronary artery disease in men. *Am J Clin Nutr* 1996;64:202–209.

27 Connor WE. The decisive influence of diet upon the progression and reversibility of coronary heart disease. *Am J Clin Nutr* 1996;64:253–254.

28 Lin DS, Connor WE, Spenler CW. Are dietary saturated, monounsaturated and polyunsaturated fatty acids deposited to the same extent in adipose tissue of rabbits? *Am J Clin Nutr* 1993;58:174–179.

29 Connor WE, Hoak JC, Warner ED. Massive thrombosis produced by fatty acid infusion. *J Clin Invest* 1963;42:860–866.

30 Grundy SM, Vega GL. Plasma cholesterol responsiveness to saturated fatty acids. *Am J Clin Nutr* 1988;47:822–824.

31 Connor SL, Artaud-Wild SM, Classick-Kohn CJ, Gustafson JR, Flavell DP, Hatcher LF et al. The cholesterol/saturated-fat index: an indication of the hypercholesterolaemic and atherogenic potential of food. *Lancet* 1986;1:1229–1232.

32 Connor SL, Gustafson JR, Artaud-Wild SM, Classick-Kohn CJ, Connor WE. The cholesterol–saturated fat index for coronary prevention: background, use, and a comprehensive table of foods. *J Am Diet Assoc* 1989;89:807–816.

33 Connor SL, Connor WE. *The new American diet system*, New York: Simon & Schuster, 1991.

34 Hegsted M, Ausman LM, Johnson JA, Dallal GE. Dietary fat and serum lipids: an evaluation of the experimental data. *Am J Clin Nutr* 1993;57:875–883.

35 Mattson FH, Grundy SM. Comparison of effects of dietary saturated, monounsaturated and polyunsaturated fatty acids on plasma lipids and lipoproteins in men. *J Lipid Res* 1985;26:194–202.

36 Neuringer M, Connor WE. Omega-3 fatty acids in the brain and retina: evidence for their essentiality. *Nutr Rev* 1986;44:285–294.

37 Connor WE, Neuringer M, Reisbick S. Essential fatty acids. The importance of n-3 fatty acids in the retina and brain. *Nutr Rev* 1992;50:21–29.

38 Nordoy A, Barstad L, Connor WE, Hatcher LF. Absorption of the n-3 eicosapentaenoic and docosahexaenoic acids as ethyl esters and triglyc-erides by humans. *Am J Clin Nutr* 1991;99:1185–1190.

39 Goodnight SH, Jr, Harris WS, Connor WE, Illingworth DR. Polyunsatu-rated fatty acids, hyperlipidemia and thrombosis. *Arteriosclerosis* 1982;2:87–113.

40 Phillipson BE, Rothrock DW, Connor WE, Harris WS, Illingworth DR. Reduction of plasma lipids, lipoproteins, and apoproteins by dietary fish oils in patients with hypertriglyceridemia. *N Engl J Med* 1985;312:1210–1216.

41 Harris WS, Connor WE, Illingworth DR, Rothrock DW, Foster DM. Effect of fish oil on VLDL triglyceride kinetics in man. *J Lipid Res* 1990;31:1549–1558.

42 Nordoy A, Hatcher LF, Ullmann D, Connor WE. The individual effects of dietary saturated fat and fish oil upon the plasma lipids and lipo-proteins in normal men. *Am J Clin Nutr* 1993;57:634–639.

43 Kromhout D, Bosschieter EB, Coulander CL. The inverse relation between fish consumption and 20-year mortality from coronary heart disease. *N Engl J Med* 1985;312:1205–1209.

44 Siscovick DS, Raghunathan TE, King I et al. Dietary intake and cell membrane levels of long-chain n-3 polyunsaturated fatty acids and the risk of primary cardiac arrest. *J Am Med Assoc* 1995;274:1363–1367.

45 Burr ML, Gilbert JF, Holliday RM, Elwood PC, Fehly AM, Rogers S et al. Effects of changes in fat, fish, and fibre intakes on death and myocar-dial reinfarction: diet and reinfarction trial (Dart). *Lancet* 1989;2:756–761.

46 Weintraub MS, Zechner R, Brown A, Eisenberg S, Breslow JL. Dietary polyunsaturated fats of the ω-6 and ω-3 series reduce postprandial lipoprotein levels: chronic and acute effects of fat saturation on post-prandial lipoprotein metabolism. *J Clin Invest* 1988;82:1884–1893.

47 Connor WE. ω-3 fatty acids and heart disease. In: Kritchevsky D, Car-roll KK, eds. *Nutrition and disease update: heart disease.* Champaign, IL, American Oil Chemists' Society; 1994:7–42.

48 Ullmann D, Connor WE, Hatcher LF, Connor SL, Flavell DP. Will a high-carbohydrate, low-fat diet lower the plasma lipids and lipopro-teins without producing hypertriglyceridemia? *Arterioscler Thromb* 1991;11:1059–1067.

49 Anderson JW, Story L, Sieling B, Chen WJL, Petro MS, Story J. Hypoc-holesterolemic effects of oat-bran or bean intake for hypercholester-olemic men. *Am J Clin Nutr* 1984;40:1146–1155.

50 Jenkins D, Wolever T, Venketeshwer Rao A, Hegele R, Mitchell S, Ransom T et al. Effect on blood lipids of very high intakes of fiber

in diets low in saturated fat and cholesterol. *N Engl J Med* 1993;329:21–26.

51 Malinow MR, Connor WE, McLaughlin P, Stafford C, Lin DS, Livingston AL et al. Cholesterol and bile acid balance in Macaca fascicularis: effects of alfalfa saponins. *J Clin Invest* 1981;67:156–162.

52 Witztum JL, Steinberg D. Role of oxidized low density lipoprotein in atherogenesis. *J Lipid Res* 1985;26:194–202.

53 Princen HMG, van Poppel G, Vogelezang C, Buytenhek R, Kok FJ. Supplementation with vitamin E but not B-carotene in vivo protects low density lipoprotein from lipid peroxidation in vitro: effect of cigarette smoking. *Arterioscler Thromb* 1992;12:548–553.

54 Luc G, Fruchart JC. Oxidation of lipoproteins and atherosclerosis. *Am J Clin Nutr* 1991;53:206s–209s.

55 Frankel EN, Kanner J, German JB, Parks E, Kinsella JE. Inhibition of oxidation of human low-density lipoprotein by phenolic substances in red wine. *Lancet* 1993;341:454–457.

56 Beard CM, Barnard JR, Robbins DC, Ordovas JM, Schaefer EJ. Effects of diet and exercise on qualitative and quantitative measures of LDL and its susceptibility to oxidation. *Arterioscler Thromb* 1996;16:201–207.

57 Esterbauer H, Dieber-Rotheneder M, Striegl G, Waeg G. Role of vitamin E in preventing the oxidation of low density lipoprotein. *Am J Clin Nutr* 1991;53:314s–321s.

58 Stephens NG, Parsons A, Schofield PM, Kelly F, Cheeseman K, Mitchinson MJ. Randomised controlled trial of vitamin E in patients with coronary disease: Cambridge Heart Antioxidant Study (CHAOS). *Lancet* 1996;347:781–786.

59 Steinberg D. Antioxidant vitamins and coronary heart disease. *N Engl J Med* 1993;328:147–148.

60 Messina M, Erdman JW, Jr. First international symposium on the role of soy in preventing and treating chronic disease. *J Nutr* 1995;35:1s–567s.

61 Welsh SO, Marston RM. Review of trends in food use in the United States, 1909 to 1980. *J Am Diet Assoc* 1982;81:120–125.

62 Malinow MR, Nieto J, Szklo M, Chambless LE, Bond G. Carotid artery intimal-medial wall thickening and plasma homocysteine in asymptomatic adults. *Circulation* 1993;87:1107–1113.

63 Gleuck CJ, Show P, Lang JE, Tracey T, Sieve-Smith L, Wang Y. Evidence that homocysteine is an independent risk factor for atherosclerosis in hyperlipidemic patients. *Am J Cardiol* 1995;75:132–136.

64 Egusa G, Beltz WF, Grundy SM, Howard BV. Influence of obesity on the metabolism of apolipoprotein B in man. *J Clin Invest* 1985;76:596–603.

65 Lichtenstein AH, Ausman LM, Carrasco W, Jenner JL, Ordovas JM, Schaefer EJ. Short-term consumption of a low-fat diet beneficially affects plasma lipid concentrations only when accompanied by weight loss. *Arterioscler Thromb* 1994;14:1751–1760.

66 McMurry MP, Cerqueira MT, Connor SL, Connor WE. Changes in lipid and lipoprotein levels and body weight in Tarahumara Indians after consumption of an affluent diet. *N Engl J Med* 1991;325:1704–1708.

67 Marmot MG, Brunner E. Alcohol and cardiovascular disease – the status of the U shaped curve. *Scott Med J* 1991;303:565–568.

68 Hennekens CH, Rosner B, Cole DS. Daily alcohol consumption and coronary heart disease. *Am J Epidemiol* 1978;107:196–200.

69 Hegsted DA, Ausman LM. Diet, alcohol and coronary heart disease in men. *J Nutr* 1988;118:1184–1189.

70 Suh II, Shaten BJ, Cutler JA, Kuller LH. Alcohol use and mortality from coronary heart disease: the role of high-density lipoprotein cholesterol. *Ann Intern Med* 1992;116:881–887.

71 Fry MM, Spector AA, Connor SL, Connor WE. Intensification of hypertriglyceridemia by either alcohol or carbohydrate. *Am J Clin Nutr* 1973;26:798–802.

72 Kudzma DJ, Schonfeld G. Alcoholic hyperlipidemia: induction by alcohol but not by carbohydrate. *J Lab Clin Med* 1970;77:384–395.

73 Ginsberg H, Olefsky J, Farquhar JW et al. Moderate ethanol ingestion and plasma triglyceride levels – a study in normal and hypertriglyceridemic persons. *Lancet* 1990;335:1235–1237.

74 Zock PL, Katan MB, Merkus MP, van Dusseldorp M, Harryvan JL. Effect of a lipid-rich fraction from boiled coffee on serum cholesterol. *Lancet* 1990;335:1235–1237.

75 Fried RE, Levine DM, Kwiterovich PO, Diamond EL, Wilder LB, Moy TF et al. The effect of filtered-coffee consumption on plasma lipid levels. Results of a randomized clinical trial. *J Am Med Assoc* 1992;267:811–815.

76 Peterson VE, Crapo PA, Weininger J et al. Quantification of plasma cholesterol and triglyceride levels in hypercholesterolemic subjects receiving ascorbic acid supplements. *Am J Clin Nutr* 1975;2835:584–587.

77 Beveridge JMR, Connell WF, Mayer GA. The nature of the substances in dietary fat affecting the level of plasma cholesterol in humans. *Can J Biochem Physiol* 1957;35:257–270.

78 Parthasarathy S, Steinberg D, Witztum JL. The role of oxidized low-density lipoproteins in the pathogenesis of atherosclerosis. *Ann Rev Med* 1992;43:219–225.

79 Connor SL, Connor WE. *The new American diet*, New York: Simon & Schuster, 1986.

80 Connor SL, Gustafson JR, Sexton GJ, Becker N, Artaud-Wild SM, Connor WE. Diet habit survey: a new method of dietary assessment that relates to plasma cholesterol changes. *J Am Diet Assoc* 1992;92:41–47.

81 Hegsted DM, McGandy RB, Myers ML, Stare FJ. Quantitative effects of dietary fat on serum cholesterol in man. *Am J Clin Nutr* 1965;17:281–295.

82 Connor WE, Connor SL. The dietary treatment of hyperlipidemia: rationale, technique and efficacy. In Havel RJ, ed. *Lipid disorders*, 66th ed. Med Clin North Am, 1982:485–518.

83 Connor SL, Connor WE. Coronary heart disease: prevention and treatment by nutritional change. In: Carroll KK, ed. *Diet, nutrition, and health*. Montreal: McGill-Queen's University Press, 1990:33–72.

84 Illingworth DR, Connor WE. Disorders of lipid metabolism. In: Felig P, Baxter JD, Broadus AE, Frohman LA, eds. *Endocrinology and metabolism*. New York: McGraw-Hill Publ. Co., 1981:917–956.

85 Lin DS, Connor WE. The long-term effects of dietary cholesterol upon the plasma lipids, lipoproteins, cholesterol absorption and the sterol balance in man: the demonstration of feedback of inhibition of cholesterol biosynthesis and increased bile acid excretion. *J Lipid Res* 1980;21:1042–1052.

86 Wolf P. High-fat, high-cholesterol diet raises plasma HDL cholesterol: studies on the mechanism of this effect. *Nutr Rev* 1996;54:34–35.

87 Connor WE, Cerqueira MT, Connor RW, Wallace RB, Malinow MR, Casdorph HR. The plasma lipids, lipoproteins and diet of the Tarahumara Indians of Mexico. *Am J Clin Nutr* 1978;31:1131–1142.

88 Knuiman JF, Hermus RJ, Hautvast JGAJ. Serum total and high density lipoprotein (HDL) cholesterol concentrations in rural and urban boys from 16 countries. *Atherosclerosis* 1980;36:529–537.

89 Miller GJ, Miller NE. Dietary fat, HDL cholesterol, and coronary disease: one interpretation. *Lancet* 1982;2:1270–1271.

90 Brinton EA, Eisenberg S, Breslow JL. A low-fat diet decreases high density lipoprotein (HDL) cholesterol levels by decreasing HDL apolipoprotein transport rates. *J Clin Invest* 1990;85:144–151.

91 Expert Panel on Detection, Evaluation, and Treatment of High Blood Cholesterol in Adults: Summary of the second report of the National Cholesterol Education Program (NCEP) expert panel on detection, evaluation, and treatment of high blood pressure in adults (adult treatment panel II). *J Am Med Assoc* 1993;269:3015–3023.

Diet and Selected Health Problems

S. GEORGE CARRUTHERS

Diet and Hypertension

Introduction

This review of diet and hypertension has been written to complement Kaplan's excellent paper (1), and the reader should refer to it for relevant background. Additional references are provided to selected recent publications. The emphasis is on studies that provide epidemiological, mechanistic, or interventional evidence linking diet to the pathophysiology or management of hypertension in humans.

Objectives

1 To appreciate the role of diet in the epidemiology, pathophysiology, and treatment of hypertension.
2 To define the relative importance of obesity, alcohol consumption, dietary fibre, and minerals in hypertension.
3 To understand the relative importance of non-pharmacological dietary interventions in the treatment of hypertension.

I am grateful to my former colleague, Carl Abbott, MD, FRCPC, of Dalhousie University, and the publishers of Medicine North America for permission to reproduce part of reference 6.

Genetic, Perinatal, and Environmental
Influences on Blood Pressure

At a recent public lecture the distinguished Canadian geneticist Charles Scriver eloquently made the point that although it is customary to think of scurvy as a disorder of the environment (dietary deficiency of vitamin C) and phenylketonuria as a genetic disorder (deficiency of the enzyme necessary to metabolize phenylalanine), it is entirely rational to take the opposite perspective. Among mammals only humans and guinea pigs lack the genetic metabolic capacity to synthesize ascorbic acid from glucose and are entirely dependent on external sources. Individuals deprived of dietary phenylalanine do not exhibit the mental retardation associated with phenylketonuria and develop normally. While it is customary to define certain risks of developing hypertension as genetic or environmental, we do well to recognize the interdependence of the hereditary and dietary factors linked to hypertension.

Danish school children with a family history of hypertension already demonstrate higher blood pressure (BP) and cardiac hypertrophy before the age of 10 years (2). This appears to be associated with increased likelihood of obesity and lower physical fitness. Perhaps the obesity and lesser fitness were associated with differing family lifestyles rather than genetic traits, but the trend to higher BP persisted even when adjusted for weight and fitness. Genetic influences on BP and cardiac structure are evident as early as the first decade of life.

The study of twins also permits an understanding of the genetic and environmental factors that influence the pathogenesis of hypertension. Monozygotic (identical) twins and dizygotic (fraternal) twins differ in their genetic constitution, the former being genetically identical while the latter are similar to other pairs of siblings. In adulthood environmental factors commonly change for all twins as they leave the parental home and establish separate lives, lifestyles, and families of their own. Elderly twins who become hypertensive provide a natural biological experiment that permits insight to the development of the factors influencing elevated BP.

Genetic factors tend to diminish with ageing for systolic BP, but the modest genetic influence on diastolic BP is similar before and after 65 years of age (3).

An American study of World War II identical-twin veterans concluded that genetic influences were important in the development of hypertension, but discordance (one twin hypertensive, the other normotensive) was commonly explained by lifestyle differences such as adult-onset weight gain and alcohol consumption (4). These results emphasize the earlier inference that a genetic predisposition to hypertension need not lead to elevated BP if adult weight gain can be avoided and alcohol consumption is curtailed.

Studies of migration and urbanization, sometimes referred to as acculturation, also give us insights to the interaction of hereditary and environmental factors. Sadly a recent Chinese study of hypertension prevalence according to latitude and urbanization provides little new information on lifestyle influences on the pathogenesis and prevalence of hypertension (5). There is a terrible sense of *déja vu* as one notes that the factors that influence hypertension and dyslipidemia among the Chinese of Beijing and Guangzhou are the same as those that have been known to promote these disorders in Europeans and North Americans for several decades: age, obesity, and alcohol consumption. There is not much we can do about the ageing process, but obesity and alcohol consumption are clearly within our potential control.

Obesity and Hypertension

In his chapter Kaplan (1) introduced the issue of obesity and insulin resistance associated with dyslipidemia and elevated blood pressure. In Western society this disorder is linked increasingly to type II diabetes mellitus, hypertriglyceridemia, and hypertension. Its associated risks, pathogenesis, and management have been investigated further and were reviewed recently (6). The key points are reiterated.

Insulin resistance (IR), with compensatory hyperinsulinemia as a cardiovascular disease (CVD) risk factor, may play a central role in the evolution of coronary artery disease exclusive of its role in obesity, non-insulin-dependent diabetes mellitus (NIDDM), and essential hypertension (EH). Evidence is accumulating that CVD risk is programmed during early (intra-uterine) growth and low birth weight may be a marker for IR in adult life (7,8). IR appears to be at least a marker for many modifiable CVD risk factors.

IR implies that increased amounts of insulin are required to maintain glucose homeostasis. Although IR is usually viewed as a defect of glucose homeostasis, insulin receptors are found in tissues such as the ovary, skin, and cardiovascular smooth muscle, where high insulin level effects may be seen. Intracellular calcium and magnesium are increased in IR, another possible link to the roles of these minerals in the regulation of blood pressure.

The IR syndrome is known by other designations: the metabolic syndrome, the (metabolic) Syndrome X, the deadly quartet, the plurimetabolic syndrome, dyslipidemic hypertension, and Reaven's syndrome. Reaven has reviewed the relationship between IR and coronary artery disease (9). Visceral obesity is seen more frequently in males than females because of larger amounts of visceral fat, even though total body fat is greater in females. It is unclear why HDL-cholesterol levels are usually low but abnormalities in lipoprotein lipase or hepatic lipase action may be the cause. Weight loss in obesity reverses the markers for IR, especially hypertriglyceridemia.

Accelerated CVD is the leading cause of death in NIDDM and 80% of patients with NIDDM are obese. IR occurs in obesity, especially with the visceral type, and in NIDDM patients (whether obese or not), where the degree of IR is usually more marked.

Weight loss can improve IR and glycemic control in obese NIDDM, but usually does not correct the dyslipidemia. Lipoprotein(a) tends to be elevated in poorly controlled diabetes mellitus (both insulin-dependent and NIDDM) and since these levels are primarily determined by genetic factors, they persist even with improvement in IR (10).

EH may be associated with a primary defect in insulin-stimulated glucose uptake of skeletal muscle and is another cause of IR, like obesity and NIDDM (11). Since obese hypertensive subjects have a greater degree of IR compared to obese normotensives, obesity cannot be the only explanation. NIDDM has an additive effect on IR in obese hypertensive subjects (12) and clustering of other risk factors is additive. In fact many of the recognized CVD risk factors are often found with EH. Many forms of secondary hypertension are not associated with IR so hypertension itself is not the cause of IR in EH.

Fasting insulin levels have been directly correlated with both systolic and diastolic BPs. It has been very difficult to demonstrate a significant, persistent elevation of BP with insulin infusions in most animals and humans, perhaps due to the vasodilator action of insulin. Hyperinsulinemia has a direct effect on the adrenergic nervous system. Insulin increases muscle sympathetic outflow, raises circulating norepinephrine, and usually decreases skeletal muscle blood flow. Insulin also stimulates secretion of endothelin-1 from endothelial cells. Endothelin, a potent vasoconstrictor, also processes mitogenic properties on vascular smooth muscle. Other endothelial-derived vasoactive peptides might also increase vascular resistance in response to hyperinsulinemia. Bradykinin, a vasodilator, is secreted in reduced amounts in some diabetics and in EH (9,12,13).

Hyperinsulinemia also decreases renal tubular sodium excretion, which may contribute to high BP. Glucose-induced vascular smooth muscle dysfunction may result from protein kinase C–induced ionic or pressor receptor changes. Finally, insulin promotes arteriolar smooth muscle hypertrophy, leading to increased peripheral vascular resistance. IR can be demonstrated in offspring of hypertensive parents before the onset of hypertension. IR in EH has been well reviewed by Ferrannini and Natali (13).

In summary there is evidence for a link between IR and several modifiable CVD risk factors (hypertension, diabetes mellitus, dyslipidemia, physical inactivity, visceral obesity, smoking, and left ventricular hypertrophy). IR is likely genetically determined as offspring of parents with EH may show hyperinsulinemia and IR, the dyslipidemia (high triglycerides, low HDL cholesterol, high LDL cholesterol) of IR, and visceral obesity before the onset of EH. Abnormal glucose tolerance and NIDDM develop when the pancreas is unable to compensate for the increasing resistance to glucose uptake and storage in muscle. IR at the adipocyte and liver contributes to the dyslipidemia and hyperglycemia.

Many of the variables in IR and CVD risk are nongenetically determined and modifiable. Regular (daily) aerobic exercise, avoidance of tobacco, control of hypertension, NIDDM, and obesity, as well as estrogen replacement in women with disorders of androgen excess and at menopause are essential and practical interventions.

Obesity, Blood Pressure, and Cardiac Function

Overweight people commonly experience disproportionate shortness of breath. Are they simply carrying too much fat, or are there cardiovascular abnormalities that result from their obesity? As discussed earlier, weight gain is associated with increased risk of hypertension, glucose intolerance, and lipid disturbances. It is assumed that these disorders lead directly or indirectly to the development of diastolic dysfunction followed by systolic dysfunction and frank cardiac decompensation. The impact of gender has also been explored in the research studies on obesity and hypertension from Sweden (14) and the United States (15).

Hemodynamics were compared between obese Swedish women and age-matched women with body mass index (mass in kg/height in m²) less than 25 kg/m² (14). Obese women had higher BPs and greater cardiac mass. There was evidence of impaired diastolic relaxation in the left ventricle, a fundamental element of so-called diastolic dysfunction. Moreover obesity was associated with a larger heart at end-diastole and with enlargement of the left atrium. The left atrium is prone to distension when it pumps against higher end-diastolic left ventricular pressures. This is a contributing factor to the development of atrial fibrillation, which further impairs the efficiency of cardiac diastolic function. Cardiac systolic function appeared well compensated to the increased afterload imposed by elevated BP.

Obesity in itself is an independent stimulus to myocardial growth, even in the presence of "normal" BPs (15). By an action as yet undefined, obesity adds to the effect of hypertension on cardiac hypertrophy such that obese hypertensives exhibit even more left ventricular hypertrophy (LVH) than obese normotensives or lean hypertensives. Women experience even more cardiac hypertrophy than men at similar levels of hypertension and overweight.

An interesting study in dogs provides a valuable perspective on this subject (16). Dogs that became 50% overweight in only four weeks on a high-fat diet became mildly hypertensive with increased cardiac output, heart rate, and left atrial pressure. The dogs were unable to complete an exercise workload with which they had no difficulty when they were lean. Impairment of cardiac diastolic function occurred very early in this canine obesity model and suggests that this is one of the primary cardiovascular changes associated with obesity, even before BP becomes seriously elevated. The cardiovascular effects of returning to a lean body mass have not been reported.

Weight Reduction for BP Control

There is increasing evidence that even modest weight reduction can be a useful alternative or adjunct to pharmacological therapy. Three Swedish publications addressed the impact of weight reduction versus drug therapy on BP control, metabolic factors such as lipids, glucose tolerance, and insulin resistance, and finally their comparative cost-effectiveness (17–19). Each approach appears to have its advantages and disadvantages. Drugs appear to be more effective and possibly more cost effective. However neglect of weight control and/or an exercise program may lead to a less than desirable overall reduction of cardiovascular risk profile.

Outcome studies that examine the co-interventions of drugs, diet, and exercise may ultimately resolve the effectiveness and overall cost effectiveness of the individual and combined approaches. In the meantime it would appear prudent to encourage weight control and physical activity in hypertensive patients, in addition to whatever pharmacological intervention is necessary. The relevance of this multifactorial approach is described later in the TOMHS review.

Alcohol Consumption and Hypertension

The association between alcohol intake and hypertension is well established in Western-style or acculturated societies. The link is causal; regular alcohol consumption increases BP within weeks. However the fact that these studies were conducted in societies with high sodium and low potassium intakes has raised questions about other dietary aspects of the alcohol/hypertension issue.

A natural experiment in human migration in China provided an opportunity to investigate the effect of alcohol intake in a society where alcohol sale is carefully monitored and where sodium intake is low and not, therefore, likely to be a confounding issue (20). Yi women do not drink. Yi men have virtually no hypertension but develop increased BPs when they migrate to cities and adopt some of the urban habits of the ethnic majority Yan people, including alcohol use. The changes in BP among migrant Yi men were in diastolic rather than systolic blood pressure (SBP) and were independent of urinary sodium, potassium, calcium, and magnesium or sodium/potassium ratio.

The epidemiological relationship between BP and alcohol is further demonstrated in a study of a rural Japanese population (21). Multiple regression analysis revealed SBP to be correlated with age, body mass index, and alcohol intake. SBP was negatively related to potassium intake. These investigators stress the need to develop a public health strategy to reduce alcohol intake in the primary prevention of hypertension.

High job stress, defined as working fast and hard with little control over the work process, appears to interact with alcohol use to increase ambulatory BP at work (22). High job stress is known to be associated with increased heart disease.

Short-term studies in humans and both short-term and long-term studies in rats demonstrate increased sympathetic nerve stimulation and increased BP following introduction of ethanol. The effects of alcohol infusion on BP, heart rate, sympathetic nerve activity, and the central release of corticotrophin-releasing hormone (CRH) were reported recently (23). On one of the two occasions that alcohol infusion was studied, the influence of central hypothalamic-pituitary control of BP in response to ethanol administration was further investigated by the suppression of CRH release by 2 mg dexamethasone daily.

Dexamethasone did not alter sympathetic responses to the Valsalva manœuvre or to immersion of the hand in ice water, but the sympathetic nerve activity stimulated by alcohol infusion was profoundly reduced in the presence of dexamethasone. With dexamethasone there was a corresponding blunting of BP elevation and an actual reduction of BP, possibly reflecting the well-known vasodilatory effect of alcohol. Instead of a mean arterial BP increase of 10 mm Hg, there was a decrease in BP of about 7 mm Hg. Plasma alcohol concentrations during this study were in the 40–80 mg/dl range, i.e., within usual legal limits for driving in most North American jurisdictions. Alcohol-induced hypertension was clearly mediated through sympathetic stimulation, in that BP response and increased vascular resistance were blunted by alpha-blockade. This study does not prove that long-term alcohol use can cause sustained hypertension, but it is consistent with animal data that demonstrate this effect (23).

The mechanism of alcohol-induced hypertension was further explored in a rat model (24). The study was designed to investigate the relation between BP and intracellular magnesium, calcium, and sodium metabolism during chronic alcohol administration. The possible role of intracellular magnesium depletion in the genesis of hypertension and the benefits of magnesium supplementation in correcting elevated BP will require further study in human hypertensives who ingest alcohol.

Modification of Alcohol Intake

Reduction of alcohol intake is recommended in the non-pharmacological management of high BP. Weight reduction is also encouraged in the obese hypertensive. In Australia approximately one-third of the adult population is overweight and 14% of men drink 5 or more drinks per day (25). It is likely that the prevalence of obesity and overuse of alcohol are similar in other Western-style societies.

Weight reduction and alcohol restriction were investigated and were found to reduce BP and to improve the metabolic abnormalities associated with obesity. Weight reduction created greater metabolic benefit than the reduction of HDL cholesterol associated with consuming less alcohol.

The benefit of reducing alcohol consumption in BP control has also been demonstrated in a group of hypertensive Britons (26). Although one-third of the initial group failed to cooperate or to comply and the study duration was only eight weeks, it was encouraging to note the good level of compliance exhibited by the responsive patients. Clearly the impact of the advice and support of a physician who encourages hypertensive patients who drink to reduce their alcohol consumption should not be underestimated.

Dietary Fibre

The effects of a dietary fibre supplement given as monotherapy for BP in mildly hypertensive patients has been investigated (27). The study was performed as a prospective randomized, double-blind, placebo-controlled trial for three months in patients attending a hospital outpatient hypertension clinic. Hypertensive patients with a minimum of two diastolic blood pressure (DBP) readings > 90 mm Hg during a two-week run-in period were included. Of the 65 patients enrolled, 63 were randomized (32 fibre, 31 placebo). Six patients did not complete the trial. Patients were treated with either fibre (beet:barley:citrus; 60:30:10, 90% insoluble) (7 g day) or matching placebo (lactose 105 mg; starch 676 mg/tablet). Based on previous studies, the a priori hypothesis was that dietary fibre supplementation could reduce BP in hypertensive patients.

Body weight was significantly reduced in the fibre group (4 kg compared with control). Dietary fibre significantly reduced DBP (4.3 mm Hg) and fasting serum insulin. However no correlation between changes in body weight and systolic BP or DBP was found. A dietary fibre supplement can lower DBP in mildly hypertensive patients independent of changes in body weight.

However, others have concluded that a low-salt diet lowered BP, while low fat intake lowered cholesterol but high fibre had no influence on BP (28) (also see below, Multiple Interventions). The independent and additive effects of sodium restriction and a low-fat, high–polyunsaturated:saturated fatty acids (P:S) ratio, high-fibre diet upon BP were investigated in a factorial study of salt restriction and a low-fat/high-fibre diet in hypertensive subjects. A randomized, parallel, double-blind, placebo-controlled (for sodium) 2 × 2 factorial trial involved 95 hypertensive subjects (mean BP, 137/83 mm Hg), mean age 53.5 years, consuming < 30 ml ethanol/day, selected from community volunteers. Seventy-nine treated and 12 untreated hypertensives completed the trial.

Subjects followed either a low-sodium, low-fat/high-fibre diet (< 60 mmol sodium/day; 30% fat energy; P:S ratio = 1; 30–50 g fibre/day) or a low-sodium, normal-fat/normal-fibre diet (< 60 mmol sodium/day; 40% fat energy; P:S ratio = 0.3; 15 g fibre/day) for eight weeks. Half of each group received 100 mmol/day NaCl and the remainder received placebo.

Sodium restriction significantly reduced standing and supine systolic BP, with no effect upon DBP. The low-fat/high-fibre diet had no effect upon BP, but significantly reduced total cholesterol, LDL cholesterol, and HDL cholesterol.

These investigators concluded that sodium restriction reduced BP and did not raise LDL cholesterol. A low-fat/high-fibre diet did not reduce BP but lowered cholesterol levels. A combination of the two regimens has the greater potential for reducing cardiovascular risk in hypertensives.

Minerals

The debate continues on the relative merits of salt (sodium) restriction, potassium supplementation, added calcium, and magnesium enrichment of the diet as means of avoiding hypertension, improving BP control, or reducing the risk of complications of hypertension such as stroke and LVH. Observational studies on sodium intake must be interpreted cautiously in the context of potassium and calcium intakes that are often high in low-sodium diets and vice versa.

Sodium intake is usually modified by altering the intake of discretionary salt and adjusting the diet to reduce salt-containing foods. There have been many short- to medium-term dietary restriction studies that suggest benefit in some but certainly not all essential hypertensives. A short-term course of moderate salt restriction in hypertensives was associated with decreased BP and diminished peripheral vascular resistance (29). Brachial artery diameter increased, but carotid dimensions were unchanged, suggesting a fundamental difference in responsiveness to sodium restriction in different vascular beds.

A BP-lowering effect of 60 mmol of potassium on systolic BP, whether supine or standing in the office or measured by ambulatory recording, was observed by Fotherby and Potter (30), who found no benefit on DBP except on clinic supine readings.

For exactly the same sodium load, a potassium, magnesium, and l-lysine-enriched salt alternative that had been shown to prolong life in hypertensive rats was found to prevent the hypertension and LVH associated with regular salt in a further set of rat experiments (31). These observations deserve further investigation as possible non-pharmacological interventions in human hypertension.

A novel approach, and one that may have some appeal to those with a powerful hedonistic salt drive, is the use of a seaweed fibre with sodium/potassium-exchanging properties (32). In an attempt to decrease sodium and increase potassium intake, 62 middle-aged patients with mild hypertension were given a potassium-loaded, ion-exchanging, sodium-adsorbing, potassium-releasing seaweed preparation (seaweed fibre, SF). The mean blood pressure (MBP) is defined as DBP plus one-third of the difference between systolic and DBP. In a double-blind crossover manner with four weeks familiarization and wash-out periods, MBP showed a significant decrease after four weeks on 12 and 24 g/day SF but not on 6 g/day or placebo treatment. Systolic BP during submaximal exercise decreased on all three SF doses. The decrease in MBP appeared to be significantly higher in sodium-sensitive (11.2 mm Hg, $p < 0.001$) than in sodium-insensitive (5.7 mm Hg, $p < 0.05$) patients and was significantly correlated in salt-sensitive patients with the increase in plasma renin activity (PRA). The urinary sodium excretion decreased, the urinary potassium increased, and the sodium/potassium urinary excretion ratio decreased, indicating that the decrease of MBP was dependent on the decreased intestinal absorption of sodium and increased absorption of potassium released from the seaweed preparation.

Could this preparation act through increasing potassium, rather than by lowering sodium? Sodium restriction, rather than potassium repletion with changes in vascular and lymphocyte beta-adrenoceptor responsiveness, appears linked (33). Feldman postulates that vascular sensitivity to the vasodilating effect of beta-adrenergic stimulation is improved by sodium depletion in both borderline and older hypertensives (34). This is consistent with the hypothesis that there is an imbalance of alpha-receptor (constricting) and beta-receptor (dilating) influences associated with ageing and suggests a possible mechanism for the BP-lowering action of sodium restriction.

A general community cohort of 89 boys and girls, aged 3–6 years, from the Framingham Children's Study was investigated with respect to nutrient data from multiple food diaries (a mean of 9.6 days of recording for each subject) (35). At the beginning of the second year of the study, anthropometric data and up to five BP readings (mean, 4.5) were obtained on each child at a single sitting. The range of subjects' average daily calcium intake was 4.9 to 19.6 mmol per 4200 kJ, with a mean of 12.8 mmol per 4200 kJ. Subjects' average systolic BP ranged from 73 to 129 mm Hg, with a mean of 95.9 mm Hg; for DBP the range was from 37 to 78 mm Hg, with a mean of 54.6 mm Hg. Multiple linear regression analysis, adjusted for the effects of sex, height, body mass index, and heart rate, showed that for each increment of 2.5 mmol of dietary calcium per 4200 kJ per day, systolic BP was 2.27 mm Hg lower (95% confidence interval, 0.63 to 3.91 mm Hg; p = 0.008). No such association with DBP was found. Dietary calcium appears inversely related to systolic BP in young children.

An intervention trial was undertaken to determine if calcium carbonate supplementation could reduce BP in an older population that had mildly increased pressure and if BP reduction could be maintained over the course of 1 year with continued supplementation (36). Volunteers 50–80 years of age were included if their systolic BP (when not taking antihypertensive medication) was consistently greater than or equal to 140 mm Hg or if DBP was greater than or equal to 90 mm Hg during a 4-week baseline period. Each subject then received placebo tablets for 4 weeks followed by 1 g calcium carbonate tablets for 12 weeks in a single-blinded fashion.

Supine and standing systolic and diastolic BP did not change significantly with 12 weeks of calcium carbonate as compared to placebo. There is no evidence in this study for general use of calcium supplementation to reduce BP in an older population. However a Japanese study conducted in elderly, hospitalized patients came to the contrary conclusion (37). Patients treated with an oyster shell electrolysate exhibited reduced BP, increased free serum calcium, and reduced parathyroid hormone. The metabolic balance of Ca^{++} in these Japanese patients at study entry must be questioned.

Multiple Interventions

Various combinations of dietary salt modification and oil supplements were studied in an ambulatory population of non-hypertensive Australian seniors (38). Most impact on both systolic and diastolic BP was observed with a low sodium/fish oil combination.

The investigators of Treatment of Mild Hypertension Study (TOMHS) report the results of this randomized, parallel, placebo-controlled evaluation of antihypertensive drugs in a setting of weight loss, exercise, and restriction of sodium and alcohol (39). All participants engaged in a strict regimen of hygienic, non-pharmacological management and were randomized to placebo or one of five major therapeutic classes of antihypertensive drugs. Their choice of diuretic was chlorthalidone 15 mg; beta-blocker, acebutolol 400 mg; alpha-1 blocker, doxazosin 1 mg/day for one month then 2 mg; calcium antagonist, amlodipine 5 mg; ACE inhibitor, enalapril 5 mg. All medications or placebo were given once daily. All participants received advice on dietary and lifestyle modification. There were two specific questions. 1. Do the drug-treatment groups differ from placebo or from one another with respect to influences on quality of life, side effects, blood lipid measurements, and echocardiographic and electrocardiographic (ECG) changes over 4 years? 2. Does use of drug treatment together with nutritional-hygienic intervention reduce the 4-year incidence of cardiovascular morbidity and mortality compared with nutritional-hygienic intervention alone?

The TOMHS investigators were interested in comparing the individual drugs in terms of cardiovascular outcomes, but recognized the lack of power in this protocol and are currently examining this issue in a new large-scale trial that does not include intensive nutritional-hygienic intervention. The average age of participants was 55 years; 38% were women and 20% were black. Mean entry BP was 140/91. A little over 60% had been on antihypertensive therapy, and there was little difference between active treatments. Quality of life improved most on the diuretic and beta-blocker. Early adverse lipid effects of the diuretic were not observed at 4 years. Doxazosin produced favourable long-term lipid changes. Only one-third of placebo-treated patients required active treatment, a benefit attributed to the success of nutritional-hygienic intervention. However all active treatments were superior to placebo.

There are clear metabolic gains from weight reduction with a reduced fat diet, alcohol restriction, and exercise that must be stressed. There are likely benefits from the high potassium/sodium ratio in this dietary regimen. It seems unlikely that supplementation of calcium beyond the 1–1.5 g recommended will modify BP to an important extent.

It is dubious if most hypertensives can be persuaded to pursue the rigorous non-pharmacological protocol of TOMHS within the setting of usual office practice. However those who do will likely be rewarded by modest BP reduction and additional benefits from low-dose concurrent pharmacotherapy, as needed.

The matter of primary prevention of hypertension deserves greater attention as a public health issue. Even minor changes in BP for the population, which might be considered clinically irrelevant for the individual patient, could create substantial effects on incidence of myocardial infarction and stroke. The Canadian Consensus Conference on Non-pharmacological Approaches to the Management of High Blood Pressure (40) and the Joint National Committee on Detection, Evaluation, and Treatment of High Blood Pressure (JNC V) (41) have taken the first steps to evaluate the information on this subject and to introduce guidelines for practising physicians. It is hoped that there will be updates from both agencies in the near future.

REFERENCES

1 Kaplan NM. Diet and hypertension. In: Carroll KK, ed. *Diet, nutrition, and health*. Montreal: McGill-Queen's University Press, 1989:93–102.
2 Hansen HS, Nielsen JR, Hyldebrandt N, Froberg K. Blood pressure and cardiac structure in children with a parental history of hypertension: the Odense Schoolchild Study. *J Hypertens* 1992;10:677–682.
3 Hong Y, de Faire U, Heller DA, McClearn GE, Pedersen N. Genetic and environmental influences on blood pressure in elderly twins. *Hypertens* 1994;24:663–670.
4 Carmelli D, Robinette D, Fabsitz R. Concordance, discordance and prevalence of hypertension in World War II male veteran twins. *J Hypertens* 1994;12:323–328.
5 Huang Z, Wu X, Stamler J, Rao X, Tao S et al. A north-south comparison of blood pressure and factors related to blood pressure in the People's Republic of China: a report from the PRC-USA collaborative study of cardiovascular epidemiology. *J Hypertens* 1994;12:1103–1112.
6 Abbott EC, Carruthers SG. Insulin resistance: a risk factor for coronary artery disease. *Med North America* 1995;Oct:846–854.
7 Fall CHD, Vijayakumar M, Barker DJO, Osmond C, Dugglesby S. Weight in infancy and prevalence of coronary heart disease in adult life. *Br Med J* 1995;310:17–19.
8 Martyn CN, Barker DJP, Jespersen S, Greenwald S, Osmond C, Berry C. Growth in utero, adult blood pressure and arterial compliance. *Br Heart J* 1995;73:116–121.
9 Reaven GM. Role of insulin resistance in human disease (syndrome X): an expanded definition. *Ann Rev Med* 1993;44:121–131.

10 Ramirez LC, Arauz-Pacheco C, Lackner C, Albright G, Adams B, Raskin R. Lipoprotein (a) levels in diabetes mellitus: relationship to metabolic control. *Ann Intern Med* 1992;117:42–47.

11 Ferrannini E, Buzzigoli G, Bonadonna R, Giorica MA et al. Insulin resistance in essential hypertension. *N Engl J Med* 1987;317:350–357.

12 Steiner G. Update on the syndrome of insulin resistance and lipoprotein metabolism. *Can J Cardiol* 1994;10(suppl B): 23B–26B.

13 Ferrannini E, Natali A. Essential hypertension, metabolic disorders and insulin resistance. *Am Heart J* 1991;121:1274–1282.

14 Wikstrand J, Pettersson P, Bjorntorp P. Body fat distribution and left ventricular morphology and function in obese females. *J Hypertens* 1993;11:1259–1266.

15 de Simone G, Devereux RB, Roman MJ, Alderman MH, Laragh JH. Relation of obesity and gender to left ventricular hypertrophy in normotensive and hypertensive adults. *Hypertens* 1994;23:600–606.

16 Mizelle HL, Edwards TC, Montani J. Abnormal cardiovascular responses to exercise during the development of obesity in dogs. *Am J Hypertens* 1994;7:374–378.

17 Fagerberg B, Berglund A, Andersson OK, Berglund G. Weight reduction versus antihypertensive drug therapy in obese men with high blood pressure: effects upon plasma insulin levels and association with changes in blood pressure and serum lipids. *J Hypertens* 1992;10:1053–1061.

18 Nilsson PM, Lindholm LH, Scherstén BF. Lifestyle changes improve insulin resistance in hyperinsulinaemic subjects: a one-year intervention study of hypertensives and normotensives in Dalby. *J Hypertens* 1992;10:1071–1078.

19 Johannesson M, Fagerberg B. A health-economic comparison of diet and drug treatment in obese men with mild hypertension. *J Hypertens* 1992;10: 1063–1070.

20 Klag MJ, He J, Whelton PK, Chen J et al. Alcohol use and blood pressure in an unacculturated society. *Hypertens* 1993;22:365–370.

21 Choudhury SR, Okayama A, Kita Y, Ueshima H et al. The associations between alcohol drinking and dietary habits and blood pressure in Japanese men. *J Hypertens* 1995;13:587–593.

22 Schnall PL, Schwartz JE, Landsbergis PA, Warren K, Pickering TG. Relation between job strain, alcohol, and ambulatory blood pressure. *Hypertens* 1992;19:488–494.

23 Randin D, Vollenweider P, Tappy L, Jéquier E, Nicod P, Scherrer U. Suppression of alcohol-induced hypertension by dexamethasone. *N Engl J Med* 1995;332:1733–1737.

118   Diet and Selected Health Problems

24 Hsieh S, Sano H, Saito K, Kubota Y, Yokoyama M. Magnesium supplementation prevents the development of alcohol-induced hypertension.
Hypertens 1992;19:175–182.
25 Puddey IB, Parker M, Beilin LJ, Vandongen R, Masarei JRL. Effects of
alcohol and caloric restrictions on blood pressure and serum lipids in
overweight men. *Hypertens* 1992;20:533–541.
26 Maheswaran R, Beevers M, Beevers DG. Effectiveness of advice to
reduce alcohol consumption in hypertensive patients. *Hypertens*
1992;19:79–84.
27 Eliasson K, Ryttig KR, Hylander B, Rossner S. A dietary fibre supplement in the treatment of mild hypertension. *J Hypertens* 1992;10:195–
199.
28 Sciarrone EG, Beilin LJ, Rouse IL, Rogers PB. A factorial study of salt
restriction and a low-fat/high fibre diet in hypertensive subjects.
J Hypertens 1992;10:287–298.
29 Safar ME, Asmar RG, Benetos A, London GM, Levy BI. Sodium, large
arteries and diuretic compounds in hypertension. *J Hypertens* 1992;10:
S133–S136.
30 Fotherby MD, Potter JF. Potassium supplementation reduces clinic and
ambulatory blood pressure in elderly hypertensive patients. *J Hypertens* 1992;10:1403–1408.
31 Mervaala EM, Himberg JJ, Laakso J, Tuomainen P, Karpannen H. Beneficial effects of a potassium- and magnesium-enriched salt alternative.
Hypertens 1992;19:535–540.
32 Krotkiewski M, Aurell M, Holm G, Grimby G, Szczepanik J. Effects of
a sodium-potassium ion–exchanging seaweed preparation in mild
hypertension. *Am J Hypertens* 1991;4: 483–488.
33 Feldman RD. Defective venous beta-adrenergic response in borderline
hypertensive subjects is corrected by a low sodium diet. *J Clin Invest*
1990;85:647–652.
34 Feldman RD. A low-sodium diet corrects the defect in beta- adrenergic
response in older subjects. *Circulation* 1992; 85:612–618.
35 Gillman MW, Oliveria SA, Moore LL, Ellison RC. Inverse association
of dietary calcium with systolic blood pressure in young children.
JAMA 1992;267:2340–2343.
36 Morris CD, McCarron DA. Effect of calcium supplementation in an
older population with mildly increased blood pressure. *Am J Hypertens*
1992;5:230–237.
37 Takagi Y, Fukase M, Takata S, Fujimi T, Fujita T. Calcium treatment of
essential hypertension in elderly patients evaluated by 24 h monitoring. *Am J Hypertens* 1991;4:836–839.

38 Cobiac L, Nestel PJ, Wing LMH, Howe PRC. A low-sodium diet supplemented with fish oil lowers blood pressure in the elderly. *J Hypertens* 1992;10:87–92.
39 Neaton JD, Grimm RH, Jr, Prineas RJ, Stamler J et al. Treatment of
   mild hypertension study: final results. *JAMA* 1993;270:713–724.
40 Chockalingham A, Abbott D, Mass M et al. Recommendations from
   the Consensus Conference on Non-pharmacologicical Approaches to
   the Management of High Blood Pressure. *Can Med Assoc J* 1990;142:
   1397–1409.
41 The fifth report of the Joint National Committee on Detection, Evaluation, and Treatment of High Blood Pressure (JNC V). *Arch Intern Med*
   1993;153:154–183.

BERTRAM L. KASISKE

The Role of Diet in Chronic Renal Disease Progression

Introduction

Renal disease often seems to progress in a predictable manner that is independent of the original cause of injury. Although the mechanisms for this non-specific disease progression are poorly understood, a large number of experimental and clinical trials have examined the effects of diet on renal disease progression. Several different diet interventions have been suggested to retard the rate of renal disease progression, including low protein and phosphorous, low cholesterol and fat, and low salt. However only low-protein and low-phosphorous diets have been extensively studied in clinical trials, and unfortunately many of these trials have suffered from poor study design. Nevertheless clinicians must advise patients on diet, using the best available information. Therefore it is important to consider the possible benefits and risks of altering diet in patients with renal disease. This review will consider diets designed to slow the rate of progression in patients with mild to moderate renal insufficiency, and will not address diet therapy designed to ameliorate signs and symptoms of uremia.

Low Protein and Low Phosphorous

Animal studies have unequivocally demonstrated that altering dietary protein intake can modulate the degree of renal injury. In particular, studies in the rat remnant kidney model have shown that altering dietary phosphorous and/or protein affects proteinuria, glomerular filtration rate (GFR), and the amount of glomerular sclerosis (1–3). However it is difficult to compare the amounts of protein and phosphorous fed to rats with the amounts consumed by humans. It is also impossible to know whether the effects of dietary phosphorous and protein on rat kidneys can be extrapolated to humans. Therefore well-designed clinical trials are of paramount importance.

A large number of clinical trials have examined the effects of a low-protein and low-phosphorous diet. Unfortunately many of these trials have been poorly designed. Many have been too small to draw firm conclusions. Most have been inadequately controlled, and how closely patients adhered to prescribed diets was often not well documented. Endpoints have also been problematic. Studies using the onset of dialysis as an endpoint cannot distinguish the effects of low-protein diet on uremic signs and symptoms from those on renal function. Many studies have used change in serum creatinine or slope of inverse creatinine as an endpoint, and these endpoints do not accurately reflect changes in GFR. Few studies have closely examined the nutritional adequacy of the dietary interventions.

Fouque and co-workers published a meta-analysis of studies on protein restriction in 1992 (4). They screened 46 investigations and combined the results of six randomized, controlled trials examining the effects of low-protein diet in patients with non-diabetic renal disease. The endpoint was death, dialysis, or transplantation. Of the six studies selected, one was not published. The length of follow-up was 12–24 months. Baseline renal function varied from mild to severe. The degree of protein restriction was quite variable between studies. The number of patients studied also varied – 19, 50, 65, 72, 228, and 456, respectively, in the six studies. In only one study were the odds of renal death significantly less in the low-protein group compared to control. However with all studies combined, the odds of renal death were significantly less than 1.0 (0.59, with 95% confidence interval 0.37 to 0.79). The authors of this meta-analysis concluded that the clinical trials strongly supported the effectiveness of low-protein diets in delaying the onset of end-stage renal disease.

The United States Congress mandated (in Public Laws 95–292 and 96–499) that a demonstration project be carried out to determine "the extent to which the commencement of nutritional therapy in early renal failure, utilizing (but not limited to) controlled protein substances, can retard or arrest the progression of the disease with a resultant substantive deferment of dialysis" (5). As a result of this mandate the multicentre Modification of Diet in Renal Disease (MDRD) study was carried out. This project consisted of a feasibility phase and a full-scale trial. In the feasibility study 96 patients were randomly allocated to protein intakes of 1.3, 0.575, and 0.28 g/kg body weight/day. Patients receiving 0.28 g/kg/day also received amino acids, or keto analogues. This feasibility study found that: 1) serum creatinine and the slope of reciprocal serum creatinine were poor markers of renal function and disease progression; 2) compliance with diet was relatively poor; 3) blood pressure was a major correlate of the rate of progression; and 4) there were no differences in the slope of the glomerular filtration rate between diet and control groups (5).

Based on the results of the feasibility trial, the full-scale MDRD study was designed to test whether a low-protein, low-phosphorus diet would retard the rate of renal disease progression, whether the diets were nutritionally adequate and acceptable to patients, and whether lowering mean arterial blood pressure to < 92 mm Hg would reduce the rate of progression (5). Two groups of patients were studied (6). In study 1, patients with GFR 25–55 ml/min/1.73m² were assigned to usual or low- protein diet (1.2 or 0.58 g/kg/day) and to usual or low blood pressure (107 or 92 mm Hg mean arterial pressure). In study 2, patients with GFR 13–24 ml/min/1.73m² were assigned to low-protein or very low-protein diet (0.58 or 0.28 g/kg/day with keto-acid/amino acid supplement) and usual or low blood pressure. There were 585 and 255 patients in studies 1 and 2, respectively. Mean follow-up was 2.2 years. In study 1 there was a slower rate of decline in GFR in the protein-restricted group, compared to the control group that started four months after diet was begun, but the difference in GFR at 3 years was not statistically significant. In study 2 diet did not slow the progression of renal disease.

Following publication of the MDRD trial results, Pedrini and co-workers carried out another meta-analysis of studies examining the effects of low-protein diet on renal disease progression (7). This meta-analysis examined diabetic and non-diabetic renal disease. For non-diabetic renal disease, five studies were included. Two studies used by Fouque and co-workers were excluded from this analysis due to the fact that one study was never published and the other did not have an adequate control group. The meta-analysis included the results of the MDRD trial. The combined relative risk of renal failure or death was 0.67 (95% confidence interval was 0.50 to 0.89; n = 1434 patients) (figure 1).

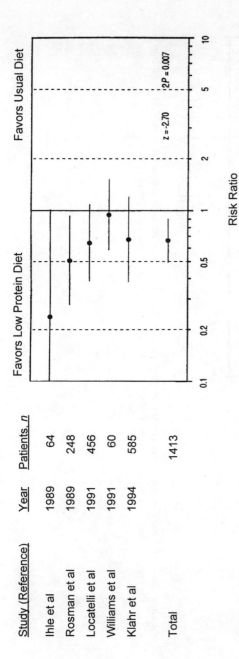

Figure 1. Effect of dietary protein restriction on progression of nondiabetic renal diseases. Data presented as risk ratios with 95% CIs on log scale. Reprinted with permission, Pedrini MT et al. *Ann Intern Med* 1996;124:627–632.

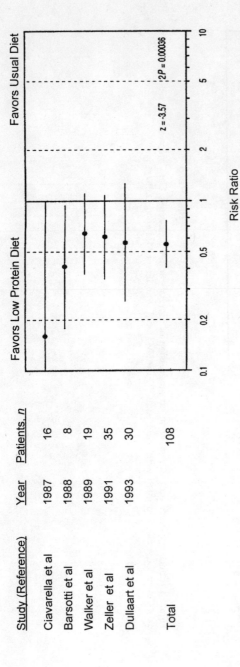

Figure 2. Effect of dietary protein restriction on progression of diabetic renal disease. Data presented as risk ratios with 95% CIs on log scale. Reprinted with permission, Pedrini MT et al. *Ann Intern Med* 1996;124:627–632.

Pedrini and co-workers also combined the results of five studies of insulin-dependent, diabetic renal disease (figure 2) (7). Unfortunately all of the studies on diabetic renal disease were small (8–35 patients per study, total 108). The endpoint was a decline in GFR (or creatinine clearance) greater than 1.2 ml/min/year, or an increase of greater than 10% from baseline in urinary albumin excretion rate. The relative risk of a decline in function or increase in albuminuria was 0.56 (95% confidence interval was 0.40 to 0.77) and the authors concluded that dietary protein restriction "effectively slows the progression of both diabetic and non-diabetic renal disease."

The results of this meta-analysis and the studies that were combined should be interpreted with caution. In the studies of diabetic renal disease the numbers of patients included were very small. With regard to non-diabetic renal disease the interpretation of the endpoints is unavoidably problematic. Dietary protein restriction in patients with severe renal dysfunction can ameliorate the signs and symptoms of uremia without altering renal structure or function. It is plausible that dialysis or transplantation was delayed in patients on low-protein diets without a substantial change in renal function. If true this could confound interpretation of whether dietary protein restriction delays the onset of end-stage renal disease.

It has recently been shown that a low serum albumin is associated with increased mortality in patients on hemodialysis (8,9). It would be counter-productive if low-protein diets left patients nutritionally compromised before or after developing end-stage renal disease. Unfortunately, few studies have adequately addressed the long-term nutritional effects of low-protein diets in patients with renal insufficiency. The MDRD study carefully assessed nutrition in the feasibility trial (10). None of the treatment groups developed protein-calorie malnutrition. However patients with lower GFRs tended to lose body mass during the study and had lower than prescribed energy intakes. Thus this study highlighted the risk of worsening nutrition by diet in patients with renal disease. Moreover the degree of diet counseling available to patients in the MDRD study may not be available to patients in other clinic settings, again raising concerns about the effect of low-protein diets on nutrition.

Low Cholesterol and Low Fat

Data from animal models suggest that hyperlipidemia may contribute to renal injury and decreased renal function. Specifically, cholesterol and high-fat diets have been shown to cause renal injury in normal rats, rats with surgical reduction in renal mass (the remnant kidney model), and rats with aminonucleoside nephrosis (11–14). Rabbit, guinea pig, and mouse models also manifest increased renal injury in response to lipogenic diets (15–18). These and other experimental data support the notion that diet-induced alterations in circulating lipoproteins may modulate renal injury.

Clinical, epidemiologic data supporting the lipid-renal injury hypothesis are largely circumstantial. Certainly lipoprotein abnormalities are common in patients with renal disease. Some rare forms of hyperlipidemia cause spontaneous renal failure (19–21). Although it is less clear whether more common forms of hyperlipidemia cause renal injury (22,23), it is interesting that lipid abnormalities have been linked to albuminuria in the general population and in patients with essential hypertension (24–26). Nevertheless it is not known whether reducing cholesterol and fat in the diet of patients with renal disease will help slow the rate of decline in renal function.

It should be mentioned, however, that there is another compelling reason to limit the dietary intake of cholesterol and fat in patients with renal disease. Cardiovascular disease is a common cause of morbidity and mortality among patients with renal disease. There are no controlled trials showing that diet can reduce cardiovascular disease complications in this population. Nevertheless, there is no reason to believe that the favourable effects of lipid-lowering diets in the general population would not be seen in patients with renal disease.

It should also be mentioned that experimental data in animal models suggest it may be possible to reduce renal injury by adding polyunsaturated fatty acids (PUFA) to the diet. Diets rich in omega-6 PUFA have been shown to reduce renal injury in animal models of progressive renal disease (27–30). Likewise dietary supplementation with omega-3 PUFA, or fish oils, has been shown to be efficacious in several animal models (27,28,30–32). Similarly, flaxseed oil rich in alpha-linolenic PUFA has been shown to reduce renal injury (33). A number of mechanisms in addition to lipid lowering have been suggested to explain the beneficial effects of PUFA diets, but there are few definitive data supporting one over another.

There are few clinical trials examining the effects of PUFA diet supplements in patients with renal disease. Donadio and co-workers carried out a randomized controlled trial of fish oil supplements in patients with IgA nephropathy (34). They found that patients given fish oil capsules had a better outcome compared to placebo controls.

The mechanism is unclear, however omega-3 PUFA may have both immune and non-immune mediated effects that could have reduced the amount of renal injury.

Salt Restriction

There is unequivocal evidence from clinical trials that hypertension accelerates renal disease progression, and that antihypertensive agents preserve renal function in patients with renal insufficiency (35). There is also evidence that hypertension in patients with renal failure is, as a rule, volume dependent (36). Unfortunately, few clinical trials have examined the effects of a reduced salt diet on hypertension in patients with renal insufficiency. It is reasonable to speculate that salt restriction, with and without antihypertensive agents, may help control blood pressure and thereby reduce the rate of progression of renal disease. It is also possible that the effects of salt restriction may act synergistically with some antihypertensive agents. It has been shown, for example, that both the antihypertensive and antiproteinuric effects of angiotensin-converting enzyme inhibitors are potentiated by diuretics or a low-salt diet.

Dietary salt restriction has also been shown to reduce renal injury in the rat remnant kidney model of chronic progressive renal disease, by unknown mechanisms (37). Moreover, the reno-protective effects of antihypertensive agents in the remnant kidney model are greater with salt restriction (38). There are no clinical data examining the possible effects of salt restriction on renal disease progression, with or without blood pressure reduction. However, there are probably few adverse effects from moderate salt restriction, so that any benefit would be high in proportion to risk.

Diabetic Diet

To the extent that diet may help achieve optimal blood sugar control in patients with diabetes, and to the extent that diabetic control may help retard the development and progression of nephropathy, adherence to a diabetic diet seems prudent. Guidelines for a diabetic diet are available and a detailed discussion of the optimal diet for diabetic control is beyond the scope of this review. The diabetes control and complications trial demonstrated that tight control of blood sugar by any means, including diet, reduced the incidence of microalbuminuria and reduced the incidence of clinical proteinuria in patients who already had microalbuminuria (39). Although the exact contribution of diet to achieving tight blood glucose control is unclear, it would seem to be a prudent option (40).

Summary

Although renal disease often seems to progress in a predictable manner, the mechanisms leading to progressive declines in function are poorly understood. Nevertheless, studies in animal models and in humans have suggested that diet might slow the rate of renal disease progression. For example, data from animal models and clinical trials suggest that protein and phosphorous restriction may slow the rate of renal disease progression. However the magnitude of the effect of diet in clinical trials has not been great, and concerns about adequate nutrition require close patient monitoring. Data from experimental models suggest that lowering plasma lipids may reduce renal injury. In any case patients with renal disease have a high incidence of cardiovascular disease complications, and a diet low in cholesterol and saturated fat may reduce the risk of cardiovascular disease. Lowering blood pressure appears to slow the rate of renal disease progression. Since hypertension is often volume dependent in patients with renal disease, it may be prudent to restrict sodium chloride. Finally data suggest that tight blood sugar control may help ameliorate diabetic renal disease. To the extent that it may improve diabetes control, a diabetic diet may, therefore, be beneficial in patients with diabetic nephropathy. In summary, reductions in dietary protein, cholesterol, fat, and salt, along with a diabetic diet when appropriate, seem reasonable strategies for slowing the rate of renal disease progression.

REFERENCES

1 Ibels LS, Alfrey AC, Haut L, Huffer WE. Preservation of function in experimental renal disease by dietary restriction of phosphate. *N Engl J Med* 1978;298:122–126.
2 Lumlertgul D, Burke TJ, Gillum DM, Alfrey AC, Harris DC, Hammond WS, Schrier RW. Phosphate depletion arrests progression of chronic renal failure independent of protein intake. *Kidney Int* 1986;29:658–666.
3 Hostetter TH, Meyer TW, Rennke HG, Brenner BM, Noddin JA, Sandstrom DJ. Chronic effects of dietary protein in the rat with intact and reduced renal mass. *Kidney Int* 1986;30:509–517.

4 Fouque D, Laville M, Boissel JP, Chifflet R, Labeeuw M, Zech PY. Controlled low protein diets in chronic renal insufficiency: meta-analysis. *Br Med J* 1992;304:216–220.

5 Klahr S. The modification of diet in renal disease study. *N Engl J Med* 1989;320:864–866.

6 Klahr S, Levey AS, Beck GJ, Caggiula AW, Hunsicker L, Kusek JW, Striker G. The effects of dietary protein restriction and blood-pressure control on the progression of chronic renal disease. *N Engl J Med* 1994;330:877–884.

7 Pedrini MT, Levey AS, Lau J, Chalmers TC, Wang PH. The effect of dietary protein restriction on the progression of diabetic and nondiabetic renal diseases: a meta-analysis. *Ann Intern Med* 1996;124:627–632.

8 Lowrie EG, Lew NL. Death risk in hemodialysis patients: the predictive value of commonly measured variables and an evaluation of death rate differences between facilities. *Am J Kidney Dis* 1990;15:458–482.

9 Iseki K, Kawazoe N, Fukiyama K. Serum albumin is a strong predictor of death in chronic dialysis patients. *Kidney Int* 1993;44:115–119.

10 Kopple JD, Berg R, Houser H, Steinman TI, Teschan P. Nutritional status of patients with different levels of chronic renal insufficiency. *Kidney Int* 1989;36(suppl 27):s184–s194.

11 Peric-Golia L, Peric-Golia M. Aortic and renal lesions in hypercholesterolemic adult, male, virgin Sprague-Dawley rats. *Atherosclerosis* 1983;46: 57–65.

12 Kasiske BL, O'Donnell MP, Schmitz PG, Kim Y, Keane WF. Renal injury of diet-induced hypercholesterolemia in rats. *Kidney Int* 1990;37:880–891.

13 Gröne HJ, Gröne E, Luthe H, Weber MH, Helmchen U. Induction of glomerular sclerosis by a lipid-rich diet in male rats. *Lab Invest* 1989;60:4433–4460.

14 Diamond JR, Karnovsky MJ. Exacerbation of chronic aminonucleoside nephrosis by dietary cholesterol supplementation. *Kidney Int* 1987;32:671–677.

15 Wellmann KF, Volk BW. Renal lesions in experimental hypercholesterolemia in normal and in subdiabetic rabbits. II. Long term studies. *Lab Invest* 1971;24:144–155.

16 French SW, Yamanaka W, Ostwald R. Dietary induced glomerulosclerosis in the guinea pig. *Arch Pathol Lab Med* 1967;83:204–210.

17 Al-Shebeb T, Frohlich J, Magil AB. Glomerular disease in hypercholesterolemic guinea pigs: a pathogenetic study. *Kidney Int* 1988;33:498–507.

18 Kelley VE, Izui S. Enriched lipid diet accelerates lupus nephritis in NZBXW mice. Synergistic action of immune complexes and lipid in glomerular injury. *Am J Pathol* 1983;111:288–297.

19 Imbasciati E, Paties C, Scarpioni L, Mihatsch MJ. Renal lesions in familial lecithin-cholesterol acyltransferase deficiency. *Am J Nephrol* 1986;6: 66–70.

20 Saito T, Sato H, Kudo K, Oikawa S, Shibata T, Hara Y, Yoshinaga K, Sakaguchi H. Lipoprotein glomerulopathy: glomerular lipoprotein thrombi in a patient with hyperlipoproteinemia. *Am J Kidney Dis* 1989;13:148–153.

21 Oikawa S, Suzuki N, Sakuma E, Saito T, Namai K, Kotake H, Fujii Y, Toyota T. Abnormal lipoprotein and apolipoprotein pattern in lipoprotein glomerulopathy. *Am J Kidney Dis* 1991;18:553–558.

22 Amatruda JM, Margolis S, Hutchins GM. Type III hyperlipoproteinemia with mesangial foam cells in renal glomeruli. *Arch Pathol Lab Med* 1974;98:51–54.

23 Smellie WSA, Warwick GL. Primary hyperlipidaemia is not associated with increased urinary albumin excretion. *Nephrol Dial Transplant* 1991;6:398–401.

24 Metcalf P, Baker J, Scott A, Wild C, Scragg R, Dryson E. Albuminuria in people at least 40 years old: effect of obesity, hypertension, and hyperlipidemia. *Clin Chem* 1992;38:1802–1808.

25 Bianchi S, Bigazzi R, Valtriani C, Chiapponi I, Sgherri G, Baldari G, Natali A, Ferrannini E, Campese VM. Elevated serum insulin levels in patients with essential hypertension and microalbuminuria. *Hypertension* 1994;23(part 1):681–687.

26 Bigazzi R, Bianchi S, Baldari G, Campese VM. Clustering of cardiovascular risk factors in salt-sensitive patients with essential hypertension: role of insulin. *Am J Hypertens* 1996;9:24–32.

27 Kasiske BL, O'Donnell MP, Lee H, Kim Y, Keane WF. The impact of dietary fatty acid supplementation on renal injury in obese Zucker rats. *Kidney Int* 1991;39:1125–1134.

28 Clark WF, Parbtani A, Philbrick D, McDonald JWD, Smallbone B, Reid B, Holub BJ, Kreeft J. Comparative efficacy of dietary treatments on renal function in rats with sub-total nephrectomy: renal polyunsaturated fatty acid incorporation and prostaglandin excretion. *Clin Nephrol* 1990;33:25–34.

29 Heifets M, Morrisey JJ, Purkerson ML, Morrison AR, Klahr S. Effect of dietary lipids on renal function in rats with subtotal nephrectomy. *Kidney Int* 1987;32:335–341.

30 Barcelli UO, Miyata J, Ito Y, Gallon L, Laskarzewski P, Weiss M, Hitzemann R, Pollak VE. Beneficial effects of polyunsaturated fatty acids in partially nephrectomized rats. *Prostaglandins* 1986;32:211–219.

31 Clark WF, Parbtani A, Philbrick DJ, Holub BJ, Huff MW. Chronic effects of ω-3 fatty acids (fish oil) in a rat 5/6 renal ablation model. *J Am Soc Nephrol* 1991;1:1343–1353.

32 Kelley VE, Ferretti A, Izui S, Strom TB. A fish oil diet rich in eicosapentaenoic acid reduces cyclooxygenase metabolites, and suppresses lupus in MRL-1pr mice. *J Immunol* 1985;134:1914–1919.

33 Ingram AJ, Parbtani A, Clark WF, Spanner E, Huff MW, Philbrick DJ, Holub BJ. Effects of flaxseed and flax oil diets in a rat-5/6 renal ablation model. *Am J Kidney Dis* 1995;25:320–329.

34 Donadio JV, Jr, Bergstralh EJ, Offord KP, Spencer DC, Holley KE. A controlled trial of fish oil in IgA nephropathy. Mayo Nephrology Collaborative Group. *N Engl J Med* 1994;331:1194–1199.

35 Maki DD, Ma JZ, Louis TA, Kasiske BL. Long-term effects of antihypertensive agents on proteinuria and renal function. *Arch Intern Med* 1995;155:1073–1080.

36 Galla JG, Luke RG. Hypertension in renal parenchymal disease. In: Brenner BM, ed. *The kidney*, 5th ed. Philadelphia:W.B. Saunders Company, 1996:2126–2147.

37 Lax DS, Benstein JA, Tolbert E, Dworkin LD. Effects of salt restriction on renal growth and glomerular injury in rats with remnant kidneys. *Kidney Int* 1992;41:1527–1534.

38 Terzi F, Beaufils H, Laouari D, Burtin M, Kleinknecht C. Renal effect of anti-hypertensive drugs depends on sodium diet in the excision remnant kidney model. *Kidney Int* 1992;42:354–363.

39 The Diabetes Control and Complications Research Group. Effect of intensive therapy on the development and progression of diabetic nephropathy in the Diabetes Control and Complications Trial. *Kidney Int* 1995;47:1703–1720.

40 American Diabetes Association. Position statement: implications of the Diabetes Control and Complications Trial. *Diabetes* 1993;42:1555–1558.

ANGELO TREMBLAY, SYLVIE ST-PIERRE,
and JEAN-PIERRE DESPRÉS

Diet and Obesity

Obesity is a condition characterized by excess body fat deposition, which is the consequence of the inability to match energy intake to expenditure or vice versa for a long period of time. It is generally accepted that obesity is explained by both environmental and genetic factors as well as their interaction (1). A significant part of the effect of environment on body fat deposition depends on dietary factors whose effects have been emphasized by numerous studies. This paper describes recent progress in this area of research and related clinical implications in the prevention and treatment of obesity.

Energy and Macronutrient Balance

The use of whole-body indirect calorimetry contributed to the demonstration that energy balance occurs when the respiratory quotient (RQ)/food quotient (FQ) ratio equals 1.0, i.e., when the composition of the fuel mix oxidized corresponds to the composition of the fuel mix ingested (2). Thus body weight stability occurs when both energy and macronutrient balances are achieved.

Experimental evidence has also emphasized that the equilibrium between substrate intake and oxidation is not the same for each macronutrient. Protein and carbohydrate have been shown to exert a greater suppressing effect than fat on subsequent energy intake (3,4). It has also been demonstrated that protein and carbohydrate promote their utilization to a greater extent than fat (2,5). Furthermore in the context of prolonged overfeeding imposing a large

excess in macronutrient intake over oxidation, protein and carbohydrate metabolism can ultimately rely on gluconeogenesis and lipo-
genesis to maintain the stability of their stores. However such a
possibility does not exist for lipid, so that most of body energy that
is stored in response to experimental overfeeding is deposited in the
form of fat (6).

In summary these observations suggest that fat balance cannot be
precisely regulated. Since protein and carbohydrate balances are
maintained stable under free living conditions, energy balance is
equivalent to fat balance. Therefore the predisposition to obesity
probably reflects the inability to maintain fat balance under free
living conditions.

Fat Intake and Body Weight Stability

The industrialization that occurred in many countries over this century has been associated with changes in lifestyle favouring body fat
accumulation. Despite the numerous interventions of health agencies
to promote more healthy habits, the prevalence of obesity has continued to increase during recent years. The increase in dietary fat intake
is an important factor that has contributed to this phenomenon.

It is now well established that spontaneous overfeeding occurs
when one has free access to high-fat foods (7–9). As illustrated in
figure 1, the *ad libitum* intake of a diet containing more than 40% of
dietary energy as fat is associated with a considerable increase in
daily energy intake compared to conditions where fat intake con-
forms to nutritional recommendations. Accordingly many epidemiological data have demonstrated that a high fat intake is associated
with an increase in body fatness (8,10,11).

The mechanisms explaining the hyperphagic effect of a high-fat
dietary regimen have been the topic of many investigations. A likely
explanation of this overfeeding is the high energy density of high-fat
foods. Indeed an increase in the energy density of foods has been
shown to increase spontaneous energy intake (12,13). An alternative
explanation refers to the weak ability of fat to promote its own oxidation acutely (5) and to inhibit carbohydrate oxidation. This would
result in a greater carbohydrate depletion and an increased risk of
excess energy intake (2). However recent experimental data do not
support this hypothesis (14).

A high-fat pre-meal load has also been shown to be characterized
by a reduced ability to inhibit subsequent energy intake (3,15). This

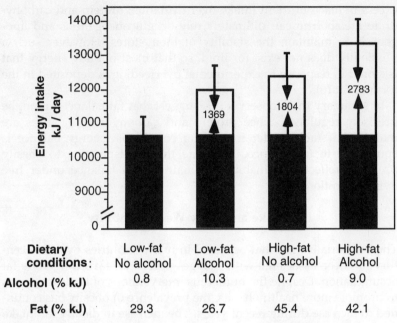

Dietary conditions:	Low-fat No alcohol	Low-fat Alcohol	High-fat No alcohol	High-fat Alcohol
Alcohol (% kJ)	0.8	10.3	0.7	9.0
Fat (% kJ)	29.3	26.7	45.4	42.1

Figure 1. Mean daily increase in energy intake (open bars) above the value (black bars) observed in the low-fat, placebo condition. Values are presented in relation to the mean percentage of energy as alcohol and fat in each condition. Reprinted from Tremblay et al. (9) with permission.

is in agreement with the demonstration that dietary fat has a reduced capacity to favour satiety (16–18). Taken together these observations tend to demonstrate that under free living conditions it is difficult to reach satiety without excess intake of calories and fat. The long-term consequence is a gain in body fat which is described in a subsequent section of this chapter as a necessary adaptation to restore energy and fat balance.

Alcohol and Fat Balance

Alcohol is an energy substrate that also has the potential to modify energy and fat balance substantially. Its impact on daily energy intake has been investigated in many epidemiological studies, whose subjects had to report their habitual food intake. Colditz et al. (19) observed a negative association between alcohol and carbohydrate intake, suggesting that alcohol intake is to some extent compensated by a decrease in carbohydrate intake. In moderate alcohol drinkers Jones et al. (20) found a reduced intake of all macronutrients. This may provide an explanation for the absence of a significant relationship between alcohol intake and body weight in the First National Health and Nutrition Examination Survey (21). This observation is, however, not concordant with results of many other studies showing that energy and macronutrient intakes are not affected by alcohol consumption, which thus represents an excess energy intake (22–25).

The use of indirect calorimetry helped to better characterize the metabolic effects of alcohol. Several years ago Suter et al. (26) reported that alcohol intake transitorily inhibits fat oxidation. For the nutritionist this finding means that drinking alcohol may be equivalent to eating fat if its suppressing effect on fat oxidation is not compensated by a concomitant decrease in fat intake. Our recent experiments confirmed that alcohol intake does not inhibit fat intake acutely under free living conditions, suggesting that alcohol induces a positive fat and energy balance (9). As illustrated in figure 1, our data showed that alcohol intake was associated with an increase in daily energy intake that was additive to the hyperphagic effect of a high-fat diet.

We investigated this issue further in a more recent study that was aimed at evaluating the extent to which the overfeeding resulting from the intake of high-fat foods and alcohol might depend on their high energy density (27). As depicted in figure 2, we measured the impact of two appetizers of comparable weight and energy density on *ad libitum* energy intake for the rest of the meal served at lunch time. According to results of the above referenced study (9), spontaneous energy intake following the high fat–alcohol appetizer exceeded by about 0.8 MJ the value observed after the high-carbohydrate appetizer (27). These observations thus suggest that alcohol accentuates the hyperphagic effect of a high-fat diet and that this effect is not mainly explained by the high energy density of these substrates.

Exercise and Fat Balance

Aerobic exercise is known to influence fat and energy balance because of its enhancing effect on fat oxidation and energy expenditure. Since this chapter pertains to the theme of diet and obesity, the only point that will be discussed here is the effect of dietary composition on the ability of exercise to promote a negative fat and energy

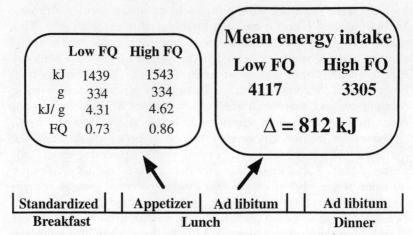

Figure 2. Effect of high-fat-alcohol (low FQ) and high carbohydrate (high FQ) appetizers on mean *ad libitum* energy intake at lunch time. Adapted from Tremblay and St-Pierre (27).

balance. In a recent study we investigated this issue by subjecting adult males to a protocol requiring *ad libitum* eating in the laboratory for two days after having completed a 60-minute exercise bout (28). In one case exercise was followed by a two-day protocol while subjects had free access to high-fat foods. In the other two sessions foods that were available for *ad libitum* intake after exercise were characterized by either a moderate- or low-fat content. The sessions were randomly assigned to subjects. As shown in table 1, exercise induced an energy deficit of 6.4 MJ over two days when the subjects had free access to low-fat foods, which had a fat content conforming to nutritional recommendations. This deficit was explained by an increase in energy expenditure of 2.2 MJ during exercise and by a deficit of 4.2 MJ during the two days that followed exercise. At the opposite, a slight energy excess was observed under the high-fat diet condition because the post-exercise increase in energy intake was greater than the surplus of energy expended both during and after exercise. These results are concordant with recent data obtained in a comparable experimental context (29).

Changes in Adiposity and Fat Balance

Several decades ago Kennedy (30) proposed a lipostatic theory, suggesting that adipose tissue–related factors affect the regulation of

Table 1
Effect of Dietary Composition on the Impact of Exercise on Energy Balance

	Diet Composition		
	Low-Fat	Mixed	High-Fat
Δ energy cost of exercise* (MJ/h)	–2.2	–2.2	–2.2
Postexercise energy balance (MJ/48h)	–4.2	–2.3	3.1
Overall energy balance (MJ/49h)	–6.4	–4.5	0.9

* Surplus of energy expended during exercise above 2 METS (i.e., n × RMR)
Adapted from Tremblay et al. (28)

energy intake and balance. This hypothesis is still valid and was recently reinforced by the discovery of leptin, which is synthetized in adipocytes and which inhibits food intake in rodents (31). Numerous human studies have also provided support for the idea of a lipostatic mechanism involved in the regulation of energy balance. Björntorp et al. (32) demonstrated that resistance to further loss of body fat during a weight-reducing program occurred in obese subjects when their fat cell size was decreased to the level of their lean controls. We have investigated factors associated with resistance to fat loss in ex-obese runners and found that their inability to lose weight was associated with a decrease in fat cell lipolysis (33). More recently Schutz et al. (34) emphasized the role of fat oxidation on the regulation of energy and fat balance. Their results showed that when an individual loses body fat a decrease in fat oxidation is observed, which contributes to a progressive re-equilibration of fat balance at a reduced level of adiposity. At the opposite, a gain in body fatness is associated with an increase in the fat content of the substrate mix, which contributes to reaching a new fat balance at an increased level of body fat stores. In other words body fat gain might be viewed as the price to pay to re-establish fat balance in a context of excess fat intake.

As discussed above the adherence to a lifestyle characterized by high-fat and alcohol intake and sedentariness is sufficient to induce a large body fat accumulation. We have recently investigated the impact of these lifestyle habits on subcutaneous adiposity and found that high-fat and alcohol intake and sedentariness were associated with a preferential storage of trunk fat (35). It is, however, important to emphasize that there are individual variations in the response of body fat to a lifestyle promoting a positive energy and fat balance.

Experimental evidence suggests that individuals predisposed to obesity are characterized by a reduced fat oxidation when their body weight is normal (36–38). Recent data also showed that the ability to increase fat oxidation in response to a high-fat diet is lower in obese than in lean subjects (39). These observations demonstrate that individuals predisposed to obesity display a decreased potential to oxidize lipid as well as a reduced ability to increase fat oxidation when exposed to a positive fat balance.

Clinical Implications for the Treatment of Obesity

Nutritional recommendations agree with the observations presented above, which emphasize the importance of modifying factors that influence fat balance in a weight-reducing program. A decrease in fat and alcohol intake should thus be important components of this program, which should also promote an increased participation in physical activities. We tested this approach several years ago in obese women, who were supervised over a 29-month period (40). This protocol included a first phase of aerobic exercise for 15 months and a low-fat diet, plus exercise, for the remaining 14 months. As depicted in figure 3, a substantial decrease in percent body fat was observed after the first 15 months. A further fat loss was noted for the following six months (months 15–21), which followed the incorporation of the low-fat diet into the program. At this time mean cumulative body fat loss reached 14 kg and subjects experienced further resistance to lose fat, although their adiposity remained much higher than in their lean controls.

Figure 3 also shows that a normalization of the glucose and insulin responses to oral glucose was achieved by the end of the weight-reducing program (40). A substantial improvement of the lipid-lipoprotein profile of the subjects was also observed. Beyond these beneficial metabolic changes, it is also relevant to emphasize that the reduced insulinemia observed at the end of the program could also potentially be related to subjects' inability to lose further body fat. Indeed hyperinsulinemia with euglycemia has been shown to increase plasma norepinephrine concentration (41) and muscle sympathetic nerve activity (42). An increase in plasma insulin is also associated with an increase in postprandial energy expenditure in the context of experimental overfeeding (43) and a reduced body fat gain during a follow-up of several years (44). Furthermore experimental data demonstrated that hyperinsulinemia decreases the level

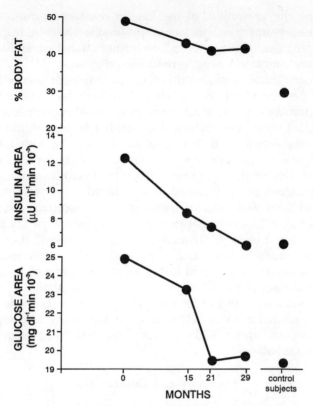

Figure 3. Percent body fat and plasma insulin and glucose responses to oral glucose (insulin and glucose area) before, during, and after a 29-month treatment including exercise training (months 0–15) and exercise training plus low-fat diet (months 15–29). Adapted from Tremblay et al. (40).

of neuropeptide Y (NPY) in the arcuate nucleus and its gene expression (45). Since this peptide exerts orexigenic effects, its inhibition by insulin might be one mechanism by which body weight stability is ultimately reached under conditions of positive energy balance. Taken together these observations suggest that insulin is involved in a sequence of biological events contributing to the regulation of energy balance.

The clinical significance of changes in insulinemia is important for the post-obese individual. The decrease in plasma insulin and the increase in insulin sensitivity that generally occur in response to a weight-reducing program are associated with many beneficial effects favouring the prevention of the insulin resistance syndrome (46). However this improved metabolic profile may also be responsible for the progressive resistance to lose further fat that generally occurs during the course of a weight-reducing program.

Another clinical implication of the macronutrient-energy balance concept pertains to the effect of changes in body fat on fat oxidation. This is particularly relevant for programs based on very low caloric diet (VLCD) which can induce a substantial fat loss in most obese individuals. As shown by Schutz et al. (34), a 10-kg body fat loss is associated with an estimated decrease in resting fat oxidation of 20 g/day. This implies that once a VLCD treatment is interrupted, fat balance cannot be maintained at a reduced body weight if pre-treatment food and activity habits are not modified. Indeed the maintenance of body weight stability is not physiologically possible for the reduced obese individual if changes in lifestyle do not have an impact on fat balance that is equivalent to the decrease in fat oxidation induced by weight loss. This can be achieved by modifying diet composition and physical activity participation, provided that the reducing effect of fat loss on fat oxidation is not too large. On the other hand if these changes are not sufficient to compensate for the decrease in fat oxidation, fat regain will be necessary to re-establish fat balance.

Summary and Conclusions

A successful dietary treatment for obesity must take into account the impact of macronutrients on energy balance. Diet should not have a high-fat and alcohol content, since these substrates do not seem to induce satiety without excess energy intake. An increase in physical activity participation is also relevant, since a low-fat diet represents a nutritional context that increases the ability of exercise to induce a negative energy balance. Experimental data show that a long-term compliance to a healthy lifestyle is associated with a substantial decrease in body fat and an improvement of the metabolic condition in obese individuals. A decrease in plasma insulin is one of the most noticeable effects of fat loss, but evidence suggests that this effect may also be responsible for the progressive development of resistance to lose fat. These observations do not necessarily discard VLCD as an approach to treat obese individuals. If one selects this therapeutic approach, changes in dietary composition and participation in physical activities will be necessary at the end of the treatment to prevent body fat regain. However major changes in fat and alcohol intake and participation in physical activities may not always be sufficient to prevent body weight regain if VLCD induces a large decrease in body fat and fat oxidation. This emphasizes the importance of designing a body weight and fat loss program that will be commensurate to the ability to prevent relapse to obesity.

REFERENCES

1 Bouchard C, Pérusse L. Genetics of obesity. *Ann Rev Nutr* 1993;13:337–354.
2 Flatt JP. Dietary fat, carbohydrate balance, and weight maintenance: effects of exercise. *Am J Clin Nutr* 1987; 45:296–306.
3 Walls EK, Koopmans HS. Effect of intravenous nutrient infusions on food intake in rats. *Physiol Behav* 1989;45:1223–1226.
4 Walls EK, Koopmans HS. Differential effects of intravenous glucose, amino acids, and lipid on daily food intake in rats. *Am J Physiol* 1992;262:R225–R234.
5 Flatt JP, Ravussin E, Acheson KJ, Jéquier E. Effects of dietary fat on post-prandial substrate oxidation and on carbohydrate and fat balances. *J Clin Invest* 1985;76:1119–1124.
6 Tremblay A, Després JP, Thériault G, Fournier G, Bouchard C. Effect of long-term overfeeding and energy expenditure in humans. *Am J Clin Nutr* 1992;56:857–862.
7 Lissner L, Levitsky DA, Strupp BJ, Kalkwarf HJ, Roe DA. Dietary fat and regulation of energy intake in human subjects. *Am J Clin Nutr* 1987;46:886–892.
8 Tremblay A, Plourde G, Després JP, Bouchard C. Impact of dietary fat content and fat oxidation on energy intake in humans. *Am J Clin Nutr* 1989;49:799–805.
9 Tremblay A, Wouters E, Wenker M, St-Pierre S, Bouchard C, Després JP. Alcohol and high-fat diet: a combination favoring overfeeding. *Am J Clin Nutr* 1995;62:639–644.
10 Dreon DM, Frey-Hewitt B, Ellsworth N, Williams PT, Terry RB, Wood PD. Dietary fat: carbohydrate ratio and obesity in middle-aged men. *Am J Clin Nutr* 1988;47:995–1000.
11 Romieu I, Willett WC, Stampfer MJ, Colditz GA, Sampson L, Rosner B, Hennekens CH, Speizer FE. Energy intake and other determinants of relative weight. *Am J Clin Nutr* 1988;47:406–412.
12 Duncan KH, Bacon JA, Weinsier RL. The effects of high and low energy density diets on satiety, energy intake, and eating time of obese and nonobese subjects. *Am J Clin Nutr* 1983;37:763–767.

13 Porikos KP, Booth G, Van Italie TB. Effect of covert nutritive dilution on the spontaneous food intake of obese individuals: a pilot study. *Am J Clin Nutr* 1977;30:1638–1644.

14 Stubbs RJ, Murgatroyd PR, Goldberg GR, Prentice AM. Carbohydrate balance and the regulation of day-to-day food in humans. *Am J Clin Nutr* 1993;57:897–903.

15 Rolls BJ, Kim-Harris S, Fischman MW, Foltin RW, Moran TH, Stoner SA. Satiety after preloads with different amounts of fat and carbohydrate: implications for obesity. *Am J Clin Nutr* 1994;60:476–487.

16 Lawton CL, Burley VJ, Wales JK, Blundell JE. Dietary fat and appetite control in obese subjects; weak effects on satiety. *Int J Obes* 1993;17:409–416.

17 Blundell J.E. Dietary fat and control of energy intake: evaluating the effects of fat on meal size and postmeal satiety. *Am J Clin Nutr* 1993;57:772s–778s.

18 Blundell JE, Green S, Burley V. Carbohydrates and human appetite. *Am J Clin Nutr* 1994;59:728s–734s.

19 Colditz GA, Giovannucci E, Rimm ER, Stampfer MJ, Rosner B, Speizer YE, Gordis E, Walter CW. Alcohol intake in relation to diet and obesity in women and men. *Am J Clin Nutr* 1991;54:49–55.

20 Jones BR, Barrett-Connor E, Criqui MH, Holbrook MJ. A community study of calorie and nutrient intake in drinkers and nondrinkers of alcohol. *Am J Clin Nutr* 1982;35:135–139.

21 Liu S, Serdula MK, Williamson DF, Mokdad AH, Byers T. A prospective study of alcohol intake and change in body weight among US adults. *Am J Epidemiol* 1994;140:912–920.

22 Bebb HT, Houser HB, Witschi JC, Litell AS, Fuller RK. Calorie and nutrient contribution of alcoholic beverages to the usual diets of 155 adults. *Am J Clin Nutr* 1971;24:1042–1052.

23 Gruchow HW, Sobocinski KA, Barboriak JJ, Scheller JG. Alcohol consumption, nutrient intake and relative body weight among US adults. *Am J Clin Nutr* 1985;42:289–295.

24 Veenstra J, Schenkel JAA, Erp-Baart AMJv, Brants HAM, Hulshof KFAM, Kistemaker C, Schaafsma G, Ockhuizen T. Alcohol consumption in relation to food intake and smoking habits in the Dutch National Food Consumption Survey. *Eur J Clin Nutr* 1993;47:482–489.

25 de Castro JM, Orozco S. The effects of moderate alcohol intake on the spontaneous eating patterns of humans: evidence of unregulated supplementation. *Am J Clin Nutr* 1990;52:246–253.

26 Suter PM, Schutz Y, Jéquier E. The effect of ethanol on fat storage in healthy subjects. *New Engl J Med* 1992;326:983–987.

27 Tremblay A, St-Pierre S. The hyperphagic effect of high-fat and alcohol persists after control for energy density. *Am J Clin Nutr* 1996;63:479–482.

28 Tremblay A, Alméras N, Boer J, Kranenbarg EK, Després JP. Diet composition and postexercise energy balance. *Am J Clin Nutr* 1994;59:975–979.

29 King NA, Blundell JE. High-fat foods overcome the energy expenditure due to exercise after cycling and running. *Eur J Clin Nutr* 1995;49:114–123.

30 Kennedy GC. The role of depot fat in the hypothalamic control of food intake in the rat. *Proc Royal Society* (London) 1952;140B:578–592.

31 Zhang Y, Proenca R, Maffei M, Barone M, Leopold L, Friedman JM. Positional cloning of the mouse obese gene and its human homologue. *Nature* 1994;372:425–432.

32 Björntorp P, Carlgren G, Isaksson B, Krotkiewski M, Larsson B, Sjostrom L. Effect of an energy-reduced dietary regimen in relation to adipose tissue cellularity in obese women. *Am J Clin Nutr* 1975;28:445–452.

33 Tremblay A, Després JP, Bouchard C. Adipose tissue characteristics of ex-obese long-distance runners. *Int J Obes* 1984;8:641–648.

34 Schutz Y, Tremblay A, Weinsier RL, Nelson KM. Role of fat oxidation in the long-term stabilization of body weight in obese women. *Am J Clin Nutr* 1992;55:670–674.

35 Tremblay A, Buemann B, Thériault G, Bouchard C. Body fatness in active individuals reporting low lipid and alcohol intake. *Eur J Clin Nutr* 1995;49:824–831.

36 Lean MEJ, James WPT. Metabolic effects of isoenergetic nutrient exchange over 24 hours in relation to obesity in women. *Int J Obes* 1988;8:641–648.

37 Buemann B, Astrup A, Madsen J, Christensen NJ. A 24-hr energy expenditure study on reduced-obese and non-obese women: effect of β-blockade. *Am J Clin Nutr* 1992;56:662–670.

38 Buemann B, Astrup A, Christensen NJ, Madsen J. Effect of moderate cold exposure on 24-h energy expenditure: similar response in post obese and nonobese women. *Am J Physiol* 1992;263:E1040–E1045.

39 Thomas CD, Peters JC, Reed GW, Abumrad NN, Sun M, Hill JO. Nutrient balance and energy expenditure during ad libitum feeding of high-fat and high-carbohydrate diets in humans. *Am J Clin Nutr* 1992;55:934–942.

40 Tremblay A, Després JP, Maheux J, Pouliot MC, Nadeau A, Moorjani PJ, Lupien PJ, Bouchard C. Normalization of the metabolic profile in obese women by exercise and a low fat diet. *Med Sci Sports Exerc* 1991;23:1326–1331.

41 Rowe JW, Young JB, Minaker KL, Steven AL, Pallotta J, Lansberg L. Effect of insulin and glucose infusions on sympathetic nervous system activity in normal man. *Diabetes* 1981;30:219–225.
42 Berne C, Fagius J, Pollare T, Hemjdahl P. The sympathetic response to euglycaemic hyperinsulinemia. *Diabetologia* 1992;35:873–879.
43 Tremblay A, Nadeau A, Després JP, Bouchard C. Hyperinsulinemia and regulation of energy balance. *Am J Clin Nutr* 1995;61:827–830.
44 Schwartz MW, Boyko EJ, Kahn SE, Ravussin E, Bogardus C. Reduced insulin secretion: an independent predictor of body weight gain. *J Clin Endocrinol Metab* 1995;80:1571–1576.
45 Schwartz MW, Sipols AJ, Marks JL, Sanacora G, White JD, Scheurink A, Kahn SE, Baskin DG, Woods SC, Figlewicz DP, Porte D. Inhibition of hypothalamic neuropeptide Y gene expression by insulin. *Endocrinology* 1992;130:3608–3616.
46 Reaven GM. Role of insulin resistance in human disease. *Diabetes* 1988;37:1495–1507.

THOMAS M.S. WOLEVER

Diet and Diabetes

Diabetes is a major socio-economic problem because of its high frequency, high morbidity and mortality, and high cost (1–3). The incidence of diabetes varies around the world from nearly 50% of the population in the Pima Indians of southern Arizona, to virtually zero in parts of rural Africa. In Canada about 5% of the population is known to have diabetes and another 5% is undiagnosed. The incidence increases with age, and 15–20% of the population over the age of 65 has diabetes (4). Diabetes is the number one cause of blindness (5), end-stage renal disease (6), and gangrene and amputation of the lower limb (7), and is a major risk factor for cardiovascular disease (8). The cost of diabetes health care is over $1.5 billion per year in Canada and at least 10 times that amount in the United States (9).

The different kinds of diabetes can be divided into two broad categories: type I, or insulin-dependent diabetes mellitus (IDDM), and type II, or non-insulin-dependent diabetes mellitus (NIDDM). IDDM, which makes up 5–10% of all diabetes, is usually first diagnosed in individuals less than 30 years of age, and is associated with leanness, ketosis proneness, low or absent plasma insulin levels, and an absolute requirement for insulin treatment. NIDDM accounts for over 85% of diabetes. It usually presents in adults over the age of 50, though in aboriginal North American populations it can occur in teenagers. NIDDM is associated with obesity and insulin resistance and the absence of ketosis. It can be treated by diet alone or with oral agents or insulin (10).

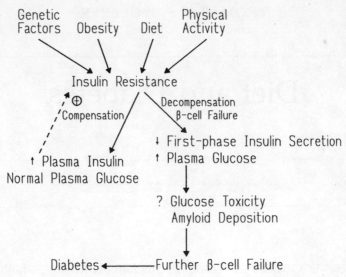

Figure 1. Current concepts on the pathogenesis of non-insulin-dependent diabetes. See text for explanation.

Since the last symposium on diet, nutrition, and health in 1987, there have been significant advances in our understanding of the cause of diabetes and its complications. Many believe that the basic defect underlying the pathogenesis of many forms of NIDDM is insulin resistance (11,12). However others argue that reduced first phase insulin secretion is present before the development of fasting hyperglycemia and may be the predominant pathophysiologic mechanism, at least in some individuals (13). Insulin sensitivity is the ability of insulin to stimulate the uptake of glucose by peripheral tissues (primarily muscle) and to shut off glucose release from the liver. In the presence of insulin resistance, a high blood insulin concentration is needed to achieve a normal rate of whole body glucose disposal (figure 1). Insulin resistance is partly genetically determined and is also influenced by physical activity (14), fat intake (15), obesity, and the distribution of body fat (16,17). Hyperinsulinemia can be considered a normal compensatory response to insulin resistance, but may lead to a vicious cycle because high blood insulin down-regulates insulin receptors resulting in an exacerbation of insulin resistance (18). In the presence of insulin resistance blood glucose rises after meals are enhanced and prolonged, but the fasting blood glucose concentration can be maintained in the normal range as long as the pancreas can secrete large amounts of insulin. Eventually, however, insulin secretion can no longer be maintained at such high levels, possibly because of the effects of glucose toxicity (19) or amyloid deposition within islets (13). At this point fasting blood glucose begins to rise and diabetes develops (11).

Another landmark was the publication of the results of the Diabetes Control and Complications Trial (DCCT) which was designed to answer the question as to whether "tight" blood glucose control could prevent complications in IDDM (20). The results of the trial were astounding: intensive insulin therapy, which improved mean glycosylated hemoglobin (HbA1c) levels from about 9% to 7.5%, was associated with 50–75% reductions in the incidence of retinopathy (eye disease), with similar reductions in nerve and kidney complications. Although only subjects with IDDM were studied it is generally felt that the results can be extrapolated to NIDDM (21) because raised blood glucose *per se* leads to the accumulation of advanced glycation end products (AGE), which have been implicated strongly in the pathogenesis of diabetes complications (22). However definitive proof that improved glucose control prevents complications in NIDDM will have to await the results of current trials examining this issue.

Dietary Recommendations for Diabetes in the Late 1980s

At the time of the last Diet, Nutrition, and Health Symposium, there was a broad consensus of agreement about the dietary guidelines for the management of diabetes in North America and Europe which was reflected in the position statements of the American (ADA) (23), British (24), and Canadian (CDA) Diabetes Associations (25). For example the ADA position at that time was that protein intake should be 0.8 g/kg body weight, an amount that is sufficient for needs but not exessive; carbohydrate should comprise 55–60% of energy and total fat less than 30% of energy, with saturated fat less than 10% of energy and polyunsaturated fat 6–8% of energy. It was recognized that dietary fibre could improve carbohydrate and lipid metabolism, and recommended that fibre intake be doubled, with particular emphasis on sources of soluble fibre and whole grains such as legumes, wholegrain cereals, root vegetables, tubers, and leafy vegetables. It was also recognized that the blood glucose-raising potential of equivalent amounts of different carbohydrate foods varies. The glycemic index

(GI) is a classification of foods according to their blood glucose–raising potential (26). It is defined as follows: $GI = 100 \times F/S$, where F is the incremental area under the blood glucose response curve (AUC) after consuming 50 g carbohydrate from the food and S is the AUC after the same subject consumes 50 g carbohydrate from a standard. Originally the standard was glucose (27), but more recently white bread is preferred (26). In 1986 the ADA position was that the glycemic index may be useful in principle, but that more research was needed before it could be recommended for general application.

Support for the recommendation of a high-carbohydrate diet in the management of diabetes was, however, not universal (28). The rationale for replacing dietary saturated fat with carbohydrate was to reduce serum LDL cholesterol and hence reduce the risk for cardiovascular disease. However there was concern that a high-carbohydrate diet increased postprandial glucose and insulin concentrations, increased serum triglycerides, and reduced HDL cholesterol (29). Over the last 10 years research in this area has focused on the role of monounsaturated fat in the diabetes diet (30–32). The conclusions drawn from these studies are that replacing saturated fat with monounsaturated fat achieves the same reduction in LDL cholesterol as a high-carbohydrate diet, but with lower postprandial glucose and insulin, lower triglycerides, and a higher HDL cholesterol. Current dietary recommendations for diabetes reflect this.

Current Dietary Recommendations for Diabetes

ADA published revised dietary guidelines for diabetes in 1994 (33) and the Diabetes and Nutrition Study Group (DNSG) of the European Association for the Study of Diabetes published guidelines in 1995 (34) (table 1). The CDA guidelines (table 2) were last published in 1989 and are currently being revised. The current ADA position is that carbohydrate plus monounsaturated fat should together contribute 60–70% of energy, with the exact proportion of each being individualized according to the clinical situation and tastes of people with diabetes. The ADA also changed its position on fibre and the glycemic index; it now recognizes no specific role for fibre in the treatment of diabetes, and does not mention the glycemic index. The glycemic index values of common foods vary over a three- to four-fold range, nevertheless the ADA position is that the priority for carbohydrate is amount rather than source.

I have four concerns about the current ADA position: 1) It ignores much evidence that changing the source of dietary carbohydrate,

Table 1
Current Dietary Guidelines for Diabetes in U.S.A. vs Europe

Dietary Component	American Diabetes Association (33)	Diabetes and Nutrition Study Group of EASD*
Protein	10–20% energy: if nephropathy, 0.8 g/kg	10–20% energy: if nephropathy, 0.7–0.9 g/kg
Total fat	< 30–40% energy	–
SFA	< 7–10% energy	< 10% energy
MUFA	< 10–20% energy	–
PUFA	< 10% energy	< 10% energy
Cholesterol	< 300 mg/d	–
Carbohydrate plus MUFA	60–70% energy	Individualized
Sucrose	No suggested amount: substitute for other carbohydrate foods	< 10% energy; include with meals and in diet prescription
Dietary fibre	Insignificant effect on glycemic control: 20–35 g/day	Use foods rich in soluble fibre
Glycemic Index	Priority is amount of carbohydrate rather than source	Low glycemic index foods may help improve glycemic control

* EASD = European Association for the Study of Diabetes (34).
SFA = saturated fatty acids; MUFA = monounsaturated fatty acids; PUFA = polyunsaturated fatty acids.

Table 2
Current Dietary Guidelines for Diabetes in Canada (25)

Dietary Component	Recommendation
Protein	0.8 g/kg
Total fat	< 30% energy
SFA	< 10% energy
MUFA	total minus (SFA + PUFA)
PUFA	< 10% energy
Cholesterol	Concomitant with reduced animal fat
Carbohydrate	balance of energy
Sucrose	in moderation; part of carbohydrate allowance
Dietary fibre	40 g/d may be beneficial; sources of soluble fibre to be emphasized
Glycemic index	use of low GI foods may be beneficial: systematic calculation of GI is not appropriate or necessary for practical application

SFA = saturated fatty acids; MUFA = monounsaturated fatty acids; PUFA = polyunsaturated fatty acids.

with no change in amount, can reduce blood glucose, insulin, cholesterol, and triglycerides; 2) High-fat diets lead to obesity, but controlling body weight is a major goal for the prevention and treatment
of NIDDM; 3) A realistic increase in monounsaturated fat intake has
only a small effect on triglycerides and no proven effect on overall
glucose control; 4) The practicality of basing dietary advice on the
amount of nutrients is questioned.

Role of Source of Carbohydrate in the Diabetes Diet

The ADA states that the first priority is the amount of carbohydrate
rather than the source. There is no indication by the ADA that source
of carbohydrate has any specific role in the management of diabetes;
the glycemic index is not mentioned. Immediately preceding the
ADA position statement there is a technical review (35) upon which,
presumably, the nutrition recommendations are based. In this review
it is acknowledged that different sources of carbohydrate, when fed
as individual foods, have different glycemic effects. However it is
noted that "...questions have arisen as to the clinical utility of these
data." It is stated that recommending only foods with a low glycemic
response severely limits food choices and it is suggested that the
glycemic index may not be useful for meal planning.

Three papers are cited as evidence that the glycemic index has
questionable clinical utility (36–38). Of all the studies that could have
been cited, the conclusions of these papers are the most negative.
Nevertheless the results of even these studies provide some support
for the application of the glycemic index to mixed meals. When all
the data are considered together, the correlation coefficient between
the observed glycemic response and the expected meal glycemic
index is nearly significant, r = 0.524 (n = 13, p = 0.066). There are at
least three other better-designed studies that provide very strong
support for the application of the glycemic index in mixed meals
(39–41). In every individual study the correlation between observed
glycemic response and expected meal glycemic index was statistically significant, and when pooled (n = 24) the correlation coefficient
is very good (r = 0.923, p < 0.0001, figure 2).

The ADA also ignored at least eight studies in which low glycemic
index diets were used in the treatment of diabetes for periods of from
two weeks to three months (42–49). In these studies the amount of
fat, protein, and carbohydrate in the diet remained constant; only the
source of carbohydrate was changed. The study with the smallest

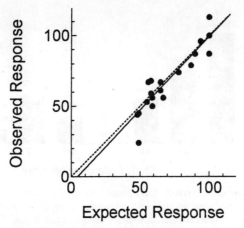

Figure 2. Relationship between expected and observed glycemic responses to mixed meals in groups of normal and diabetic subjects from 3 studies (39–41) not cited by the ADA in considering the clinical utility of the glycemic index (35). Expected response was calculated from the glycemic index of the foods in the meals; observed response is the mean incremental area under the curve. Expected and observed responses in each group of subjects are expressed as a percentage of the meal with the highest expected response. Dotted line is the line of identity; solid line is the regression line (r = 0.923, r² = 0.85, p < 0.0001).

change in diet glycemic index (45,50) was unable to detect a change in HbA1c over a four-week treatment period, which is not surprising because changes in HbA1c occur quite slowly; it takes at least four to eight weeks for a sustained change in glucose control to be reflected in a reduction of HbA1c (51,52). However every one of the other seven studies showed that a low glycemic index diet significantly improved overall blood glucose control, measured by glycosylated albumin or HbA1c (figure 3). Considering all eight studies, the average improvement in overall blood glucose control seen with the use of low glycemic index foods, 9%, is about half that achieved with intensified insulin therapy during the DCCT (20). In addition reducing diet glycemic index has been shown to reduce insulin secretion and to lower serum cholesterol and triglyceride concentrations with no change in HDL cholesterol in both diabetic and non-diabetic individuals (48–54). Thus I believe that the concept of the glycemic index has a role to play, at least in principle, in the management of diabetes. In addition low glycemic index foods may have a role to play in preventing NIDDM.

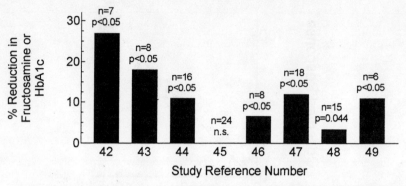

Figure 3. Improvement in overall blood glucose control, expressed as the percentage reduction of glycosylated albumin (fructosamine) or glycosylated hemoglobin (HbA1c) in diabetic subjects treated with a low glycemic index diet. Data from 8 studies.

It has been suggested that high glycemic index foods, which stimulate high postprandial insulin responses, may be at least in part responsible for causing NIDDM (55). This is compatible with our current understanding of the role of insulin resistance and hyperinsulinemia in the pathogenesis of NIDDM (figure 1). It has recently been demonstrated in Sprague-Dawley rats, which spontaneously develop insulin resistance as they age, that the rate of development of insulin resistance is promoted by feeding a diet containing high glycemic index starch (56). It has also been shown in humans with impaired glucose tolerance that reducing postprandial glucose and insulin responses, using an alpha-glucosidase inhibitor, improves insulin sensitivity (57). However it remains to be demonstrated whether altering the nature of the carbohydrate foods will improve insulin resistance in humans, and whether this in turn will delay or prevent the onset of NIDDM.

Dietary Fat and Obesity

A major concern about increasing monounsaturated fat intake at the expense of carbohydrate is that it may promote weight gain. Obesity is associated with insulin resistance (58) and is a major factor predisposing to the development of NIDDM (59). Most patients with NIDDM are obese, and one of the major aims of diet therapy in NIDDM in these individuals is to achieve and maintain ideal body weight. A number of strategies are possible to promote weight loss, including reducing energy intake, reducing fat intake, and increasing physical activity. Amongst dietary strategies it has been found that restriction of fat and energy intake promotes equivalent or greater weight loss, with greater acceptability, than just restricting energy intake (60,61). In one study of weight changes over two years in 303 women, weight loss was more strongly associated with a reduction in percentage of energy from fat than with change in total energy intake (62).

High-fat diets are associated with obesity (63,64). Dietary fat appears to promote weight gain not only because it promotes excess energy intake (65), but also because it is inefficiently oxidized. The body has little storage capacity for carbohydrate and protein and intake of these substrates promotes their oxidation. On the other hand fat stores are large and almost infinitely expandable. Thus under conditions of positive energy balance, carbohydrate and protein are preferentially oxidized and fat is preferentially stored. Dietary fat is absorbed as chylomicrons which deposit their load of fat directly into adipose tissue. Dietary fat cannot be oxidized unless it is released from adipose tissue in the form of free fatty acids. Free fatty acid release is proportional to fat mass. Thus, with positive energy balance, dietary fat continues to be stored until the adipose tissue mass has increased enough so that fat oxidation has increased to match fat intake (66).

Dietary fat appears to promote obesity and prevent weight loss, but there is little information as to whether all kinds of fat have this effect. There is some evidence that polyunsaturated fat is oxidized more readily than saturated fat (67,68), but the relative rate of oxidation of monounsaturated fat is unknown. A few studies have shown that weight loss can be achieved on a diet high in monounsaturated fat, but these are short term and involve subjects consuming pre-weighed very low-calorie diets (69,70). The long-term effects of a high-monounsaturated-fat diet on body weight are not known.

Effects of Monounsaturated Fat in Diabetes

The early studies promoting the use of monounsaturated fat came from Garg et al. and involved diets containing 50% or more of energy from fat (31). These studies found that a high-monounsaturated-fat diet, compared to a high-carbohydrate diet, resulted in the same reduction in LDL cholesterol, but a higher HDL cholesterol, lower serum triglycerides, and lower postprandial glucose and insulin responses. The most recent study from Garg et al. (32) was a large, well-designed, multi-centre trial that looked at the effect of more realistic diets with 45% energy from fat (25% energy from monoun-saturated fat) and 40% carbohydrate versus a diet containing 30% fat and 55% carbohydrate. In this study no significant effect on HDL cholesterol was seen, but there was a highly significant increase in serum triglycerides. During a day when the subjects ate foods pro-vided to them, plasma glucose and insulin concentrations during the day were higher on the high-carbohydate diet than the high-monounsaturated-fat diet, but there was no significant difference in overall long-term blood glucose control, as measured by HbA1c.

Monounsaturated Fat and Blood Glucose

When considering the effect on blood glucose of replacing dietary carbohydrate with monounsaturated fat, two factors besides the amount of fat need to be considered. The first is that a high-carbohydrate diet may have different effects in different subjects. Recently it has been shown that, compared to a diet containing 40% carbohydrate (29% monounsaturated fat), a 60% carbohydrate diet (13% monounsat-urated fat) significantly increased postprandial glucose and insulin in subjects treated with glibenclamide, but had no significant effect in subjects with mild diabetes treated by diet alone (71).

The other factor that may alter the response to monounsaturated fat is the type of carbohydrate it replaces. Replacing high glycemic index–carbohydrate foods with low glycemic index foods has effects on blood glucose and lipids similar to those of exchanging carbohydrate with monounsaturated fat, ie., reduced postprandial glucose and insu-lin, and reduced serum cholesterol and triglycerides. The diets in the studies from Garg et al. (32) are typical North American diets contain-ing high glycemic index carbohydrate. Replacement of low glycemic index carbohydrate with monounsaturated fat may not benefit blood glucose and lipids, or may even be deleterious; there are no long-term studies examining this issue. However in the acute situation it is known that both source and amount of carbohydrate influence post-prandial blood glucose and insulin responses. Thus the reduction in postprandial glucose response on high-monounsaturated-fat diets may simply be due to the reduction in carbohydrate intake.

We recently studied the effect of isocaloric exchange of fat and carbohydrate on acute blood glucose and insulin in subjects with NIDDM (72). Isocaloric test meals were designed containing 30, 50, or 70 g carbohydrate from a high glycemic index food (bread) or a low

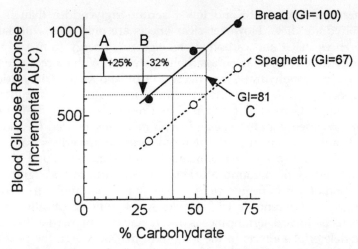

Figure 4. Theoretical effects of altering the source and amount of carbohydrate on postprandial glycemic responses in NIDDM. Data from (72). Points represent mean incremental areas under the curve (AUC) of 7 subjects with NIDDM who consumed isocaloric test meals of bread or spaghetti containing 29, 49, or 69% of energy from carbohydrate. Lines through points represent regression lines. See text for explanation.

glycemic index food (spaghetti), to which margarine and cheese were added to vary the fat content while holding protein constant. For both bread and spaghetti test meals, the ratio %carbohydrate:%fat varied from 29:55 to 69:16. For both bread and spaghetti test meals, blood glucose and insulin response areas increased as the amount of carbohydrate increased. According to regression lines drawn to fit the glucose response data (figure 4), increasing carbohydrate intake from bread from 40% to 55% increases postprandial glucose by 25% (A on figure 4), similar to the increase in postprandial glucose seen by Garg et al. (32) when carbohydrate intake was increased from 40% to 55%. However consumption of spagetti instead of bread at 55% carbohydrate reduces postprandial glucose by 32% (B on figure 4). An increase in carbohydrate intake from 40% to 55% energy can, theoretically, be accomplished with no change in postprandial glucose response by reducing glycemic index from 100 (e.g., white bread) to 81 (e.g., white rice; C on figure 4).

Monounsaturated Fat and Blood Lipids

One of the major reasons why high-monounsaturated-fat diets have been promoted in the treatment of diabetes is that they may result in higher HDL cholesterol and lower serum triglycerides than high-carbohydrate diets. However clear effects are only seen with large differences in fat and carbohydrate, e.g., 50% energy from fat, 35% carbohydrate vs 25% fat, 60% carbohydrate (31). With more moderate changes in carbohydrate, the effects on HDL and serum triglycerides are generally quite small and sometimes not statistically significant. For example Garg et al. (32) found that reducing carbohydrate from 55 to 40% energy and replacing it with monounsaturated fat had no significant effect on HDL, and reduced serum triglycerides from 2.19 to 1.75 mmol/l (p < 0.001). Similarly Parillo et al. (73) found no significant effect of monounsaturated fat on HDL, but a significant reduction of serum triglycerides from 1.37 to 1.16 mmol/l (p < 0.01). Though the difference in triglycerides was highly statistically significant, its biological significance is questionable. A higher-fat diet may have deleterious effects in the long-term that outweigh the possible benefit of the difference in triglycerides. For example low-income Mexicans in Mexico City have a higher-carbohydrate diet, 65% energy, than low-income Mexican-Americans living in San Antonio, Texas, 49% energy (74). Although the San Antonio residents have lower mean serum triglycerides, they are more obese, have higher serum cholesterol, and have a 36% higher prevalence of diabetes than the Mexico City residents (74) (figure 5).

Practicality of Dietary Advice for Diabetes.

Traditional dietary guidelines for diabetes focus on controlling the amounts of nutrients ingested. Current ADA guidelines are specific in this respect in stating that the amount of carbohydrate is of greater priority than the source. However it is difficult for individuals with diabetes to make long-term changes in their diet, and there is evidence that dietary advice based on amounts of nutrients influences neither the nature of the diet consumed nor the clinical outcome. When 70 subjects with NIDDM were randomized to receive a weight-reducing diet, a modified-fat diet, or a high-carbohydrate diet and followed for 18 months, there were virtually no differences between dietary prescriptions with respect to nutrient intakes, body weight, or blood glucose or lipid control (75). By contrast there is some evidence that dietary advice based on the glycemic index, i.e., advice focused on the source of carbohydrate foods, results in higher carbohydrate and fibre intakes, reduced blood lipids, and improved glucose control in individuals with newly diagnosed diabetes,

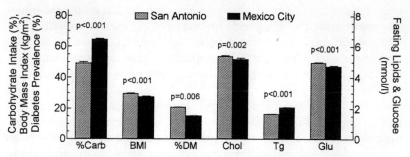

Figure 5. Carbohydrate intake as percentage of energy, body mass index (BMI), age- and sex-adjusted prevalence of diabetes (%DM), fasting serum cholesterol (Chol) and triglycerides (Tg), and fasting plasma glucose (Glu) in 1138 35- to 64-year-old, low-income Mexican-Americans living in San Antonio, Texas, and 646 similarly aged, low-income Mexicans living in Mexico City (74).

compared to standard dietary advice based on amount of carbohydrate (76). In subjects who received low glycemic index advice, there was a significant fall in serum triglycerides despite a higher carbohydrate intake. This study was only three months long, and longer-term studies are required to confirm its results. Nevertheless the results are in direct contrast to the current ADA position that the first priority with respect to carbohydrate is amount rather than source. Focusing the dietary prescription for diabetes on the amount of carbohydrate and other nutrients, for example by teaching carbohydrate exchanges, may not be the best approach to achieving recommended nutrient intakes and improving therapeutic outcome. Perhaps other approaches may be more successful, and more research is needed on how best to implement nutritional recommendations.

Conclusions

The past decade has seen major advances in the understanding of the pathogenesis of diabetes and its complications. New dietary guidelines for diabetes stress greater individualization of the dietary prescription to enhance compliance and improve clinical outcome. A major emphasis of nutrition research in diabetes has been the role of monounsaturated fat as a way of avoiding the tendency of high-carbohydrate diets to raise postprandial glucose and insulin, raise fasting triglycerides, and lower HDL cholesterol. However the benefits of moderate changes in monounsaturated fat intake on serum triglycerides are not great, there is no proven benefit on overall blood glucose control, and the effects on body weight are not known. Large increases in monounsaturated fat intake, such that the total fat content of the diet is over 30%, have greater effects on serum triglycerides and HDL, but would not be consistent with dietary guidelines for the general public (77), nor with dietary guidelines to prevent cancer (78) and heart disease (79). It should not be forgotten that modifying the source of carbohydrate, for example by using low glycemic index foods, can have the same beneficial effects as monounsaturated fat on postprandial glucose, insulin, and serum triglycerides, with none of the potential problems of increased fat intake. Therefore the use of soluble fibre and low glycemic index foods should continue to be an option in the dietary management of diabetes. More research is needed to improve the strategy used to implement dietary guidelines in clinical practice.

REFERENCES

1 Tan MH, Wornell CM. Diabetes mellitus in Canada. *Diabetes Res Clin Pract* 1991;14(suppl 2):s3–s8.
2 Huse DM, Oster G, Killen AR, Lacey MJ, Colditz GA. The economic costs of non-insulin-dependent diabetes mellitus. *JAMA* 1989;262:2708–2713.
3 Harris MI. Summary. In: *Diabetes in America*, 2nd ed. National Institutes of Health, National Institute of Diabetes and Digestive and Kidney Diseases. NIH publication no 95-1468, 1995:1–13.
4 Kenny SJ, Aubert RE, Geiss LS. Prevalence and incidence of non-insulin-dependent diabetes. In: *Diabetes in America*, 2nd ed. National Institutes of Health, National Institute of Diabetes and Digestive and Kidney Diseases. NIH publication no 95-1468, 1995:47–67.
5 Klein R, Klein BEK. Vision disorders in diabetes. In: *Diabetes in America*, 2nd ed. National Institutes of Health, National Institute of Diabetes and Digestive and Kidney Diseases. NIH publication no 95-1468, 1995:293–338.
6 Nelson RG, Knowler WC, Pettit DJ, Bennett PH. Kidney diseases in diabetes. In: *Diabetes in America*, 2nd ed. National Institutes of Health, National Institute of Diabetes and Digestive and Kidney Diseases. NIH publication no 95-1468, 1995:349–400.
7 Palumbo PJ, Melton LJ. Peripheral vascular disease and diabetes. In: *Diabetes in America*, 2nd ed. National Institutes of Health, National Institute

of Diabetes and Digestive and Kidney Diseases. NIH publication no 95-1468, 1995:401–428.

8 Wingard DL, Barrett-Connor E. Heart disease and diabetes. In: *Diabetes in America*, 2nd ed. National Institutes of Health, National Institute of Diabetes and Digestive and Kidney Diseases. NIH publication no 95-1468, 1995:429–448.

9 Javitt JC, Chiang YP. Economic impact of diabetes. In: *Diabetes in America*, 2nd ed. National Institutes of Health, National Institute of Diabetes and Digestive and Kidney Diseases. NIH publication no 95-1468, 1995:601–611.

10 American Diabetes Association Position Statement. Office guide to diagnosis and classification of diabetes mellitus and other categories of glucose intolerance. *Diabetes Care* 1996;19(suppl 1):s4.

11 DeFronzo RA. Lilly Lecture 1987: the triumvirate: -cell, muscle, liver: a collusion responsible for NIDDM. *Diabetes* 1988;37:667–687.

12 DeFronzo RA, Ferrannini E. Insulin resistance: a multifaceted syndrome response for NIDDM, obesity, hypertension, dyslipidemia and atherosclerotic cardiovascular disease. *Diabetes Care* 1991;14:173–194.

13 Porte D, Jr. Banting Lecture 1990: – cells in type II diabetes mellitus. *Diabetes* 1991;40:166–180.

14 Manson JE, Rimm EB, Stampfer MJ, Colditz GA, Willett WC, Krolewski AS, Rosner B, Hennekens CH, Speizer FE. Physical activity and incidence of non-insulin-dependent diabetes mellitus in women. *Lancet* 1991;338:774–778.

15 Howard BV, Abbott WGH, Swinburn BA. Evaluation of metabolic effects of substitution of complex carbohydrates for saturated fat in individuals with obesity and NIDDM. *Diabetes Care* 1991;14:786–795.

16 Després JP, Nadeau A, Tremblay A, Ferland M, Moorjani S, Lupien PJ, Thériault G, Pinault S, Bouchard C. Role of deep abdominal fat in the association between regional adipose tissue distribution and glucose tolerance in obese women. *Diabetes* 1989;38:304–309.

17 Pouliot MC, Després JP, Nadeau A, Moorjani S, Prud'Homme D, Lupien PJ, Tremblay A, Bouchard C. Visceral obesity in men: associations with glucose tolerance, plasma insulin, and lipoprotein levels. *Diabetes* 1992;41:826–834.

18 Del Prato S, Leonetti F, Simonson DC, Sheehan P, Matsuda M, DeFronzo RA. Effect of sustained physiologic hyperinsulinaemia and hyperglycaemia on insulin secretion and insulin sensitivity in man. *Diabetologia* 1994;37:1025–1035.

19 Rossetti L, Gaiccari A, DeFronzo RA. Glucose toxicity. *Diabetes Care* 1990;13:610–630.

20 The Diabetes Control and Complications Trial Research Group. The effect of intensive treatment of diabetes on the development and progression of long-term complications in insulin-dependent diabetes mellitus. *New Eng J Med* 1993;329:977–986.

21 Lasker RD. The diabetes control and complications trial: implications for policy and practice. *New Eng J Med* 1993;329:1035–1036.

22 Brownlee M. Glycation products and the pathogenesis of diabetic complications. *Diabetes Care* 1992;15:1835–1843.

23 American Diabetes Association Position Statement. Nutrition recommendations and principles for individuals with diabetes mellitus: 1986. *Diabetes Care* 1987;10:126–132.

24 The Nutrition Sub-Committee of the British Diabetic Association's Medical Advisory Committee. Dietary recommendations for diabetics for the 1980s – a policy statement by the British Diabetic Association. *Hum Nutr App Nutr* 1982;36A:378–394.

25 Canadian Diabetes Association Position Statement. Guidelines for the nutritional management of diabetes mellitus in the 1990s. *Beta Release* 1989;13(3):8–17.

26 Wolever TMS, Jenkins DJA, Jenkins AL, Josse RG. The glycemic index: methodology and clinical implications. *Am J Clin Nutr* 1991;54:846–854.

27 Jenkins DJA, Wolever TMS, Taylor RH, Barker HM, Fielden H, Baldwin JM, Bowling AC, Newman HC, Jenkins AL, Goff DV. Glycemic index of foods: a physiological basis for carbohydrate exchange. *Am J Clin Nutr* 1981;34:362–366.

28 National Institutes of Health. Consensus Development Conference on diet and exercise in non-insulin-dependent diabetes mellitus. *Diabetes Care* 1987;10:639–644.

29 Reaven GM. Dietary therapy for non-insulin-dependent diabetes mellitus. *New Eng J Med* 1988;319:862–864.

30 Garg A, Bonanome A, Grundy SM, Zhang ZJ, Unger RH. Comparison of a high-carbohydrate diet with a high-monounsaturated-fat diet in patients with non-insulin-dependent diabetes mellitus. *New Eng J Med* 1988;319:829–834.

31 Garg A, Grundy SM, Unger RH. Comparison of effects of high and low carbohydrate diets on plasma lipoproteins and insulin sensitivity in patients with mild NIDDM. *Diabetes* 1992;41:1278–1285.

32 Garg A, Bantle JP, Henry RR, Coulston AM, Griver KA, Raatz SK, Brinkley L, Chen YDI, Grundy SM, Huet BA, Reaven GM. Effects of varying carbohydrate content of diet in patients with non-insulin-dependent diabetes mellitus. *JAMA* 1994;271:1421–1428.

33 American Diabetes Association. Nutritional recommendations and principles for people with diabetes mellitus. *Diabetes Care* 1994;17:519–522.

34 Diabetes and Nutrition Study Group (DNSG) of the European Associa-
    tion for the Study of Diabetes (EASD), 1995. Recommendations for the
    nutritional management of patients with diabetes mellitus. *Diabetes
    Nutr Metab* 1995;8:186–189.
35 Franz MJ, Horton ES, Sr, Bantle JP, Beebe CA, Brunzell JD, Coulston
    AM, Henry RR, Hoogwerf BJ, Stacpoole PW. Technical review: nutri-
    tion principles for the management of diabetes and related complica-
    tions. *Diabetes Care* 1994;17:490–518.
36 Nuttall FQ, Mooradian AD, DeMarais R, Parker S. The glycemic effect
    of different meals approximately isocaloric and similar in protein, car-
    bohydrate and fat content as calculated using the ADA exchange lists.
    Diabetes Care 1983;6:432–435.
37 Laine DC, Thomas W, Levitt MD, Bantle JP. Comparison of predictive
    capabilities of diabetic exchange lists and glycemic index of foods.
    Diabetes Care 1987;10:387–394.
38 Hollenbeck CB, Coulston AM, Reaven GM. Comparison of plasma glu-
    cose and insulin responses to mixed meals of high-, intermediate-, and
    low-glycemic potential. *Diabetes Care* 1988;11:323–329.
39 Collier GR, Wolever TMS, Wong GS, Josse RG. Prediction of glycemic
    response to mixed meals in non-insulin-dependent diabetic subjects.
    Am J Clin Nutr 1986;44:349–352.
40 Chew I, Brand JC, Thorburn AW, Truswell AS. Application of the glyce-
    mic index to mixed meals. *Am J Clin Nutr* 1988;47:53–56.
41 Indar-Brown K, Norenberg C, Madar Z. Glycemic and insulinemic
    responses after ingestion of ethnic foods by NIDDM and healthy sub-
    jects. *Am J Clin Nutr* 1992;55:89–95.
42 Collier GR, Giudici S, Kalmusky J, Wolever TMS, Helman G, Wesson V,
    Ehrlich RM, Jenkins DJA. Low glycaemic index starchy foods improve
    glucose control and lower serum cholesterol in diabetic children. *Diabe-
    tes Nutr Metab* 1988;1:11–19.
43 Fontvielle AM, Acosta M, Rizkalla SW, Bornet F, David P, Letanoux M,
    Tchobroutsky G, Slama G. A moderate switch from high to low glycaemic-
    index foods for 3 weeks improves the metabolic control of type I (IDDM)
    diabetic subjects. *Diabetes Nutr Metab* 1988;1:139–143.
44 Brand JC, Colagiuri S, Crossman S, Allen A, Roberts DCF, Truswell
    AS. Low glycemic index foods improve long term glycemic control
    in non-insulin-dependent diabetes mellitus. *Diabetes Care* 1990;14:95–
    101.
45 Calle-Pascual AL, Gomez V, Leon E, Bordiu E. Foods with a low glyce-
    mic index do not improve glycemic control of both type 1 and type 2
    diabetic patients after one month of therapy. *Diabete Metab* (Paris)
    1988;14:629–633.

46 Jenkins DJA, Wolever TMS, Buckley G, Lam KY, Giudici S, Kalmusky J, Jenkins AL, Patten RL, Bird J, Wong GS, Josse RG. Low glycemic index starchy foods in the diabetic diet. *Am J Clin Nutr* 1988;48:248–254.

47 Fontvielle AM, Rizkalla SW, Penfornis A, Acosta FRJ, Slama G. The use of low glycaemic index foods improves metabolic control of diabetic patients over five weeks. *Diabetic Med* 1992;9:444–450.

48 Wolever TMS, Jenkins DJA, Vuksan V, Jenkins AL, Buckley GC, Wong GS, Josse RG. Beneficial effect of a low-glycaemic index diet in type 2 diabetes. *Diabetic Med* 1992;9:451–458.

49 Wolever TMS, Jenkins DJA, Vuksan V, Jenkins AL, Wong GS, Josse RG. Beneficial effect of low-glycemic index diet in overweight NIDDM subjects. *Diabetes Care* 1992;15:562–566.

50 Wolever TMS. Glycaemic index revisited. In: Marshall SM, Home PD, Alberti KGMM, Krall LP, eds. *The diabetes annual/7.* Amsterdam: Elsevier Science Publishers BV, 1993:258–272.

51 Dunn PJ, Cole RA, Soeldner JS, Gleason RE, Kwa E, Firoozabadi H, Younger D, Graham CA. Temporal relationship of glycosylated haemoglobin concentrations to glucose control in diabetics. *Diabetologia* 1979;17:213–220.

52 Jones IR, Owens DR, Williams S, Ryder REJ, Birtwell AJ, Jones MK, Gicheru K, Hayes TM. Glycosylated serum albumin: an intermediate index of diabetic control. *Diabetes Care* 1983;6:501–503.

53 Jenkins DJA, Wolever TMS, Kalmusky J, Guidici S, Giordano C, Patten R, Wong GS, Bird JN, Hall M, Buckley G, Csima A, Little JA. Low-glycemic index diet in hyperlipidemia: use of traditional starchy foods. *Am J Clin Nutr* 1987;46:66–71.

54 Jenkins DJA, Wolever TMS, Collier GR, Ocana A, Rao AV, Buckley G, Lam KY, Meyer A, Thompson LU. The metabolic effects of a low glycemic index diet. *Am J Clin Nutr* 1987;46:968–975.

55 Brand Miller JC, Colagiuri S. The carnivore connection: dietary carbohydrate in the evolution of non-insulin-dependent diabetes. *Diabetologia* 1994;37:1280–1286.

56 Byrnes SE, Brand Miller JC, Denyer GS. Amylopectin starch promotes the development of insulin resistance in rats. *J Nutr* 1995;125:1430–1437.

57 Chiasson J-L, Josse RG, Leiter LA, Mihic M, Nathan DM, Palmason C, Cohen RM, Wolever TMS. The effect of acarbose on insulin sensitivity in subjects with impaired glucose tolerance. *Diabetes Care* 1996;19:1190–1193.

58 Chung JW, Suh KI, Joyce M, Ditzler T, Henry RR. Contribution of obesity to defects of intracellular glucose metabolism in NIDDM. *Diabetes Care* 1995;18:666–673.

59 Chan JM, Rimm EB, Colditz GA, Stampfer MJ, Willett WC. Obesity, fat distribution, and weight gain as risk factors for clinical diabetes in men. *Diabetes Care* 1994;17:961–969.

60 Shah M, McGovern P, French S, Baxter J. Comparison of a low-fat, ad libitum complex-carbohydrate diet with a low-energy diet in moderately obese women. *Am J Clin Nutr* 1994;59:980–984.

61 Pascale RW, Wing RR, Butler BA, Mullen M, Bononi P. Effects of a behavioural weight loss program stressing calorie restriction versus calorie plus fat restriction in obese individuals with NIDDM or a family history of diabetes. *Diabetes Care* 1995;18:1241–1248.

62 Sheppard L, Kristal AR, Kushi LH. Weight-loss in women participating in a randomized trial of low fat diets. *Am J Clin Nutr* 1991;54:821–828.

63 Romieu I, Willett WC, Stampfer MJ, Colditz GA, Sampson L, Rosner B, Hennekens CH, Speizer FE. Energy intake and other determinants of relative weight. *Am J Clin Nutr* 1988;47:406–412.

64 Hill JO, Prentice AM. Sugar and body weight regulation. *Am J Clin Nutr* 1995;62(suppl):264S–274S.

65 Lissner L, Levitsky DA, Strupp BJ, Kalkwarf HJ, Roe DA. Dietary fat and the regulation of energy intake in human subjects. *Am J Clin Nutr* 1987;46:886–892.

66 Flatt JP. McCollum Award Lecture, 1995: Diet, lifestyle, and weight maintenance. *Am J Clin Nutr* 1995;62:820–836.

67 Jones PJH, Schoeller DA. Polyunsaturated:saturated ratio of diet fat influences energy substrate utilization in the human. *Metabolism* 1988;37:145–151.

68 Ackman RG, Cunnane SC. Long-chain polyunsaturated fatty acids: sources, biochemistry and nutritional/clinical applications. In: Padley FB, ed. *Advances in applied lipid research*, vol 1. London: JAI Press, 1992:161–215.

69 Lehmann T, Golay A, James RW, Pometta D. Effects of two hypocaloric diets, fat restricted or rich in monounsaturated fat, on body weight loss and plasma lipoprotein distribution. *Nutr Metab Cardiovasc Dis* 1995;5:290–296.

70 Low CC, Grossman EB, Gumbiner B. Potentiation of effects of weight loss by monounsaturated fatty acids in obese NIDDM patients. *Diabetes* 1996;45:569–575.

71 Parillo A, Giacco R, Ciardullo AV, Rivellese AA, Riccardi G. Does a high-carbohydrate diet have different effects in NIDDM patients treated with diet alone or hypoglycemic drugs? *Diabetes Care* 1996;19:498–500.

72 Wolever TMS, Jenkins DJA, Vuksan V, Katzman L, Jenkins AL, Josse RG. Variation in meal fat does not affect the relative blood glucose

response of spaghetti in subjects with type 2 diabetes. *Diabetes Nutr Metab* 1992;5:191–197.

73 Parillo M, Rivellese AA, Ciardullo AV, Capaldo B, Giacco A, Genovese S, Riccardi G. A high-monounsaturated-fat/low-carbohydrate diet improves peripheral insulin sensitivity in non-insulin-dependent diabetic patients. *Metabolism* 1992;41:1373–1378.

74 Stern MP, Gonzalez C, Mitchell BD, Villalpando E, Haffner SM, Hazuda HP. Genetic and environmental determinants of type II diabetes in Mexico City and San Antonio. *Diabetes* 1992;41:484–492.

75 Milne RM, Mann JI, Chisholm AW, Williams SM. Long-term comparison of three dietary prescriptions in the treatment of NIDDM. *Diabetes Care* 1994;17:74–80.

76 Frost G, Wilding J, Beecham J. Dietary advice based on the glycaemic index improves dietary profile and metabolic control in type 2 diabetic patients. *Diabetic Med* 1994;11:397–401.

77 US Department of Agriculture and US Department of Health and Human Services. *Nutrition and your health: dietary guidelines for Americans*, 3rd ed., USDA, 1990.

78 Butrum RR, Clifford CK, Lanza E. NCI dietary guidelines: rationale. *Am J Clin Nutr* 1988;48:888–895.

79 Expert Panel on Detection, Evaluation, and Treatment of High Blood Cholesterol in Adults. Summary of the second report of the National Cholesterol Education Program (NCEP) Expert Panel on detection, evaluation, and treatment of high blood cholesterol in adults (adult treatment panel 2). *JAMA* 1993;269:3015–3023.

Diet and Health Maintenance

JONATHAN D. ADACHI, ALEXANDRA
PAPAIOANNOU, and GEORGE IOANNIDIS

Diet in Relation to Osteoporosis

Diet and nutritional supplements, specifically the administration of calcium and vitamin D, can play a crucial role in preventing osteoporosis by developing and sustaining bone mass throughout an individual's life. However proper nutrition may not prevent osteoporosis in many individuals. To understand the relationship between diet and osteoporosis, it is first necessary to review our understanding of osteoporosis.

Osteoporosis

Osteoporosis is defined as a systemic skeletal disorder characterized by a decrease in bone mass and microarchitectural deterioration of bone tissue, with a resultant increase in bone fragility and susceptibility to fracture (1). It is a major cause of morbidity and mortality in society today, significantly affecting an estimated 1.8 million women in Canada in 1993 (2). Osteoporosis frequently results in fractures of the spine, hip, and wrist. The estimated numbers of osteoporosis–related fractures in Canada in 1993 were as follows: 6,628 vertebral fractures in males and 20,446 in females; 4,033 wrist fractures in males and 23,657 in females; 5,236 hip fractures in males and 16,066 in females (2). Hip fractures are a major cause of disability and death. For Canadians over the age of 75 years, 345 males and 594 females died because of hip fractures (2). Hip fractures also account for the bulk of medical costs relating to osteoporotic fractures (2). In Canada it is estimated that $333 million was spent on the treatment of hip fractures (2). The total cost of osteoporosis in

Canada, including long-term care, may have been as high as $1.3 billion in 1993 (2). The indirect costs of hip fracture have not been accurately measured, yet should include lost productivity due to morbidity, mortality, institutionalization of a dependent spouse, and negative social impact. The negative social impact of fractures should include pain and suffering, decreased functional ability and quality of life, and loss of independence (3).

PATHOPHYSIOLOGY

Bone is composed of metabolically active cells, with bone turnover occurring at discrete sites in the skeleton known as bone remodeling units. The osteoclast is the cell responsible for bone resorption and the osteoblast for bone formation (4). Under normal circumstances there is a coupled equilibrium of bone formation and bone resorption with an initiating signal sent to activate bone resorption. A resorption pit is created and subsequently filled in by the osteoblast laying down new bone. When bone formation is equivalent to bone resorption, bone mass is maintained, however when resorption exceeds formation, osteoporosis results (4).

CLINICAL PRESENTATION

Osteoporosis is a silent thief, stealing bone until there is an increase in fracture susceptibility. Fractures typically involve the hip, wrist, proximal humerus, ribs, and vertebrae (5). Rib fractures may occur after coughing or from a simple hug from a loved one. Fractures of the hip and wrist typically occur after a fall. Hip fractures have a 20% mortality within the first three months following fracture (6). Vertebral fractures may be asymptomatic, however this is the exception rather than the rule. On the other hand patients with osteoporosis do not have back pain due to osteoporosis unless they begin to fracture. Vertebral fractures typically occur in clusters and the presence of a fracture in any vertebra is a significant risk factor for further fractures. When multiple vertebral fractures occur patients may become quite kyphotic, and are typically described as having a dowager's hump. In rare instances after multiple vertebral fractures the rib cage may sit upon the iliac crest. Abdominal bloating, early satiety, and symptoms of reflux then come into play. Respiratory failure may be precipitated in those with underlying lung disease. Acute back pain is often replaced by more chronic pain, usually because of increasing pressure being placed on the posterior elements of the spine.

Bone mass is the major determinant of osteoporotic fractures. Bone mass increases during childhood and adolescence, peaks in the second to third decade, and declines thereafter at a rate of 0.5 to 1% per year until the menopause, when accelerated rates of bone loss occur. During the first five years after the menopause it is not uncommon to see rates of loss averaging 3–5% per year. Lifetime losses may reach as high as 30–40% in women and 20–30% in men (5).

Those characteristics said to present greatest risk for osteoporosis are as follows (7,8):

a) postmenopause and estrogen deficiency states including:
   i) premature menopause either as a result of a natural menopause or oophorectomy
   ii) anorexia nervosa
   iii)hyperprolactinemia
   iv)excessive exercise
b) thin, small stature
c) positive family history
d)cigarette smoking
e) alcohol abuse
f) sedentary lifestyle
g)poor dietary calcium intake
h)white or Asian race
i) drug use including
   i) anticonvulsants
   ii) corticosteroids

Falls are a major risk factor for fractures, therefore anything that precipitates falls increases fracture risk (5). Neurologic diseases such as Parkinson's disease, poor vision, and drugs such as long half–life sedative medication are examples.

Nutrition and Osteoporosis

CALCIUM

Adequate dietary calcium intake is required for the development and maintenance of a normal skeleton. Matkovic et al. (9) initiated interest in the idea that lifelong dietary calcium intake may be important in attaining higher peak bone mass and reduced hip fracture rates.

For example in a randomized, control trial Johnston et al. (10) examined the effects of supplemental calcium in young healthy twins. They found that calcium supplementation increased bone mass in prepubertal children with adequate dietary calcium intake, when compared to their placebo-treated twins. They suggested that if this increase were maintained and translated into an increased peak bone mass, fracture rates could be reduced in later life. In a 4 year, prospective, non-intervention study in women between the ages of 20 and 30 years, Recker et al. (11) found that lumbar spine bone mineral density (BMD) was positively correlated with an individual's calcium/protein intake ratio. In addition a 16.4% increase in lumbar spine BMD was found in women with the highest calcium intake (2,106 mg/d) compared to a 1.5% decrease in women with the lowest calcium intake (220 mg/d). The investigators concluded that modest increases in calcium intake in women aged in the third decade may significantly reduce the fracture risk later in life (11). In perimenopausal women calcium supplementation is probably of benefit, but the effects of calcium are outweighed by the effects of estrogen deficiency (12). In postmenopausal women calcium supplementation decreases rates of bone loss and may be particularly important in those whose dietary calcium intake is poor (13,14). Chapuy et al. (15) in a randomized trial of 1,200 mg calcium per day and 800 IU vitamin D_3 per day, versus double placebo, were able to demonstrate increases in hip bone density and reductions in hip and non–vertebral fracture rates in the elderly, whose average age was 84 years. These studies demonstrate the importance of calcium throughout life and of vitamin D in maintaining bone health.

Calcium is a "threshold" nutrient, so that intake below the required threshold will not promote or maintain optimal bone mineralization, while intake significantly exceeding the threshold will not lead to increased skeletal benefit (16). Therefore it is important to maintain a daily intake of calcium that does not fall below the threshold specified by age and sex, which increases risk of osteoporosis occurrence. The risks of high intakes of dietary calcium are few (17). The previous belief that high intake of dietary calcium increases the risk of kidney stones has been reversed recently (17). Table 1 shows the recommended calcium intake published by the Osteoporosis Society's 1993 consensus conference.

The best sources of calcium are food sources such as milk and dairy products, so that bone tissue receives balanced nutrition. Pharmaceutical supplements can provide roughly the equivalent calcium of milk and can be similarly absorbed when taken with food in divided doses (17).

VITAMIN D

Given that vitamin D metabolites maintain calcium absorption, vitamin D deficiency is another factor contributing to human bone disease (18). Dietary vitamin D sources include fish oils, liver, and milk. As well vitamin D can be obtained from exposure to sunlight, which stimulates its production in the skin (17). Thus vitamin D deficiency tends to occur in the housebound elderly, especially during the winter months (19). The Osteoporosis Society of Canada proposes that the recommended daily intake of vitamin D, 200 IU for adults, should probably be increased to 400 to 800 IU in order to prevent fractures more reliably.

Controversy exists over the use of calcitriol, an active metabolite, in the treatment of osteoporosis. In separate, well-designed, randomized, controlled trials using bone density as the primary outcome measure, Gallagher and Goldgar (20) demonstrated benefit, while Ott and Chestnut (21) concluded that it was not effective in postmenopausal osteoporosis. In a recent study, though, Tilyard et al. (22) found that calcitriol, 0.25 mg twice a day, reduced both vertebral and non–vertebral fracture rates when compared to those supplemented with 1,000 mg per day of calcium. Hypercalcemia and hypercalciuria are potential complications that need to be monitored (20,21). As outlined earlier, Chapuy et al. (15) found that a combination of 800 IU per day vitamin D_3 and 1,200 mg per day calcium reduced hip and non–vertebral fracture rates.

OTHER FACTORS

Although calcium and vitamin D are the primary nutritional factors affecting bone density and osteoporosis, other factors have been studied for their respective effects on osteoporosis. Many of these factors remain controversial and continue to be reviewed for their harmful or preventative effects. Increased urinary calcium excretion has been attributed to high intake of animal proteins, which contain phosphates as well as sodium (23). However a recent study suggests that increased protein in the diets of the malnourished elderly leads to improved bone mass, since protein intake is associated with a growth hormone (IGF-I) that exerts anabolic effects on bone even in adulthood (24). This positive connection between increasing protein intake and bone mass should be considered in light of the fact that a decline in calcium intake is associated with a decline in protein energy intake in the first place. Thus diets that contain no animal products are potentially harmful to bone health if they offer little calcium to be absorbed. Bonjour et al. (24) suggest that vitamin K deficiency may contribute to bone fragility; they propose that vitamin K may influence bone metabolism and reduce urinary excretion of calcium, although further investigation is required.

The effects of acute and lifelong caffeine consumption on BMD has also been examined. Harris and Dawson-Hughes (25) found that daily consumption of caffeine in amounts equal to or greater than two or three servings of brewed coffee may accelerate lumbar spine and total body bone loss in postmenopausal women. In addition in a retrospective study of lifelong caffeine use in postmenopausal women, Barrett-Connor et al. (26) found an association between increasing lifetime caffeine intake and decreasing BMD at both the hip and spine, independent of several other factors. In contrast other studies have not shown an association between caffeine and BMD (27,28).

A women's weight may also influence fracture rates and osteoporosis. Cummings et al. (29) conducted a study that assessed potential risk factors in postmenopausal women. They showed that the more weight a women had gained since the age of 25 the lower her risk of hip fracture. Furthermore women who weighed less than they had at 25 had a double risk of hip fracture. However the high correlation between weight change and current weight to the risk of hip fracture did not permit the investigators to determine which of these factors affected the risk of hip fracture to a greater extent.

Another controversial area is the effect of exercise on osteoporosis prevention. Although it has been shown that bedridden individuals lose bone mass, the specific effect of exercise on bone density remains unclear. A stronger relationship exists between exercise, a high-calcium diet, and increased bone density (30). Whether or not exercise has an affect on BMD may depend on several factors, such as the type of exercise performed (endurance vs strength training) and a woman's level of fitness before she starts an exercise program. Nonetheless all healthy women should be encouraged to exercise because it has been shown that women who maintain higher levels of physical activity have a lower incidence of hip fractures (31). This may be indirectly due to improved strength, coordination, and flexibility, which may decrease the likelihood of falling (31,32).

Table 1
Recommendations by the Osteoporosis Society of Canada

Age (years)	Recommended Calcium Intake (mg/day) (17)
7–9	700
10–12 (boys)	900
10–12 (girls)	1200–1400*
13–16	1200–1400
17–18	1200
19–49	1000
50+	1000–1500**

 * Girls go through their adolescent growth spurt 2 years earlier than boys on average.
** A minimum of 1000 mg is recommended, but higher intakes may be advisable if the risk of osteoporosis is high.

RECOMMENDATIONS BY THE OSTEOPOROSIS SOCIETY OF CANADA (17)

The following recommendations outline nutritional guidelines for preventing osteoporosis and resulting fractures:

1 To ensure optimal bone health, Canadians should consume adequate amounts of calcium throughout life. Recent evidence suggests that current recommended intakes of calcium are too low; intakes recommended by the Osteoporosis Society's consensus panel are listed in table 1. These intakes should reduce bone loss and protect against osteoporotic fractures on the basis of currently available data.

2 Canadians should attempt to meet their calcium requirements principally through food sources. However if it is not possible to achieve an adequate intake of calcium from food alone, because of either intolerance to dairy foods or dietary preferences, the use of pharmaceutical calcium supplements should be considered either in addition to calcium-containing food sources or as a major source of calcium.

3 Strict vegetarians who do not consume milk products should take special care to ensure they are receiving adequate amounts of calcium, and if necessary they should seek professional advice from a qualified nutritionist. A pharmaceutical calcium supplement may not be required.

4 Further research is necessary before recommending the general use of calcium supplements by adolescents.

5 Calcium supplementation cannot substitute for hormone therapy in the prevention of postmenopausal bone loss and fractures. While it does have a preventive effect of its own, other preventive strategies such as hormone therapy in menopausal women and a physically active lifestyle are also of major, independent importance in prevention of osteoporotic fractures.

6 Adequate amounts of vitamin D are also necessary for optimal calcium absorption and bone health. While many Canadians obtain sufficient vitamin D through the effects of sunlight, adequate dietary sources of vitamin D are particularly important for seniors or for individuals who customarily use heavy sunscreen preparations. A dietary intake of 400 to 800 units per day is recommended for such individuals.

Conclusion

Many factors influence bone health and the occurrence of osteoporosis. Although individuals may be genetically predisposed to osteoporosis, environmental factors can also play a significant role (23). Diet is one factor that can be altered to provide sufficient calcium and vitamin D, thus maximizing bone density. This approach seems to be most effective prior to puberty and in attaining peak adult bone mass prior to menopause. Once osteoporosis has been detected, clinical treatments of calcium and vitamin D in combination with other treatments are more likely to improve or maintain bone health than diet alone.

REFERENCES

1 Consensus development conference: diagnosis, prophylaxis and treatment of osteoporosis. *Am J Med* 1991;90:107–10.
2 Goeree R, O'Brien B, Pettitt D, Cuddy L, Ferraz, Adachi J. An assessment of the burden of illness due to osteoporosis in Canada. *J Soc Obstet Gynaecol Can* 1996;(suppl July)18: 15–24.
3 Narod S, Spasoff RA. Economic and social burden of osteoporosis. In: Jaworski G, ed. *Current concepts in bone fragility.* New York: Springer Verlag, 1986:391–401.
4 Parfitt AM. Bone remodeling: relationship to the amount and structure of bone, and the pathogenesis and the prevention of fractures. In: Riggs BL, Melton LJ, III, eds. *Osteoporosis: etiology, diagnosis and management.* New York: Raven Press, 1988:45–93.

5 Riggs BL, Melton LJ, III. Involutional osteoporosis. *N Engl J Med* 1986;314:1676–1686.

6 Kleerekoper M, Avioli LV. Evaluation and treatment of postmenopausal osteoporosis. In: Favus MJ, ed. *Primer on the metabolic bone diseases and disorders of mineral metabolism.* Richmond:William Bird Press, 1990:151– 154.

7 Cumulative development conferences. Diagnosis, prophylaxis and treatment of osteoporosis. *Am J Med* 1993;94:646–650.

8 Ross PD. Osteoporosis frequency, consequences, and risk factors. *Arch Intern Med* 1996;156:1399–1411.

9 Matkovic V, Kostial K, Siminovic I, Buzina R, Brodarec A. Bone status and fracture rates in two regions of Yugoslavia. *Am J Clin Nutr* 1979;32:540–549.

10 Johnston CC, Jr, Miller JZ, Slemenda CW, Reister TK, Hui S, Christian JC, Peacock M. Calcium supplementation and increases in bone mineral density in children. *N Engl J Med* 1992;327:82–87.

11 Recker RR, Davies KM, Hinders SM, Heaney RP, Stegman MR, Kimmel DB. Bone gain in young adult women. *JAMA* 1992;268:2403–208.

12 Riis B, Thomsen K, Christiansen C. Does calcium supplementation prevent postmenopausal bone loss? *N Engl J Med* 1987;316:173–177.

13 Dawson–Hughes B, Dallal GE, Krall EA, Sadowski L, Sahyoun N, Tannenbaum S. A controlled trial of the effect of calcium supplementation on bone density in postmenopausal women. *N Engl J Med* 1990; 323:878–883.

14 Reid IR, Ames RW, Evans MC, Gamble GD, Sharpe SJ. Effect of calcium supplement on bone loss in postmenopausal women. *N Engl J Med* 1993;328:460–464.

15 Chapuy MC, Arlot ME, Dubœuf F et al. Vitamin D_3 and calcium to prevent hip fractures in elderly women. *N Engl J Med* 1992;327:1637–1642.

16 Matkovic V, Heaney RP. Calcium balance during human growth: evidence for threshold behavior. *Am J Clin Nutr* 1992;55:992–996.

17 Murray TM. Calcium nutrition and osteoporosis: report from the 1993 consensus conference of the Osteoporosis Society of Canada. *Can Med Assoc J* 1996;155:935–944.

18 Dawson-Hughes B, Harris SS, Krall EA et al. Rates of bone loss in postmenopausal women randomly assigned to one of two dosages of vitamin D. *Am J Clin Nutr* 1995;61:1140–1145.

19 Dawson-Hughes B, Dallal GE, Krall EA et al. Effect of vitamin D supplementation on wintertime and overall bone loss in healthy postmenopausal women. *Ann Intern Med* 1991;115:505–512.

20 Gallagher JC, Goldgar D. Treatment of postmenopausal osteoporosis with high doses of synthetic calcitriol. *Ann Intern Med* 1990;113:649–655.

21 Ott SM, Chestnut CH, III. Calcitriol treatment is not effective in post-
    menopausal osteoporosis. *Ann Intern Med* 1989;110:267–274.
22 Tilyard MW, Spears GFS, Thomson J, Dovey S. Treatment of postmeno-
    pausal osteoporosis with calcitriol or calcium. *N Engl J Med*
    1992;326:357–362.
23 National Institutes of Health. Optimal calcium intake. NIH Consensus
    Statement 1994;12:1–31.
24 Bonjour JP, Schurch MA, Rizzoli R. Nutritional aspects of hip fractures.
    Bone 1996;18:139s–144s.
25 Harris SS, Dawson-Hughes B. Caffeine and bone loss in healthy post-
    menopausal women. *Am J Clin Nutr* 1994;60:573–578.
26 Barrett-Connor E, Chang JC, Edelstein SL. Caffeine-associated
    osteoporosis offset by daily milk consumption. The Rancho Bernardo
    Study. *JAMA* 1994;271:280–83.
27 Eliel LP, Smith LC, Ivey J, Baylink DJ. Longitudinal changes in radial
    bone mass – dietary caffeine, milk and activity. *Calcif Tissue Int*
    1983;35(suppl):669.
28 Hansen MA, Overgaard K, Riis BJ, Christiansen C. Potential risk fac-
    tors for development of postmenopausal osteoporosis – examined over
    a 12-year period. *Osteoporos Int* 1991;1:95–102.
29 Cummings SR, Nevitt MC, Browner WS et al. Risk factors for hip frac-
    tures in white women. Study of osteoporotic fractures research group.
    N Engl J Med 1995;332:767–773.
30 Prince R, Devine A, Dick I et al. The effects of calcium supplementa-
    tion (milk powder or tablets) and exercise on bone density in post-
    menopausal women. *J Bone Miner Res* 1995;10:1068–1075.
31 American College of Sports Medicine position stand on osteoporosis
    and exercise. *Med Sci Sports Exerc* 1995;24:i-vii.
32 Krall EA, Dawson-Hughes B. Walking is related to bone density and
    rates of bone loss. *Am J Med* 1994;96:20–26.

HAROLD KALANT

Nutrition in Relation to Alcohol Use

A review of this subject nine years ago (1) dealt mainly with six topics: the question of alcohol and "empty calories," and the effects of alcohol on nutrient absorption from the intestine, vitamin storage, vitamin activation, nutrient utilization, and nutrient excretion. The progress of knowledge in this field during the past nine years is demonstrated rather strikingly by a comparison of that list with the topics covered in the present review, reflecting the major content of the recent literature:

- "empty calories" vs obesity in alcohol users
- effect of alcohol on vitamin metabolism, especially vitamin A and retinoids
- alcohol metabolism and oxidative stress in relation to organ damage and cancer
- alcohol, myocardial infarction, and the "French paradox"

These topics, which will be covered in some detail below, illustrate the degree to which the study of alcohol and nutrition has moved beyond simple description to mechanistic explanation of the basis of alcohol effects at cellular level.

The views expressed in this review are those of the author and do not necessarily reflect the policies of the Addiction Research Foundation.

"Empty Calories" and Body Weight

As pointed out in the earlier review (1), it is obvious that alcohol per se is a poor food in the sense that most alcoholic beverages are relatively poor in vitamins and other nutrients, so that the calories derived from oxidation of ethanol are as "empty" as those derived from purified sugar or fat. However the concept that calories derived from ethanol are empty in the sense that they can not be utilized metabolically is difficult to grasp. It has long been known that acetate derived from the oxidation of ethanol is indistinguishable metabolically from acetate derived from the metabolism of carbohydrates or lipids (2). Human infants receiving complete parenteral nutrition because of upper gastrointestinal obstruction were able to grow well when ethanol provided up to 16% of the total calories (3). Many earlier studies (e.g., 4,5) had shown that rats fed a liquid diet in which 35% of the calories were derived from ethanol grew almost as well as those receiving a control diet in which the ethanol had been replaced equicalorically with carbohydrate.

This was confirmed recently by Bondy and Pearson (6), but they added the important qualification that the ability of ethanol to sustain a normal growth rate depended on the nature of the rest of the diet. When the controls and the ethanol group both received liquid diets, identical except for the replacement of some carbohydrate by equicaloric ethanol, the groups grew at an identical rate. But when the ethanol group received 25% ethanol in the drinking water and both groups had unlimited access to rat chow, the controls grew rapidly whereas the ethanol group barely held constant weight. This outcome is not surprising because 25% ethanol is aversive to most rat strains, and if their total fluid intake is reduced as a result, their intake of dry food is also decreased. Appropriate controls would have been given the same volume of water as the volume of ethanol solution consumed by the ethanol group.

Unfortunately such experiments do not really mimic the dietary balance in humans who consume ethanol. Numerous studies (e.g., 7) have shown that most drinkers add ethanol to their normal diets, rather than substitute it for part of their diet. In that case their total caloric intake is increased by the ethanol consumption, and if it is metabolically utilized they should gain weight. In reality males showed no correlation between the amount of daily ethanol intake and the body mass index, and in women the body mass index actually fell as mean daily alcohol intake increased (7). In both males and females, however, when ethanol intake exceeded 50 g per day (i.e., four or more standard drinks a day) there was a trend towards increasing body mass index (7).

The pattern of alcohol intake also affects the result. For subjects consuming the same average daily amount of alcohol, those who spread it out by taking a small amount every day showed a reduction of body mass index, while those who drank on fewer days per week but drank a larger amount when they did drink showed increased body mass index (8). Various possible explanations come to mind. Regular light drinkers, for example, might have a different lifestyle than intermittent heavier drinkers, with lower fat intake, more regular exercise, or other differences reflecting a greater preoccupation with health.

The probable explanation has been suggested by several recent studies. Orozco and de Castro (9) studied two groups of healthy young women who wore cardiac monitors throughout alcohol-free baseline periods, as well as during voluntary drinking periods in which one group could drink alcohol at their individual preferred rates while the others drank only soda. The alcohol group, on the days when they did drink alcohol, showed a sustained elevation of heart rate both during the day and overnight. The elevated heart rate is suggestive of a higher level of metabolic activity. This interpretation was confirmed by Klesges et al. (10), who found a significant elevation of resting rate of energy expenditure in subjects drinking alcohol, with or without concurrent smoking, whereas no increase occurred with smoking alone, or with smoking together with food. Suter et al. (11) similarly observed that ethanol, whether simply added to the diet or replacing part of the diet, produced a small but significant increase in energy expenditure, but in addition it caused a sharp decrease in the oxidation of lipids.

Thus it appears that the end result with respect to weight gain or loss depends on the balance between the decrease in fat utilization and the increase in energy expenditure produced by alcohol consumption. This balance varies as a function of the rest of the diet, the amount of alcohol consumed on a given occasion, the basal metabolic rate, the rate of ethanol metabolism, and probably other factors not yet recognized. But the concept of empty calories appears now, as it did nine years ago, to have no scientific basis.

Effects of Ethanol on Vitamin Metabolism

Most of the questions that were under active investigation nine years ago, concerning the effects of ethanol on the uptake and metabolism of the water-soluble vitamins, appear to have been answered, and they no longer appear as major issues in the current research literature on alcohol and general nutrition. In contrast there is much interest in the interactions between ethanol and certain vitamins that have been implicated in the pathogenesis of a number of diseases long recognized as consequences of heavy alcohol consumption. These are best illustrated by current studies on the retinoids in relation to fetal alcohol syndrome and oropharyngeal cancers, and those on biotin and folate in relation to oxidative cell damage.

Most interest has been directed toward the retinoids – β-carotene, retinol, and retinoic acid. Ethanol consumption, in the range of 1 to more than 4 drinks a day, does not appear to be very closely linked to the dietary intake of β-carotene or of vitamin E, though there is a slight tendency for the intakes to decrease in both men and women with the highest levels of alcohol consumption (12). When comparisons were made over a wider range of alcohol intakes, however, the plasma levels of β-carotene showed a progressive decrease with increasing alcohol consumption, while the levels of retinol increased progressively (13). The probable explanation for these findings is that two factors contribute, viz., a significant reduction in dietary carotene intake at very high levels of alcohol consumption, and a competitive inhibition of the oxidation of retinol to the biologically active forms, retinal and retinoic acid. Retinol, the alcohol form, is normally oxidized by alcohol dehydrogenase (ADH) to the aldehyde, retinal, which is in turn oxidized by aldehyde dehydrogenase (ALDH) to retinoic acid. Ethanol competes with retinol for binding to ADH (14), and the acetaldehyde to which it gives rise competes with retinal for binding to ALDH. Thus ethanol probably has a greater effect on the metabolic activation of the carotenes than on their dietary supply.

The potential pathogenetic importance of these competitions is suggested by recent findings in the rat fetal model of the fetal alcohol syndrome. As in the plasma of the humans described above, the level of retinol was found to be significantly higher in the brains of fetuses of rats drinking alcohol solution throughout pregnancy than in those of water-drinking controls, and the levels of retinoic acid were decreased (15). The abundance of retinoic acid receptors was increased in the alcoholic fetuses, presumably reflecting an up-regulation secondary to the low levels of retinoic acid, and the cytosolic levels of free retinoic acid–binding protein were increased because there was less retinoic acid present to utilize the binding sites. Retinoic acid is known to play an important role in the maturation of the fetal neural crest, and the disturbance of retinol metabolism may thus contribute to the production of some of the nervous system defects found in the fetal alcohol syndrome (14,15). A similar increase in the levels of free and esterified retinol, and a decrease in retinoic acid, has also been found in the fetal heart in alcohol-drinking pregnant rats (16), and it has been suggested that these changes are involved in the cardiac anomalies characteristic of the fetal alcohol syndrome.

Similar changes in retinoid metabolism have also been suggested as etiological factors in the production of certain alcohol-related cancers. It has been found repeatedly that heavy drinkers have a greatly increased risk (over 13-fold) of oropharyngeal and lower esophageal cancer compared to light drinkers or abstainers (17–19). Plasma levels of β-carotene and vitamin A were significantly lower in such cancer cases than in matched controls, and conversely the relative risk of such cancers in individuals with high dietary intakes of vitamin A and vitamin C was only 40% of that in individuals with low intakes. Comparable case-control studies have also indicated an increased risk of laryngeal cancer associated with alcohol use, and an apparent protective effect of dietary carotenoids (20). A possible mechanism for the protective effect of these vitamins will be discussed below in relation to alcohol and oxidative stress.

In a comparable manner recent work on water-soluble vitamins such as biotin and folate has also been directed toward explanation of certain types of alcohol-related pathology. For example ethanol has been shown to inhibit the uptake and transport of pyridoxal and of biotin by the human placenta, the degree of inhibition being proportional to the ethanol concentration (21,22). This has led to the suggestion that impaired biotin uptake into the fetus might also contribute to the production of the fetal alcohol syndrome (22). However this seems rather unlikely to be a major factor, because significant inhibition of biotin transport occurred only at ethanol concentrations of 200 mg/dl or more, sustained for several hours (22). Therefore it seems more credible that the impairment of biotin transport is itself a consequence of alcohol-induced damage to the placenta, rather than a primary mechanism of fetal damage.

In contrast alcohol-related disturbances in folate metabolism probably do have pathogenetic significance. Human alcoholics were found to have elevated serum levels of homocysteine compared to those in non-alcoholic control subjects, but significantly lower levels of pyridoxal phosphate, vitamin B-12, and red cell folate (23). These are all involved as co-factors in reactions that methylate homocysteine to S-adenosylmethionine or that convert it to glutathione (24). The elevated serum homocysteine is actually an indication of its impaired utilization by these reactions. Glutathione plays an essential role in the protection of cells against oxidative or toxic damage, and the impairment of glutathione formation from homocysteine is probably a contributory factor in the production of various kinds of cell damage in the heavy drinker (25).

Alcohol and Oxidative Stress

The term oxidative stress is now widely applied to a metabolic state in which oxidative reactions that generate free radicals and other oxidizing molecules exceed the reducing reactions that dispose of these oxidative products (26). As a result the oxidizing molecules increase to a level at which they cause significant damage to proteins, nucleic acids, and lipids that are essential for cellular integrity and normal function.

The role of ethanol in this disturbance has been the subject of intensive study over the past decade, and there is ample evidence that the metabolism of ethanol by the cytochrome P450 system is capable of giving rise to a significant degree of oxidative stress (26,27). At low concentrations ethanol is oxidized mainly by alcohol dehydrogenase in tbe liver, being converted first to acetaldehyde, then to acetate, and finally to carbon dioxide and water (2). However at higher concentrations a progressively larger fraction of the ethanol is oxidized by CYP2E1, a specific member of the cytochrome P450 superfamily of enzymes, which produces as by-products free radicals that react with a variety of substrates to form lipid peroxides, conjugated dienes, and other oxidized products (27).

At the same time alcohol also decreases the hepatic production of the major antioxidant glutathione, increases its loss from the liver (28), and decreases the cellular levels of protein thiols, vitamin E, and vitamin C (29). As a result there is a decreased level of protection against oxidative damage to cell membranes, intracellular organelles, and nucleic acids. This damaging effect of ethanol metabolism is intensified by a high-fat diet, and affects many organs including the liver, heart, central nervous system, and testis (26). In experimental animals the oxidative damage can be decreased or prevented by dietary supplements of vitamin E (30), and some effects can also be prevented by vitamin C. Even in cultured, isolated rat fetal hepatocytes, the alcohol-induced increase in lipid peroxidation and the resulting cell damage could be prevented by pre-exposure of the cells to vitamin E (31).

Among the many molecules that can be damaged by oxidative stress are transmembrane ion transport systems such as the Ca^{2+}-ATPase, which transports excess calcium out of the cell (30). The increase in intracellular Ca^{2+} that may result from this impairment of transport may well be one of the mechanisms of certain types of alcohol-related cell damage, and it is therefore potentially important that the damage to the Ca^{2+}-ATPase was prevented by adding vitamin E and vitamin D supplements to the diet.

As noted earlier it is known that regular high intake of alcohol increases the risk of certain types of cancer, including cancers of the esophagus and oropharynx among others (17–19). It is therefore of interest that ethanol can enhance the production of experimental cancers by certain known carcinogens. For example N-nitrosomethyl-benzylamine produces esophageal cancers in mice, and it does so in a higher percentage of the animals and produces a larger number of tumours per mouse if the animals are also receiving an alcohol-containing diet (32). The increase in number of tumours was proportional to the increase in the hepatic concentration of conjugated dienes, and the effect of ethanol could be completely prevented by dietary supplementation with vitamin E. When severe oxidative damage has already been produced, vitamin E will probably not reverse it. For example patients with severe alcoholic cirrhosis were not benefited by daily supplementation of the diet with vitamin E, even though it did raise the serum levels of vitamin E (33). The main value appears to be in preventing the production of damage.

As noted above some of the oxidative stress effects of ethanol can also be reduced or prevented by the antioxidant effect of vitamin C. For example the serum of human subjects who have drunk alcohol contains a cytotoxic factor that reduces the number of viable A9 cells that adhere to the culture vessel in tissue culture; the post-alcohol serum also reduces the oxidative function of mitochondria *in vitro* (34). Both of these effects were prevented if the subjects received vitamin C together with the alcohol. The cytotoxic effects are probably due to the formation of acetaldehyde-protein adducts, which is prevented by increased vitamin C levels.

While there are numerous such examples of oxidative damage related to the metabolism of ethanol, perhaps the greatest interest has focused on the possible beneficial effect of antioxidants in the prevention of atherosclerosis, the reported protective effect of a low level of alcohol consumption in the prevention of coronary heart disease, and the so-called French paradox. Because of the wide attention paid to this topic in both the medical and scientific literature and the popular press, it is treated separately in the next section.

Alcohol and the French Paradox

It is now generally accepted that a low daily intake of alcoholic beverages, amounting to 1–2 standard drinks a day (a standard drink contains 13.6 grams of absolute ethyl alcohol, and is equivalent to 12 oz of an ordinary Canadian beer, 5 oz of an average table wine, or 1.5 oz of most distilled spirits), results in a lower risk of coronary heart attacks and a lower fatality rate than in non-drinkers (35). A recent example is the Caerphilly study (36), carried out in Wales, which showed a lower relative risk of ischemic heart disease in drinkers than in non-drinkers. Various mechanisms have been proposed for this protective effect of alcohol, including its ability to lower the plasma level of low density lipoprotein (LDL) cholesterol, to increase the level of high density lipoprotein (HDL) cholesterol, and to decrease the rate of *in vitro* blood coagulation under standard conditions (37).

The so-called French paradox, also referred to by some writers as the "European paradox" because it is not confined to France (38), consists of the fact that there is a much lower incidence of, and mortality from, coronary heart disease (CHD) in France than in most northern European and North American countries, despite a high prevalence in France of risk factors that normally predict a high rate of CHD, including high dietary intake of saturated fat, high serum cholesterol levels, high prevalence of hypertension, and much higher rates of smoking than in the U.S.A., Canada, or the U.K. (39). Several possible explanations of this "paradox" have been suggested. One possibility is under-reporting of CHD in France, but careful examination of hospital records provides no support for this hypothesis. Another possible explanation is a high French dietary intake of antioxidants. But the explanation that has attracted the most media attention is that the high intake of red wine in France provides a particularly good source of antioxidants that are primarily responsible for the cardioprotective effect (39). A recent Danish study, for example, found a significant and progressive reduction of CHD risk with increasing amount of wine consumption, no effect with beer, and *increased* CHD risk with increasing amount of spirits consumption

(40). As will be shown below, however, it is necessary to keep one's mind open to the possibility of alternative explanations.

An interesting case in point is the comparative study of diet, alcohol, and CHD in Belfast, Northern Ireland, and Toulouse, France (41). Among males in the 45–54 and 55–64 year age groups, the relative risk of CHD was more than 4 times as high in Belfast as in Toulouse, and the difference was specific for this disease. While the relative risk was somewhat higher in Belfast than in Toulouse for other types of cardiovascular disease, cancer, and all causes, the risk ratio was only between 1.2:1 and 1.8:1. A detailed analysis of the diets showed that much more than the higher French consumption of red wine appeared to be involved. The French ate significantly more meat, cheese, fresh fruits and vegetables, and polyunsaturated fat, whereas the Irish ate much more potatoes and saturated fat. There were thus several sources of higher antioxidant consumption in the French diet (38).

Experimental evidence does support the claim that bioflavonoids such as phenolic compounds in red wine, including resveratrol and quercetin, have a direct dose-related inhibitory effect on platelet aggregation induced *in vitro* by ADP or by thrombin (42). An experimental study in humans found that consumption of red wine for two weeks was accompanied by a progressive reduction in the plasma levels of lipid peroxidation products, whereas two weeks' consumption of the same amount of white wine was associated with either no change or actual increases in these levels (43). Another known risk factor for CHD is central adiposity, i.e., accumulation of fat on the trunk and in the abdominal cavity, relative to the limbs. It is often expressed in terms of the waist-to-hip ratio, a higher ratio being indicative of a greater degree of central adiposity. A recent study, comparing waist-to-hip ratios in drinkers of wine, beer, and spirits, found no beverage-related difference in very light drinkers (less than 1 drink a week), but the ratio decreased progressively in heavier drinkers of wine, while it increased progressively in heavier drinkers of either beer or spirits (44).

However it must be pointed out that the highest level of drinking examined in that study (44) was "more than 6 drinks a week," which is 1 or more drinks a day, a level that would be considered very light by most investigators. That is a level at which any alcoholic beverage (not only wine) appears to have a protective effect against CHD (35). In the Caerphilly study, for example, a clear cardioprotective effect of alcohol was seen even though the great preponderance of alcohol consumed was beer and very little wine was used by that population (36). Furthermore the claimed benefits of bioflavonoid consumption appear to be equally valid if they are obtained from dietary sources other than wine, such as tea, onions, and apples (45).

Moreover other studies have found a greater protective effect with white wine than with red, no difference among beverages, or a reversed order for spirits vs beer (35). International comparisons have shown no consistency in terms of the relative protective values of different beverages. It is therefore necessary to examine other possible explanations of the "French paradox." Recent evidence suggests that the dietary level of α-tocopherol is a very important factor. A recent comparison of public health data from 24 countries in all parts of the world revealed an inverse correlation between the cardiac death rates and the mean daily intake of dietary α-tocopherol that was at least as strong, and possibly stronger, than the inverse correlation with mean daily wine intake (38). In addition the same study showed that between 1961 and 1986 there was an excellent inverse correlation between changes in CHD incidence and in dietary α-tocopherol intake within Canada and the U.S.A., whereas there was no correlation at all between changes in CHD and in wine consumption in France. These findings are consistent with those of other international comparisons (46) and with those of the Toulouse-Belfast comparison (41), which found that the Toulouse diet was much richer than the Belfast diet in various sources of tocopherols, vitamin C and other antioxidants, and polyunsaturated fats, such as fresh fruits, vegetables, and olive oil.

Moreover most of the studies that have found a greater protective effect of wine than of other alcoholic beverages have not examined for the possible confounding effect of contributions by other factors in light wine drinkers (who tend, in North America and the U.K., to be of higher educational and socio-economic status), such as lighter diets with more fruit and vegetables, and more regular exercise (47). Thus it appears that the role of red wine is of uncertain importance. If the diet is low in other protective factors, it is conceivable that wine may be of relatively greater importance, whereas in the presence of a diet rich in antioxidants, wine may add little or no extra benefit.

One additional factor that must be noted is that those countries in southern Europe that have the highest per capita consumptions of wine are also the countries with the lowest per capita consumptions of milk and dairy products other than cheese (48). It was therefore suggested that the lower CHD death rates in countries with high wine consumption might really be due not to the wine, but to the low consumption of milk by heavier wine drinkers. The positive correlation between per capita milk consumption and CHD death rates was actually stronger than the negative correlation between per capita wine consumption and CHD death rates. A breakdown of milk constituents suggested that the harmful effect was related to consumption of non-fermented milk protein, i.e., protein other than that contained in natural cheese products. It was therefore suggested that the risk factor in milk might be lactose, which would be safely removed by bacterial fermentation in the production of cheese. A recent international comparison (49) has provided rather striking support for this suggestion: there was a positive correlation between lactose intake and CHD death rates in the 22 countries studied, with $r = 0.74$ ($p < 0.001$).

In summary, therefore, it appears unwarranted to recommend that people should drink more red wine in order to protect themselves against CHD (46). Increasing the total alcohol intake to more than 3–4 drinks a day increases the risk of morbidity or death from numerous other diseases, such as hypertensive heart disease, stroke, cirrhosis, and various types of cancer, so that the protective effect against CHD is soon more than offset by increased rates of other disease as the alcohol consumption is increased. It appears that the protective effect against CHD can be achieved by increasing the dietary intake of α-tocopherol, vitamin C, and flavonoids from food sources, and by improving the diet in other ways (possibly such as reducing lactose intake), without running the risk that is associated with increased alcohol intake.

REFERENCES

1 Kalant H. Alcohol use and nutrition. In: Carroll KK, ed. *Diet, Nutrition, and Health*. Montreal & Kingston: McGill-Queen's University Press, 1990:176–187.
2 Hawkins RD, Kalant H. The metabolism of ethanol and its metabolic effects. *Pharmacol Rev* 1972;24:67–157.
3 Wei P, Hamilton JR, LeBlanc AE. A clinical and metabolic study of an intravenous feeding technique using peripheral veins as the initial infusion site. *Can Med Assoc J* 1972;106:969–974.
4 DeCarli LM, Lieber CS. Fatty liver in the rat after prolonged intake of ethanol with a nutritionally adequate liquid diet. *J Nutr* 1967;91:331–336.

5 Khanna JM, Kalant H, Yee Y, Chung S, Siemens AJ. Effect of chronic ethanol treatment on metabolism of drugs in vitro and in vivo. *Biochem Pharmacol* 1976;25:329–335.

6 Bondy SC, Pearson KR. Ethanol-induced oxidative stress and nutritional status. *Alcohol Clin Exp Res* 1993;17:651–654.

7 Prentice AM. Alcohol and obesity. *Int J Obesity* 1995;19(suppl 5):s44–s50.

8 Istvan J, Murray R, Voelker H. The relationship between patterns of alcohol consumption and body weight. *Int J Epidemiol* 1995;24:543–546.

9 Orozco S, de Castro JM. Effect of spontaneous alcohol intake on heart rate and dietary intake of free-living women. *Pharmacol Biochem Behav* 1994;49:629–638.

10 Klesges RC, Mealer CZ, Klesges LM. Effects of alcohol intake on resting energy expenditure in young women social drinkers. *Am J Clin Nutr* 1994;59:805–809.

11 Suter PM, Schutz Y, Jequier E. The effect of ethanol on fat storage in healthy subjects. *N Engl J Med* 1992;326:983–987.

12 Rimm E, Colditz G. Smoking, alcohol, and plasma levels of carotenes and vitamin E. *Ann NY Acad Sci* 1993;686:323–333.

13 Simonetti P, Cestaro B, Porrini M, Viani P, Roggi C, Testolin G. Effect of alcohol intake on lipids and fat-soluble vitamins in blood. *Minerva Med* 1993;84:447–452.

14 Duester G. Retinoids and the alcohol dehydrogenase gene family. EXS 1994;71:279–290.

15 Grummer MA, Langhough RE, Zachman RD. Maternal ethanol ingestion effects on fetal rat brain vitamin A as a model for fetal alcohol syndrome. *Alcohol Clin Exp Res* 1993;17:592–597.

16 DeJonge MH, Zachman RD. The effect of maternal ethanol ingestion on fetal rat heart vitamin A: a model for fetal alcohol syndrome. *Pediat Res* 1995;37:418–423.

17 Day GL, Blot WJ, Austin DF, Bernstein L, Greenberg RS, Preston-Martin S, Schoenberg JB, Winn DM, McLaughlin JK, Fraumeni JF, Jr. Racial differences in risk of oral and pharyngeal cancer: alcohol, tobacco, and other determinants. *J Natl Cancer Inst* 1993;85:465–473.

18 Kabat GC, Ng SK, Wynder EL. Tobacco, alcohol intake, and diet in relation to adenocarcinoma of the esophagus and gastric cardia. *Cancer Causes Control* 1993;4:123–132.

19 Kune GA, Kune S, Field B, Watson LF, Cleland H, Merenstein D, Vitetta L. Oral and pharyngeal cancer, diet, smoking, alcohol, and serum vitamin A and β-carotene levels: a case-control study in men. *Nutr Cancer* 1993;20:61–70.

20 Freudenheim JL, Graham S, Byers TE, Marshall JR, Haughey BP, Swanson MK, Wilkinson G. Diet, smoking, and alcohol in cancer of the larynx: a case-control study. *Nutr Cancer* 1992;17:33–45.

21 Schenker S, Johnson RF, Mahuren JD, Henderson GI, Coburn SP. Human placental vitamin b6 (pyridoxal) transport: normal characteristics and effects of ethanol. *Am J Physiol* 1992;262:R966–R974.

22 Hu Z-Q, Henderson GI, Mock DM, Schenker S. Biotin uptake by basolateral membrane vesicles of human placenta: normal characteristics and role of ethanol. *Proc Soc Exp Biol Med* 1994;206:404–408.

23 Cravo ML, Gloria LM, Selhub J, Nadeau MR, Camilo ME, Resende MP, Cardoso JN, Leitão CN, Mira FC. Hyperhomocysteinemia in chronic alcoholism: correlation with folate, vitamin B-12, and vitamin B-6 status. *Am J Clin Nutr* 1996;63:220–224.

24 Anonymous. Folate, alcohol, methionine, and colon cancer risk: is there a unifying theme? *Nutr Rev* 1994;52(1):18–20.

25 Lieber CS. Alcohol and the liver: 1994 update. *Gastroenterology* 1994;106:1085–1105.

26 Nordmann R. Alcohol and antioxidant systems. *Alcohol Alcohol* 1994;29:513–522.

27 Lieber CS. Mechanisms of ethanol-drug-nutrition interactions. *J Toxicol Clin Toxicol* 1994;32:631–681.

28 Speisky H, Macdonald A, Giles G, Orrego H, Israel Y. Increased loss and decreased synthesis of hepatic glutathione after acute ethanol administration. *Biochem J* 1985;225:565–572.

29 Ribière C, Hininger I, Rouach H, Nordmann R. Effects of chronic ethanol administration on free radical defence in rat myocardium. *Biochem Pharmacol* 1992;44:1495–1500.

30 Nanji AA, Sadrzadeh SM. The effect of fish oil and vitamin E on ethanol-induced changes in membrane atpases. *Life Sci* 1994;55:PL245–PL249.

31 Devi BG, Henderson GI, Frosto TA, Schenker S. Effect of ethanol on rat fetal hepatocytes: studies on cell replication, lipid peroxidation and glutathione. *Hepatology* 1993;18:648–659.

32 Eskelson CD, Odeleye OE, Watson RR, Earnest DL, Mufti SI. Modulation of cancer growth by vitamin E and alcohol. *Alcohol Alcohol* 1993;28:117–125.

33 de la Maza MP, Petermann M, Bunout D, Hirsch S. Effects of long-term vitamin E supplementation in alcoholic cirrhotics. *J Am Coll Nutr* 1995;14:192–196.

34 Wickramasinghe SN, Hasan R. In vivo effects of vitamin C on the cytotoxicity of post-ethanol serum. *Biochem Pharmacol* 1994;48:621–624.

35 Rimm EB, Klatsky A, Grobbee D, Stampfer MJ. Review of moderate alcohol consumption and reduced risk of coronary heart disease: is the effect due to beer, wine or spirits. *Brit Med J* 1996;312:731–736.

36 Fehily AM, Yarnell JW, Sweetnam PM, Elwood PC. Diet and incident ischaemic heart disease: the Caerphilly study. *Br J Nutr* 1993;69:303–314.

37 Goldberg DM, Hahn SE, Parkes JG. Beyond alcohol: beverage consumption and cardiovascular mortality. *Clin Chim Acta* 1995;237:155–187.

38 Bellizzi MC, Franklin MF, Duthie GG, James WP. Vitamin E and coronary heart disease: the European paradox. *Eur J Clin Nutr* 1994;48:822–831.

39 Burr ML. Explaining the French paradox. *J Roy Soc Health* 1995;115:217–219.

40 Grønbæk M, Deis A, Sørensen TIA, Becker U, Schnohr P, Jensen G. Mortality associated with moderate intakes of wine, beer, or spirits. *Brit Med J* 1995;310:1165–1169.

41 Evans AE, Ruidavets JB, McCrum EE, Cambou JP, McClean R, Douste-Blazy P, McMaster D, Bingham A, Patterson CC, Richard JL et al. Autres pays, autres cœurs? Dietary patterns, risk factors and ischaemic heart disease in Belfast and Toulouse. *Quart J Med* 1995;88:469–477.

42 Pace-Asciak CR, Hahn S, Diamandis EP, Soleas G, Goldberg DM. The red wine phenolics trans-resveratrol and quercetin block human platelet aggregation and eicosanoid synthesis: implications for protection against coronary heart disease. *Clin Chim Acta* 1995;235:207–219.

43 Fuhrman B, Lavy A, Aviram M. Consumption of red wine with meals reduces the susceptibility of human plasma and low-density lipoprotein to lipid peroxidation. *Am J Clin Nutr* 1995;61:549–554.

44 Duncan BB, Chambless LE, Schmidt MI, Folsom AR, Szklo M, Crouse JR, III, Carpenter MA. Association of the waist-to-hip ratio is different with wine than with beer or hard liquor consumption. *Am J Epidemiol* 1995;142:1034–1038.

45 Hertog MG, Feskens EJ, Hollman PC, Katan MB, Kromhout D. Dietary antioxidant flavonoids and risk of coronary heart disease: the Zutphen elderly study. *Lancet* 1993;342:1007–1011.

46 Criqui MH, Ringel BL. Does diet or alcohol explain the French paradox? *Lancet* 1994;344:1719–1723.

47 Woodward M, Tunstall-Pedoe H. Alcohol consumption, diet, coronary risk factors, and prevalent coronary heart disease in men and women in the Scottish heart health study. *J Epidemiol Community Health* 1995;49:354–362.

48 Popham RE, Schmidt W, Israel Y. Variation in mortality from ischemic heart disease in relation to alcohol and milk consumption. *Med Hypoth* 1983;12:321–329.

49 Segall JJ. Dietary lactose as a possible risk factor for ischaemic heart disease: review of epidemiology. *Int J Cardiol* 1994;46:197–207.

ERNST L. WYNDER and JOSHUA E. MUSCAT

Role of Diet in Health Maintenance throughout Life

As we examine the epidemiology of youthful longevity, it becomes clear that to succeed in attaining this goal we need to conduct a healthy lifestyle since we cannot control our genetic constitution. The good news here is that most of these lifestyle variables, including smoking, alcohol abuse, drug use, unhealthy nutrition, lack of exercise, and unsafe sexual practices, have been well established as risk factors through a large number of cohort and retrospective epidemiological studies. Their establishment may be considered the good news from the point of view of causation. The bad news is that we have to intervene on these factors ourselves. Here we are faced with the well-known phenomenon of our illusion of immortality and our inability to modify a health habit that we enjoy for a possible future benefit.

Among these risk factors, and what we are discussing here, is nutrition, which has a preventive effect for health, not just by itself but also because it is so well interrelated with most other risk-taking behaviour. For instance the eating of meat is positively correlated with smoking, whereas the consumption of fruits and vegetables is negatively related (1). From the very onset then we need to recognize that as we deal with nutritional variables we deal with a number of interrelated variables. It might be said that good nutritional practices serve as an indication of other healthy lifestyle practices. What is also important is to realize that this interrelationship already exists among adolescents and that here too we find a high correlation between dietary fat intake and smoking, which, in turn, is highly correlated with other unhealthy behaviours. From the beginning, therefore, we need to emphasize that if we want to educate a population about healthy nutrition we must educate them simultaneously about a healthy lifestyle.

Nutrition in Youth

Nutritional habits have their beginning early in childhood. This is important not only from an etiological point of view but also from a habit-forming one. Finnish children, for instance, have among the highest serum cholesterol levels in the world, which correlates well with the levels among Finnish adults (2). Children of two years of age already have serum cholesterol levels of 180 mg/dl. Obesity also has its beginnings early in life with 75% of obese adults already so as children. The fact that obesity is increasing among adolescents does not bode well for the future (3).

Taste habits are also set early in life so that the foods we cherish as young children, be it peanut butter and jelly or noodles with gooseberries, are the consequence of what we enjoyed when very young. Thus nutritional education must be taught very early in life. Unfortunately this lesson is not too well appreciated by many parents and schools, nor by health professionals.

Role of Nutrition in Adulthood

The evidence that nutrition *per se* plays a role in the majority of our chronic diseases is based upon epidemiological, biological, and mechanistic data. Nutrition has a broad effect on the morbidity and mortality of a wide range of diseases. The correlation between blood lipids and coronary artery disease, first established in the 1960s is of course too well known to bear repetition here. It is also quite well established and generally accepted that caloric excesses leading to obesity are important variables for such disease entities as hypertension, arthritis, gall bladder disease, and adult-onset diabetes. The key parameter here is nutritional overload, primarily in total calories and in fat calories (4).

It has been more difficult to reach a consensus relating nutrition to such cancers as cancer of the breast, prostate, and colon. Ecological data show a high correlation between dietary fat and these cancers (5). This correlation is well supported by animal studies showing that certain types of fats are more conducive to promoting mammary gland tumours in rodents than others. Studies by Cohen et al. (6) have shown that the tumour-promoting effect in rodents is correlated with the linoleic acid content of the diet and gives relatively small increases with olive oil, a finding that correlates well with ecologic studies showing a relatively low breast cancer rate in postmenopausal women in Spain, Greece, and southern Italy. Further to fatty acids, linoleic acid in the athymic mouse model appears to accelerate tumour metastasis, as well shown by Rose et al. (7), while omega-3 fatty acids tend to have an inhibitory effect.

These data appear to be at odds with cohort and case-control studies based upon food frequency questionnaires. Studies, notably of Hunter and co-workers, show no differences in risk comparing the first and last quintiles in terms of fat or linoleic acid dietary intake (8). We have proposed that the available method for nutritional assessment leaves us at odds. Already the early studies on serum cholesterol and cardiovascular disease by Paul et al. could not show a correlation between dietary history and serum cholesterol levels, even though their dietary histories were taken in much more detail than could be done in a large cohort study (9). It has been suggested that in an homogenous population, the measurement error in taking a dietary history by question method is so large that it becomes virtually valueless to use this type of evidence to establish an association (10). Repeated interviews, even if they give a highly reproducible result, would not be acceptable. True validation, as carried out by Mertz et al. on people's food intake, was actually measured and then, when asked questions about what they had eaten, underreported by at least 20% (11). A similar degree of underreporting was shown by Martin et al., using doubly-labelled water (12). Such underreporting may even be greater when health professionals are interviewed, and may be still greater among cases of breast cancer than controls in a retrospective study, because of the greater knowledge and/or concern the cases may have, for instance, in terms of fat intake. Given that the nutritional assessment data in epidemiologic data are not in agreement with the abundant evidence from ecologic and experimental studies linking nutrition with postmenopausal breast cancer, it seems likely that the nutritional assessments are poor indicators of dietary fat intake, especially given the sizeable measurement error and the lack of heterogeneity in the diet within populations. Here we deal with an "overexposure" of the control group in that all members of a study population in Western countries consume an excess of calories and fat (13).

Intervention Studies

To provide a population with healthy nutrition demands the collaboration of several segments of our society, including that of schools where we have been involved in a comprehensive health education program for many years – a program that must have its beginning in kindergarten and preferably in preschool. Our Know Your Body School Health Education Program represents such an effort – it is multifactorial (14). The effectiveness of health education in general depends on the dose given in terms of quality, intensity, and duration. A key component of this program is a full-time health education teacher. We recommend that this type of effort should become a mandatory component of school curricula everywhere.

If we had to make just one recommendation of broad public health importance beyond that purely relating to nutrition, we would provide all children, ideally beginning in preschool, a health education program that teaches them, besides knowledge about risk-taking behaviour, the idea that they are responsible for their own health on a lifelong basis. Such a program must be started early in life because it has become increasingly evident that cognitive, emotional, and learning practices take place very early in our lives, when our brain synapses are in the best state of readiness to accept new information.

For adult intervention programs we suggest that under the aegis of managed care all individuals should know their ideal blood levels and weights and be given incentive programs to reduce them if elevated. From a public health point of view, food labelling is an additional step that needs to be enhanced. Food companies must be encouraged to lower both the fat and caloric content of their products. We have recommended a 25/25 diet – 25% calories from fat and 25 from cell fibre (15). We have developed an "Icebox" poster to assist the consumer in following our dietary recommendations. In respect to intervention studies, we are currently involved in the Women's Intervention Nutrition Study (WINS), which tests the hypothesis that a 15% low-fat diet will reduce the recurrence of breast cancer in postmenopausal women with stage I and II disease, who have received standard therapy. Our results show that women can be accrued and maintain compliance to about 15% fat and that their fat intake is significantly different from that of the controls (15). This study has to accrue 2,500 patients to have sufficient statistical power to establish the kind of differences we project between the intervention and non-intervention group. In addition to what we might expect on breast cancer recurrence we hope to show other benefits related to the cardiovascular systems and such other conditions as cancer of the colon, arthritis, and gall bladder disorders, as well as adult onset diabetes. We are about to launch a similar trial on prostate cancer for patients who have undergone prostatectomy and whose prostate-specific antigen test (PSA) has become positive. When after prostatectomy the PSA becomes 0.4 ng/ml or higher, the patient will be randomized, with the dietary intervention stopped if the PSA reaches the level of 10. The men will be divided into four groups: one on a 15% low-fat diet alone; one on a nutritional cocktail consisting of selenium (20 micrograms), vitamin E (800 IU), and a soy protein; one on both the diet and the nutritional cocktail; and a control group on a standard diet. In this study PSA will serve as the initial biomarker whose velocity we expect to positively affect through dietary intervention.

As established by Ornish, dietary intervention, not only for certain types of cancers but also for atherosclerosis, can occur (16). What must take place is that the dietary intervention has the proper dose level. In addition to modifying the level of fat, there is also a role for antioxidants – a role that for atherosclerosis has been well established for vitamin E, a vitamin that also seems to affect the development of cancer of the prostate (17). Considerable biological work has also been done on selenium as a chemopreventive agent, especially for experimental cancers of the breast and colon (17). A combination of a low-fat, low-calorie diet rich in greens, fruits, and vegetables is the ideal diet suggested on the basis of our evolutionary history.

As our grandmothers already told us, and as we concur, "we are what we eat." This is difficult to relate to on the basis of our dietary habits, which we regard as "normal," and on the basis of an age where molecular biology reigns supreme. Obstacles to improve nutrition for the general public include the "illusion of immortality" of most individuals, making them unwilling to give up a momentary pleasure for a possible long-term benefit; the fact that physicians know little about how to "optimize" diet; and the fact that the food industry has its own priorities not always conducive to health. Yet we need to recognize that nutrition can affect the expression of our genes. Perhaps as scientists begin to think how nutrition interrelates with molecular biology and gene function, more young scientists will enter the field of nutrition, recognizing that in the long run our knowledge of nutrition will teach us much about prevention of disease and youthful longevity. In the meantime, however, we all can learn what an optimal diet ought to be and recognize that throughout history disease prevention was possible long before we knew the pathogenesis and intricacies of disease – and that diet deficient in proteins, vitamins, and minerals, and assessed largely in terms of calories and fats, is detrimental to health. Proper nutrition in terms of its make-up, preparation, amount, and frequencies of consumption affects our mental and physical development and our youthful longevity, demanding therefore much more attention from the scientific, medical, and consumer communities alike. In its optimal phase it will have a significant impact on our nation's productivity and health care costs and therefore requires much more of our attention than given at present.

REFERENCES

1 Berger J, Wynder EL. The correlation of epidemiologic variables. *J Clin Epidemiol* 1994;47:941–952.

2 Puska P, Vartianen E, Pallonen U, Salonen JT, Pöyhiä P, McAlister A. The North Karelia Youth Project: evaluation of two years of intervention on health behavior and CVD risk factors among 13- to 15-year-old children. *Prev Med* 1982;11:550–570.

3 Kennedy E, Goldberg J. What are American children eating? Implications for public policy. *Nutr Rev* 1995;53:111–126.

4 Wynder EL. Nutrition and metabolic overload. *Resident and Staff Physician* February 1992:63–70.

5 Carroll KK, Khor HT. Dietary fat in relation to tumorigenesis. *Prog Biochem Pharmacol* 1975;10:308–353.

6 Cohen LA, Thompson DO, Masura Y, Choi K, Black ME, Rose DP. Dietary fat and mammary cancer. I. Promoting effect of dietary fat in N-nitrosomethylurea-induced rat mammary carcinogenesis. *J Natl Cancer Inst* 1986;77:33–42.

7 Rose DP, Connoly Liu X-H. Effect of linoleic acid on the growth and metastasis of two human breast cancer cell lines in nude mice, and the invasive capacity of these cell lines in vitro. *Cancer Res* 1994;54:6557–6562.

8 Hunter DJ, Spiegelman D, Adami H-O, Beeson L, Van Den Brandt P, Folsom AR et al. Cohort studies of fat intake and the risk of breast cancer – a pooled analysis. *New Engl J Med* 1996;334:356–361.

9 Paul O, Lepper MH, Phelan WH, Dupertuis W, Wesley G, MacMillan A et al. A longitudinal study of coronary heart disease. *Circulation* 1963;28:20–31.

10 Hegsted DM. 1985 W.O. Atwater Memorial Lecture. Nutrition. The changing scene. *Nutr Rev* 1985;43:357–367.

11 Mertz W, Tsui JC, Judd JT, Reiser S, Hallfrisch J, Morris ER et al. What are people really eating? The relationship between energy intake derived from estimated diet records and intake determined to maintain body weight. *Am J Clin Nutr* 1991;54:291–295.

12 Martin LJ, Su W, Jones PJ, Lockwood GA, Trichler DL, Boyd NF. Comparison of energy intakes determined by food records and doubly labeled water in women participating in a dietary-intervention trial. *Am J Clin Nutr* 1996;63:483–490.

13 Wynder EL, Stellman SD. The "overexposed" control group. *Am J Epidemiol* 1992;135:459–461.

14 Walter HJ, Wynder EL. The development, implementation, evaluation, and future directions of a chronic disease prevention program for children: the "Know Your Body" studies. *Prev Med* 1989;18:59–71.

15 Chlebowski RT, Blackburn GL, Buzzard M, Rose DP, Martino JD, Khandekar JD et al. Adherence to a dietary fat intake reduction program in postmenopausal women receiving therapy for early breast cancer. *J Clin Oncol* 1993;11:2072–2080.

16 Ornish D. Can life-style changes reverse coronary atherosclerosis? *Hospital Practice* 1991;26:123–126, 129–132.

17 El-Bayoumy K. The role of selenium in cancer prevention. In: Devita V, Hellman S, Rosenberg SA, eds. *Cancer prevention*. Philadelphia: Lippincott, 1991:1–15.

GUYLAINE FERLAND

Nutritional Problems of the Elderly

Introduction

As in many Western countries the population of Canada is ageing as a result of an increasing life expectancy, which at 65 is now 20 years for women and 14 years for men (1). In the year 2021 almost 20% of the Canadian population will be over 65 years of age, and over 40% of all elderly will be over 75 years. It is projected that in 2031, 1.1 million Canadians will be aged > 85 years (1). To limit the impact of these changes in demographics on the health care system, health of Canadians will have to be optimized for a greater number of years. It is now well established that nutrition plays a central role in the maintenance of health and quality of life of older adults. Nutrition has been shown to modulate various age-related organ and physiological changes, and to influence the risk of developing certain chronic diseases (2). Evidence is also accumulating that diet may have an important role in the prevention of premature morbidity and mortality amongst older adults (3). Yet the importance of nutrition has often been underestimated in both community-dwelling and institutionalized elderly (3,4).

Ageing is generally conceptualized as a progressive decline of physiological functions combined with a gradual decreased ability to withstand stress. Ageing studies point to the fact that age-related changes show great inter-individual variations (2). As a result older persons exhibit striking heterogeneity as a group, a characteristic of significant importance when it comes to nutritional considerations.

Factors Affecting the Nutritional Status of the Elderly

A broad spectrum of nutritional problems have been identified in the elderly. The nutritional status of older persons is determined by their nutrient requirements and intakes. Physiological, psychological, and socio-economic factors interact to affect the nutritional well-being of the individual.

SOCIAL, ECONOMIC AND PSYCHOLOGICAL FACTORS

Bereavement, social isolation, living alone, and being housebound have been linked to risk of malnutrition (5–8). By changing the social context of eating, widowhood can significantly alter eating behaviours and quality of the diet. When compared to still-married individuals, recently widowed persons had less appetite, poorer eating habits, lower overall and nutrient-specific quality diets, and suffered more unintentional weight loss (5). Living alone has been associated with poorer diets in a number of studies (6,7). A higher proportion of people living alone were found to have substandard intake of protein, vitamins A and C, and calcium than those living in a family (6).

Limited financial resources also add to the risk of poor diet, with money spent on food a good predictor of dietary quality and energy intake (6–8). Similarly loneliness and depression may affect dietary patterns through loss of appetite, loss of enjoyment of cooking, and decreased interest in foods (6,9). Depression was found to be associated with weight loss in ambulatory elderly patients (10).

PHYSIOLOGICAL FACTORS

The physiological changes associated with ageing can also influence the nutritional status of elderly persons by affecting food intake and nutrient metabolism. Ageing is associated with a decrease in lean body and bone mass and an increase in body fat (11). These changes, along with the observed reduction in energy expenditure due to the decline in physical activity in most elderly, result in decreased energy needs. Decreasing energy intake, however, may lead to lower intake of vitamins and minerals, adding to the risk of malnutrition.

Alterations in the sense of taste and smell and oral health problems can diminish the enjoyment of eating, decrease appetite, and reduce food intake (12). Elderly have been shown to have elevated taste and smell detection and recognition thresholds (13). Flavour concentration needs to be 2–12 times greater to induce the same flavour response as in younger adults (14). Similarly threshold for odours in the elderly can be >10 times higher than in the young (13). In a recent study involving 80 free-living women, nearly half of the participants had olfactory dysfunction (15). In this study decreased odour and flavour perception was associated with lower interest in food-related activities, lower preference for fruits and vegetables rich in vitamins A and C (e.g., citrus fruits), higher intakes of sweets, and a nutrient profile indicative of higher risk for cardiac disease (15). Thirst perception can also be decreased in elderly, a condition that can lead to dehydration (16). Proper hydration status is essential as dehydration in older adults has been associated with increased infection and mortality rates (16). Fluid recommendations for adults >65 years are 1 ml per kilocalorie of food ingested or 30 ml per kilogram of body weight (16,17).

Tooth loss and lack of or poor-fitting dentures are common in older people and can profoundly affect food choices. In Canada 70% of those >55 years of age wear full or partial dentures and only 10% have all of their natural teeth (18). Dental problems in free-living elderly have been linked to low nutrient intake in some studies (19) but not in others (20). Eating and swallowing problems are common in geriatric hospital settings and have been associated with undernutrition (12,21). In frail elderly the number of general oral health problems was found the best predictor of significant involuntary weight loss within 1 year of admission to a geriatric rehabilitation unit (22).

Alterations of the gastrointestinal tract are more common in older persons. Constipation can affect up to 70% of elderly and is usually associated with low fluid intake, diets low in fibre, decreased physical activity, and intake of constipating drugs (3). Attention to such factors should precede the prescription of laxatives as chronic or abusive laxative use can lead to nutrient malabsorption. Similarly diverticulosis is a condition that can affect up to 50% of those over 80 (23). The dietary management is similar to that for constipation. Lactose intolerance has been estimated to occur in 12% of Caucasian and 70–75% non-Caucasian seniors (23). This condition can lead to GI discomfort and may cause older persons to avoid dairy products, which represent good sources of the B vitamins as well as vitamins A and D and calcium. Another common ageing-related change in digestion is atrophic gastritis which occurs in ~30% of individuals older than 60 years and is due primarily to parietal cell malfunction

(24). Atrophic gastritis, which is associated with diminished gastric secretion of hydrochloric acid, pepsin, and intrinsic factor, may result in decreased digestion and absorption of vitamin B_{12}, folic acid, and iron. Malabsorption of vitamin B_{12} in patients with this condition appears to involve both the maldigestion of the food protein–bound vitamin B_{12} complex in the stomach and the uptake of the vitamin by the greater number of bacteria that reside in the proximal small intestine (25).

DIET-RELATED CHRONIC DISEASES

The prevalence of chronic disease increases as age advances; reports indicate that 80% of Canadian seniors have one or more chronic diseases that can impact on the nutritional status or could benefit from dietary intervention (1,3). Physical illness has been associated with increased nutritional risk (26), low energy intake (20,27), and inadequate diet (9). In a recent study involving 90 home-living people aged 73–94 years, men with chronic diseases received significantly less energy (7.5 ± 1.76 MJ) than those who did not suffer from chronic diseases (8.9 ± 2.0 MJ) (27). In another study the number and severity of physical illnesses was related to decreased intakes of vitamins A and C in a group of independently living individuals aged 60–94 years (9).

The most commonly reported chronic conditions are osteoporosis, arthritis, heart disease, hypertension, and diabetes (1). Osteoporosis affects more than 1.5 million Canadians and strikes more women than men; 15% of women will have a hip fracture and 32% a vertebral fracture after the age of 50 (28). Associated health care costs are projected to be $30 billion over the next 20 years (28). Hip fractures have been associated with a 12–15% decrease in expected survival (23). The role of diet in osteoporosis has clearly been established both from an etiological perspective, and as a mean of managing the disease. Calcium and vitamin D, the nutrients that have received the most attention with respect to this disorder, have been shown to have significant impact on bone integrity in older persons. Although the amount of dietary calcium and vitamin D to minimize bone loss and optimize bone health in the elderly is still a subject of investigation, it does appear that recommended intakes should be higher than current Recommended Nutrient Intakes (RNIs) (29). Studies involving postmenopausal women suggest that intakes of 1,000 to 1,500 mg/d of calcium and of 10–20 µg/d of vitamin D could be beneficial in the consolidation of bone mass and in the prevention of hip and non-vertebral fractures (28). For men over the age of 65 years the National Institutes of Health consensus panel recommends a calcium intake of 1,500 mg/d, nearly double the current RNI (30).

In Canada limb and joint problems have been reported by 46% of men and 63% of women (1). By restricting the mobility of afflicted individuals, arthritis may affect the ability to self feed, decrease food intake, and contribute to the risk of malnutrition. Heart disease and hypertension are estimated to affect 24–28% and 34–43% of elderly Canadians, respectively (1). The importance of food choices in reducing the risk of heart disease and its management is generally recognized in the general public including the elderly: in the Santé Québec study 40% of men and 49% of women aged 65–74 years were reported to make special food choices because of concern for heart disease (31). Modification of dietary habits was more likely for heart disease and hypertension than for other conditions such as cancer (6–10%) and osteoporosis (9–19%).

The prevalence of diabetes mellitus increases with age, affecting 10% of Canadians and 18% of Americans over 65 years of age (23,32). Diabetic patients are more likely to be hospitalized or institutionalized than non-diabetics, and to suffer clinical complications (32). Nutritional therapy is an essential component of successful diabetes management. Recent recommendations have focused on the individualization of the therapy. In addition to maintaining reasonable body weight and engaging in the practice of exercise, diabetics are generally encouraged to increase their intake of complex carbohydrate, including fibre, lower that of fat, and use concentrated sugars in moderation (32,33).

The link between mental health, food intake, and nutritional status is evident in all age groups but particularly in the elderly. In 1991 over 1/4 of a million Canadians had dementia, 64% of whom had Alzheimer's disease (34). On the basis of current demographic trends it is estimated that by the year 2031 over 3/4 of a million Canadian adults will have dementia (> 1/2 a million with Alzheimer's disease). Studies of elderly patients in psychogeriatric units have shown that patients with cognitive impairments are at the greatest risk for the development of nutrition-related problems (35). Patients with dementia and especially Alzheimer's disease have been shown to be underweight, to lose weight during the course of the illness, and to be at risk of or suffer from malnutrition (26,36–38). As many as 50% of patients with Alzheimer-type dementia suffer from protein-energy malnutrition (39). In the early stages of the disease, when the patient is living independently, weight loss may be related to memory loss, indifference to food, impaired judgement, and lack of assistance with respect to provision of food and preparation of the meals. Later on weight loss may be related to increased energy requirement due to agitation. Energy requirements have been shown to increase by 600–1,600 kcal in Alzheimer patients who pace or wander (40,41). In a recent study involving outpatients and bedridden institutionalized demented patients, energy requirement was found to be greater for Alzheimer patients than for multi-infarct or non-demented control subjects of similar size (42). This study also showed that Alzheimer patients had increased fat-free mass when compared to MID and control subjects, a finding that suggests that the elevated energy requirement of Alzheimer patients may be attributable to their increased lean body mass (42). In the final stages of the disease, patients with dementia may develop swallowing problems and become more dependent on health care providers for feeding assistance. Time allowed for feeding and adequacy of staff can then become important issues.

DEPENDENCY IN ACTIVITIES OF DAILY LIVING

Dependency in activities of daily living has been identified as a risk factor for malnutrition in various reports (3). In free-living elderly, decreased functional ability was associated with decreased energy intake (20) and inadequate intake of protein, vitamins C, B_{12}, and A, niacin, and iron (6).

MEDICATION USE

The presence of chronic disease or the coexistence of several illnesses in the elderly can result in the use of various prescription drugs, over-the-counter medication, and self-prescribed dietary supplements. In population-based cohorts prescription and non-prescription drugs were found to be used by 60–78% and 52–76% of elderly, respectively (43). In nursing home settings residents have been shown to consume an average of 7–8 medications, an amount that can increase to 10 when patients are transferred to an acute-care institution (44–46). Polypharmacy increases the susceptibility of drug-nutrient interactions. In a recent study involving three long-term-care facilities, there was a direct linear relationship between the number of drugs a patient was taking and the number of drug-nutrient interactions for which the patient was at risk (47).

Drugs can depress appetite by altering taste and smell and decrease food intake in response to gastrointestinal disturbances (47). In functionally dependent elderly living in the community, use of psychotropic drugs was negatively associated with energy intake (20). Medications can also interfere with nutrient absorption, metabolism, and excretion, increasing the risk for vitamin and mineral deficiencies (47). Nutrients whose deficiencies may occur with chronic use of common drugs include vitamins B_6, B_{12}, C, D, and K, folic acid, phosphate, potassium, calcium, magnesium, and zinc (44).

Dietary Practices of Elderly Canadians

We know from various studies that energy intake of the elderly tends to decrease with age, a phenomenon associated with overall low food consumption (23). This observation was recently confirmed in two provincial surveys (Québec and Nova Scotia) where average energy intakes were 1,394–1,511 kcal/d for women and 2,025–2,143 kcal/d for men; these intakes were below the 1,800 and 2,300 kcal recommended for women and men, respectively (29,31,48). In general men have higher energy intakes than women (49). Because elderly tend to eat less food they are at greater risk of not getting sufficient vitamins and minerals. In Canada below-recommended intakes have been commonly observed for protein, vitamins A, D, C, and B_6, β-carotene, calcium, and zinc (49,50). In a group of frail elderly receiving community services, 88–93% had energy intakes below the RNI, and more than 50% failed to meet the recommended level for protein intake (0.8 g/kg body weight) (20).

Sub-optimal nutrient intakes in elderly Canadians have been related to low consumption of grains, milk products, and fruits and vegetables (49). In the Santé Québec study between 55% and 83% of women and 33% and 77% of men aged 65–74 years did not eat the minimum number of servings recommended in Canada's Food Guide to Healthy Eating. In women below-recommended intakes were most common for milk products (83%) followed by grains (64%) and meat and alternatives (63%). In men sub-optimal intakes were mainly observed for milk products (77%). The recommended 5–10 servings/day for fruits and vegetables were met by only 45% of men and women. Average number of servings for grains, fruits and vegetables, dairy products, and meat and alternatives, were, respectively, 4.8, 5.0, 1.0, and 2.1 in women, and 7.1, 5.5, 1.3, and 3.1 in men.

Malnutrition

Long neglected by the medical profession, malnutrition is now recognized as a key determinant of morbidity and mortality in the elderly. Reports of the incidence of malnutrition in geriatric patients have ranged from 20 to 65%, depending on evaluation parameters used (21,36,37,51,52). Clinically malnutrition is often described by rapid non-intentional weight loss, low body mass index, low anthropometric measures, and a decrease in the following biochemical parameters: albumin, transferrin, hemoglobin, hematocrit, total lymphocyte count, and cholesterol (3,36,37,51). Patients with signs of malnutrition have been found to have higher mortality rates, both in hospital and following hospital discharge (51,53). The link between malnutrition and morbidity has also been clearly established with undernourished patients being more at risk of developing infections, decubitus ulcers, and life-threatening complications (37,54,55). As a consequence of their less favourable clinical outcome, malnourished patients tend to have longer mean lengths of stay in the hospital (56) and higher rates of readmission (57), both of which translate into higher hospital costs (58). In a report by Christensen (59) average charges per stay for malnourished patients were found to be roughly double those for non-malnourished patients.

Reports indicate that nutritional status of undernourished geriatric patients can be improved through proper intervention, and that such intervention can have a significant impact on clinical outcome (60). Dietary supplementation of elderly patients with fractured neck of the femur was found to reduce the number of medical complications, decrease the length of hospitalization, and reduce mortality (61). In a Canadian study (62) a weight increase of at least 5% of body weight in previously undernourished patients was associated with a decrease in the incidence of death and a reduction of morbidity events.

Given the impact of malnutrition on individuals and the health care system, nutrition screening programs have been developed in the past few years. One example of such programs, the Nutrition Screening Initiative (NSI), was initiated in 1990 in the U.S. to increase public awareness of the nutritional problems of older persons, and promote optimal nutrition with advancing age (3).

Table 1
Recommendations for Older Adults

Nutrients (RNI)		Age (years) 50–74	75 +	Suggested change
Protein (g)	M	63	59	↑ 1.0–1.25 g/kg/d
	F	54	55	
Vitamin A (μg RE)	M	1,000	1,000	↓
	F	800	800	
Vitamin D (μg)	M	5	5	↑ 10–20
	F	5	5	
Vitamin E (mg)	M	7	6	↑ 23–27*
	F	6	5	
β-carotene (mg)	M	–	–	↑ 5.2–6.0*
	F	–	–	
Vitamin C (mg)	M	40	40	↑ 217–225*
	F	30	30	
Riboflavin (mg)	M	1.2	1.0	↑ 1.3–1.7
	F	1.0	1.0	
Vitamin B_6 (mg)	M	0.95	0.89	↑ 1.90–1.96
	F	0.81	0.83	
Vitamin B_{12} (μg)	M	1.0	1.0	↑ 3.0
	F	1.0	1.0	
Folate (μg)	M	230	215	↑ 400
	F	195	200	
Calcium (mg)	M	800	800	↑ 1,000–1,500
	F	800	800	
Magnesium (mg)	M	250	230	↓
	F	210	210	

* Amounts obtained from a diet comprising at least 5 servings of fruits and vegetables per day (67).
(From references 29,63–67).

Meeting the Nutrition Needs of Elderly

An important issue related to the nutritional needs of the elderly is that of the adequacy of current RNIs (29). As in other countries Canadian RNIs for persons > 51 years have mostly been mathematical extrapolations of recommendations for younger adults. However epidemiological and clinical studies performed in the past decade suggest that many of these recommendations need to be re-evaluated (63). Nutrients whose RNIs are likely to be modified in the future are presented in table 1, along with the suggested changes.

Hence intake of protein, vitamins D, E, C, B_6, and B_{12}, folic acid, riboflavin, β-carotene, and calcium should be increased and that of vitamin A and magnesium decreased (64–67).

Recommendations for meeting the nutritional needs of the elderly will differ depending on whether they live in the community or in an institution. In community-living elderly, nutrition problems are frequently related to low food intake, so efforts should be oriented towards insuring food access and maintaining appetite. Hence assistance with transportation, shopping, and cooking may help improve the quality of the diet of those with functional limitations. Congregate meals and luncheon clubs can be suggested to those who are isolated or feel lonely. Similarly, disabled elderly may benefit from home-delivered meals (68).

In the institution efforts should be made to offer appetizing meals with high nutritive values. When intakes are insufficient, commercially available single nutrients and liquid meal replacements can help palliate the deficits. Food intake of patients can often be improved through fairly simple procedures. For instance patients with tremor or stroke disability may benefit from the use of special utensils. Similarly, proper positioning of persons with swallowing problems and discontinuation or avoidance of unnecessary restrictive diets may help increase appetite and food intake (36,51).

Conclusion

Persons over 65 represent the fastest growing segment of the Canadian population. Given the fundamental role of nutrition in maintaining health, optimizing the nutritional status of elderly should be a priority as good nutrition is likely to increase years of independent life of seniors and help contain health care costs.

REFERENCES

1 Desjardins B, Dumas J, eds. *Vieillissement de la population et personnes âgées. La conjoncture démographique.* Ottawa: Statistique Canada, cat 91-533 F hors série, 1993.
2 Casper RC. Nutrition and its relationship to aging. *Exper Gerontol* 1995;30:299–314.
3 Dwyer JT. *Screening older Americans' nutritional health. Current practices and future possibilities.* Washington: Nutrition Screening Initative, 1991.

4 Millen-Posner B, Saffel-Schrier S, Dwyer JT. Position of the American Dietetic Association: nutrition, aging, and the continuum of health care. *J Am Diet Assoc* 1993;93:80–82.

5 Rosenbloom CA, Whittington FJ. The effects of bereavement on eating behaviors and nutrient intakes in elderly widowed persons. *J Gerontol* 1993;48:223–229.

6 Bianchetti A, Rozzini R, Carabellese C et al. Nutritional intake, socio-economic conditions, and health status in a large elderly population. *J Am Geriatr Soc* 1990;38:521–526.

7 Davis MA, Murphy SP, Neuhaus JM et al. Living arrangements and dietary quality of older U.S. adults. *J Am Diet Assoc* 1990;90:1667–1672.

8 Murphy SP, Davis MA, Neuhaus JM et al. Factors influencing the dietary adequacy and energy intake of older Americans. *J Nutr Educ* 1990;22:284–291.

9 Walker D, Beauchene RE. The relationship of loneliness, social isolation, and physical health to dietary adequacy of independently living elderly. *J Am Diet Assoc* 1991;91:300–304.

10 Thompson MP, Morris LK. Unexplained weight loss in the ambulatory elderly. *J Am Geriatr Soc* 1991;39:497–500.

11 Roe DA. *Geriatric nutrition*, 3rd ed. New Jersey: Prentice Hall,1992.

12 Ship JA, Duffy V, Jones JA. Geriatric oral health and its impact on eating. *J Am Geriatr Soc* 1996;44:456–464.

13 Schiffman S. Changes in taste and smell: drug interactions and food preferences. *Nutr Rev* 1994;52:S11–S14.

14 Sekuler R, Blake R. Sensory underload. *Psychol Today* 1987;12:48–51.

15 Duffy VB, Backstrand JR, Ferris AM. Olfactory dysfunction and related nutritional risk in free-living, elderly women. *J Am Diet Assoc* 1995;95:879–884.

16 Weinberg AD, Minaker KL, Council on Scientific Affairs, American Medical Association. Dehydration. Evaluation and management in older adults. *JAMA* 1995;274:1552–1556.

17 Hoffman N. Diet in the elderly. Needs and risks. *Med Clin North Amer* 1993;77:745–756.

18 The Canadian Dental Association. *Canada health monitor report on the spring 1991 poll*. Ottawa: Canadian Dental Association, 1991.

19 Millen Posner B, Jette A, Smigelski C et al. Nutritional risk in New England elders. *J Gerontol* 1994;49:M123–M132.

20 Payette H, Gray-Donald K, Cyr R et al. Predictors of dietary intake in a functional dependent elderly population in the community. *Am J Public Health* 1995;85:677–683.

21 Keller HH. Malnutrition in institutionalized elderly: how and why? *J Am Geriatr Soc* 1993;41:1212–1218.

22 Sullivan DH, Martin W, Flaxman N et al. Oral health problems and involuntary weight loss in a population of frail elderly. *J Am Geriatr Soc* 1993;41:725–731.

23 National Institute of Nutrition. *Food and nutrition opportunities in the seniors' market. A situational analysis.* Ottawa: 1996.

24 Krasinski SD, Russell RM, Samloff IM et al. Fundic atrophic gastritis in an elderly population: effect on hemoglobin and several serum nutritional indicators. *J Am Geriatr Soc* 1986;34:800–806.

25 Suter PM, Golner BB, Goldin BR et al. Reversal of protein-bound vitamin B_{12} malabsorption with antibiotics in atrophic gastritis. *Gastroenterology* 1991;101:1039–1045.

26 Nickols-Richardson S, Johnson MA, Poon LW et al. Mental health and number of illnesses are predictors of nutritional risk in elderly persons. *Exper Aging Res* 1996:22:141–154.

27 Rissanen PM, Laakkonen EI, Suntioinen S et al. The nutritional status of Finnish home-living elderly people and the relationship between energy intake and chronic disease. *Age Ageing* 1996;25:133–138.

28 Atkinson SA. Optimizing bone health. *Rapport* 1995;10:10.

29 Health and Welfare Canada. *Nutrition recommendations: the report of the scientific review committee.* Ottawa: 1990.

30 Optimal calcium intake. NIH consensus statement. 1994;12:1–31.

31 Santé Québec, Bertrand L (sous la direction de): *Les Québécoises et les Québécois mangent-ils mieux? Rapport de l'enquête québécoise sur la nutrition, 1990.* Montréal: Ministère de la Santé et des Services sociaux, gouvernement du Québec, 1995.

32 Fonseca V, Wall J. Diet and diabetes in the elderly. *Clin Geriatr Med* 1995;11:613–624.

33 The Canadian Diabetes Association, National Nutrition Committee: *Diabetes and meal planning: a new philosophy opens choices.* Insert in *J Can Diet Assoc* 1995;56(3).

34 Canadian Study of Health and Aging Working Group. Canadian study of health and aging: study methods and prevalence of dementia. *Can Med Assoc J* 1994;150:899–913.

35 Gray GE. Nutrition and dementia. *J Am Diet Assoc* 1989;89:1795–1802.

36 Morley JE, Silver AJ. Nutritional issues in nursing home care. *Ann Intern Med* 1995;123:850–859.

37 Kerstetter JE, Holthausen BA, Fitz PA. Malnutrition in the institutionalized older adult. *J Am Diet Assoc* 1992;92:1109–1116.

38 Wolf-Klein GP, Silverstone FA. Weight loss in Alzheimer's disease: an international review of the literature. *Int Psychogeriatr* 1994;6:135–142.

39 Sandman PO, Adolfsson R, Nygren C et al. Nutritional status and dietary intake in institutionalized patients with Alzheimer's disease and multiinfarct dementia. *J Am Geriatr Soc* 1987;35:31–38.

40 Litchford MD, Wakefield LM. Nutrient intakes and energy expenditures of residents with senile dementia of the Alzheimer's type. *J Am Diet Assoc* 1987;87:211–213.

41 Rheaume Y, Riley ME, Volicer L. Meeting nutritional needs of Alzheimer patients who pace constantly. *J Nutr Elderly* 1987;7:43–52.

42 Wolf-Klein GP, Silverstone FA, Lansey SC et al. Energy requirements in Alzheimer's disease patients. *Nutrition* 1995;11:264–268.

43 Chrischilles EA, Foley DJ, Wallace RB et al. Use of medication by persons 65 and over: data from the established populations for epidemiologic studies of the elderly. *J Gerontol* 1992;47:M137–M144.

44 Varma RN. Risk for drug-induced malnutrition is unchecked in elderly patients in nursing homes. *J Am Diet Assoc* 1994;94:192–194.

45 Beers MH, Ouslander JG, Rollingher I et al. Explicit criteria for determining inappropriate medication use in nursing home residents. *Arch Intern Med* 1991;151:1825–1832.

46 Jones JK. Drugs and the elderly. In: Reichel W, ed. *Clinical aspects of aging*. Baltimore: Williams & Wilkins, 1989:41–60.

47 Lewis CW, Frongillo EA, Roe DA. Drug-nutrient interactions in three long-term-care facilities. *J Am Diet Assoc* 1995;95:309–315.

48 Nova Scotia Department of Health and Department of National Health and Welfare: *Report of the Nova Scotia Nutrition Survey, 1987.* Halifax: Nova Scotia Department of Health, 1993.

49 Yeung DL, Imbach A. Geriatric nutrition in Canada – a review. *J Nutr Elderly* 1988;7:27–45.

50 Chandra RK, Imbach A, Moore C et al. Nutrition of the elderly. *Can Med Assoc J* 1991;145:1475–1487.

51 Abbasi AA, Rudman D. Undernutrition in the nursing home: prevalence, consequences, causes and prevention. *Nutr Rev* 1994;52:113–122.

52 Fischer J, Johnson MA. Low body weight and weight loss in the aged. *J Am Diet Assoc* 1990;90:1697–1706.

53 Sullivan DH, Walls RC, Bopp MM. Protein-energy undernutrition and the risk of mortality within one year of hospital discharge: a follow-up study. *J Am Geriatr Soc* 1995;43:507–512.

54 Pinchcofsky-Devin GD, Kaminski MV. Correlation of pressure sores and nutritional status. *J Am Geriatr Soc* 1986;34:435–440.

55 Sullivan DH, Walls RC. The risk of life-threatening complications in a select population of geriatric patients: the impact of nutritional status. *J Am Coll Nutr* 1995;14:29–36.

56 Ferguson RP, O'Connor P, Crabtree B et al. Serum albumin and prealbumin as predictors of clinical outcomes of hospitalized elderly nursing home residents. *J Am Geriatr Soc* 1993;41:545–549.

57 Sullivan DH. Risk factors for early hospital readmission in a select population of geriatric rehabilitation patients: the significance of nutritional status. *J Am Geriatr Soc* 1992;40:792–798.

58 Reilly JJ, Hull SF, Albert N et al. Economic impact of malnutrition: a model system for hospitalized patients. *JPEN* 1988;12:371–376.

59 Christensen KS. Hospitalwide screening increases revenue under prospective payment system. *J Am Diet Assoc* 1986;86:1234–1235

60 Larsson J, Unosson M, Ek AC et al. Effect of dietary supplement on nutritional status and clinical outcome in 501 geriatric patients – a randomised study. *Clin Nutr* 1990;9:179–184.

61 Delmi M, Rapin C-H, Bengoa J-M et al. Dietary supplementation in the elderly patients with fractured neck of the femur. *Lancet* 1990;335:1013–1016.

62 Keller HH. Weight gain impacts morbidity and mortality in institutionalized older persons. *J Am Geriatr Soc* 1995;43:165–169.

63 Tucker K. Micronutrient status and aging. *Nutr Rev* 1995;53:S9–S15.

64 Russell RM, Suter PM. Vitamin requirements of elderly people: an update. *Am J Clin Nutr* 1993;58:4–14.

65 Wood RJ, Suter PM, Russell RM. Mineral requirements of elderly poeple. *Am J Clin Nutr* 1995;62:493–505.

66 Campbell WW, Crim MC, Dallal GE et al. Increased protein requirements in elderly people: new data and retrospective reassessment. *Am J Clin Nutr* 1994;60:501–509.

67 Lachance P, Langseth L. The RDA concept: time for a change? *Nutr Rev* 1994;52:266–270.

68 Davies L, Carr Knutson K. Warning signals for malnutrition in the elderly. *J Am Diet Assoc* 1991;91:1413–1417.

Diet and Cancer

Dietary
Mutagens and Carcinogens:
Heterocyclic Amines

1 Heterocyclic Amine Mutagenicity and Carcinogenicity

Epidemiological studies have indicated that environmental factors, especially dietary factors, are closely related to the development of human cancer (1). A variety of naturally occurring mutagens/carcinogens, such as mycotoxins, fermentation-associated compounds, pyrolysis products, and other harmful substances of plant origin, may exist in foods, and their identification must be the first step in determining their contribution to cancer in humans.

The discovery of the mutagenic potential of cooked meat and fish in *Salmonella typhimurium* TA98, in the presence of s9 mix, metabolic activation system, led us to search for the individual responsible mutagens. Monitoring of mutagenicity to *S. typhimurium* TA98 or TA1538 has now led to more than 20 heterocyclic amines (HCAs) being isolated from a variety of heated materials, including cooked food, pyrolysis products of amino acids, and proteins (2–6). The chemical names and abbreviations are listed in table 1 and the chemical structures in figure 1. They are classified into 2-amino-3-

The studies carried out at the National Cancer Center Research Institute that are discussed in this review were supported in part by Grants-in-Aid for Cancer Research from the Ministry of Health and Welfare and the Ministry of Education, Science, Sports and Culture, Japan; a Grant-in-Aid from the Ministry of Health and Welfare for the Second-Term Comprehensive 10-Year Strategy for Cancer Control, Japan; and a Research Grant from the Princess Takamatsu Cancer Research Fund.

methylimidazo[4,5-f]quinoline (IQ)-type compounds, having a 2-aminoimidazole moiety as a common structure, and non-IQ-type compounds, having a 2-aminopyridine moiety in common. All the HCAs so far identified have demonstrated higher mutagenicity in *S. typhimurium* TA98, a detector of frameshift mutations, than in *S. typhimurium* TA100, used for detecting mutations leading to base-pair changes, with S9 mix. The numbers of revertants with HCAs in TA98 range from 2 to 661,000 per μg, a 10^5-fold difference in magnitude (2,4). Some HCAs exhibit greater mutagenicity than such typical strong mutagens/carcinogens as aflatoxin B_1, 4-nitroquinoline 1-oxide, and benzo[a]pyrene. A new *Salmonella* tester strain, YG1024, which has high O-acetyltransferase level due to introduction of plasmids containing the acetyltransferase gene from *S. typhimurium* TA1538 into TA98, has been found to be much more sensitive to HCAs than TA98 itself (7). Some of the HCAs are also mutagenic in Chinese hamster lung cells with diphtheria toxin resistance (8), and induce chromosomal aberrations and sister chromatid exchanges in cultured cells *in vitro* (9–12).

The carcinogenicity of HCAs has been extensively examined in CDF_1 mice and F344 rats of both sexes, with chronic administration of pellet diets containing doses of 100–800 ppm throughout the experiments. Ten HCAs so far tested were all demonstrated to be carcinogenic (2,4,13–16). The target organs vary with the chemical and the animal species, as shown in table 2. In rats tumours were found in the liver, small and large intestines, Zymbal glands, clitoral gland, skin, oral cavity, urinary bladder, and prostate and mammary glands. In mice tumours were observed in the liver, forestomach, lung, hematopoietic system, lymphoid tissue, and blood vessels. All the HCAs except PhIP are capable of inducing tumours in the livers of rats and mice. Interestingly PhIP was found to cause colon, prostate, and mammary carcinomas in rats and lymphomas in mice (14–16). One of the HCAs, IQ, has also proven to be carcinogenic in monkeys, inducing hepatomas (17).

2 HCA Metabolic Activation and DNA Adduct Formation

HCAs are metabolically oxidized by CYP1A2 to generate N-hydroxyamino derivatives, these then being further activated by esterification with acetic acid and sulfuric acid to the ultimate reactive forms that react with DNA bases (18,19). *In vitro* N-acetoxy-2-amino-3,8-dimethylimidazo[4,5-f]quinoxaline (N-acetoxy-MeIQx), the ultimate form of MeIQx, reacts with deoxyguanosine to produce two kinds of adducts, one major, N^2-(deoxyguanosin-8-yl)-2-amino-3,8-dimethylimidazo[4,5-f]quinoxaline(dG-C8-MeIQx), and one minor, 5-(deoxyguanosin-N^2-yl)-2-amino-3,8-dimethylimidazo[4,5-f]quinoxaline(dG-N^2-MeIQx) (20,21). The dG-C8-MeIQx adduct has also been found to be produced *in vivo*, such as in the liver of rats given MeIQx (20). In contrast no data are presently available concerning dG-N^2-MeIQx *in vivo*. In the case of 2-amino-1-methyl-6-phenylimidazo[4,5-b]pyridine (PhIP), the ultimate form reacts with guanine bases of DNA to form dG-C8-PhIP both *in vitro* and *in vivo* (22–24). The metabolic pathways of MeIQx and PhIP are illustrated in figure 2.

Examination of cancers developing in rats treated with MeIQx for mutations of Ha-*ras* and *p*53 genes revealed two of six squamous cell carcinomas of the Zymbal gland to have point mutations of Ha-*ras*, one a G to T transversion in codon 13 and the other an A to T transversion in codon 61 (25). Four mutations in the *p*53 gene were also observed in three of thirteen hepatocellular carcinomas of rats (26). Three had G to T transversions and the remaining one had a C to G transversion. These results suggest that modification of guanine bases by adduct formation is involved in the gene alterations in Zymbal gland and liver cancers induced by MeIQx.

Similar analysis of rat mammary carcinomas induced by PhIP demonstrated three of seventeen carcinomas to have G to A transitions at the second position of Ha-*ras* codon 12. One of ten carcinomas examined exhibited a G to T transversion at the third position of codon 130 of the *p*53 gene (27). Especially noteworthy is the demonstration of a specific mutation of the *Apc* gene in five of eight rat colon tumours induced by PhIP. All five demonstrated deletion of a guanine base at a 5′-GGGA-3′ site (28). Thus formation of adducts at guanine bases is also most likely to be related to PhIP-induced mammary and colon carcinogenesis.

3 Human Exposure to HCAs

To evaluate the risk of HCAs for cancer causation in humans, the levels of exposure must be determined. We measured amounts in various kinds of cooked foods using a combination of blue cotton treatment and HPLC and found PhIP to be the most abundant HCA, present at levels of 0.56–69.2 ng per g. The level of 4′-OH-PhIP was second highest, at 0.28–21.0 ng per g, followed by MeIQx at 0.64–6.44 ng per g. Other HCAs were detected at levels of 0.03–4.18 ng per g (4,29).

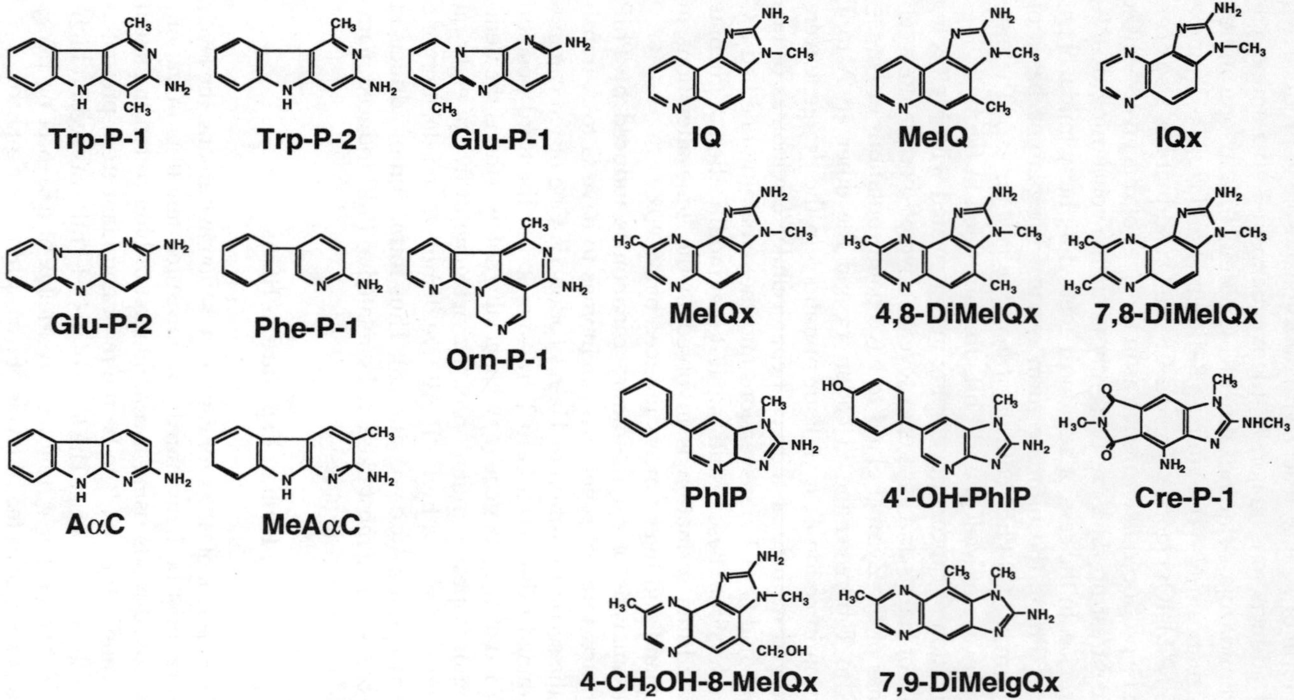

Figure 1. Structures of heterocyclic amines.

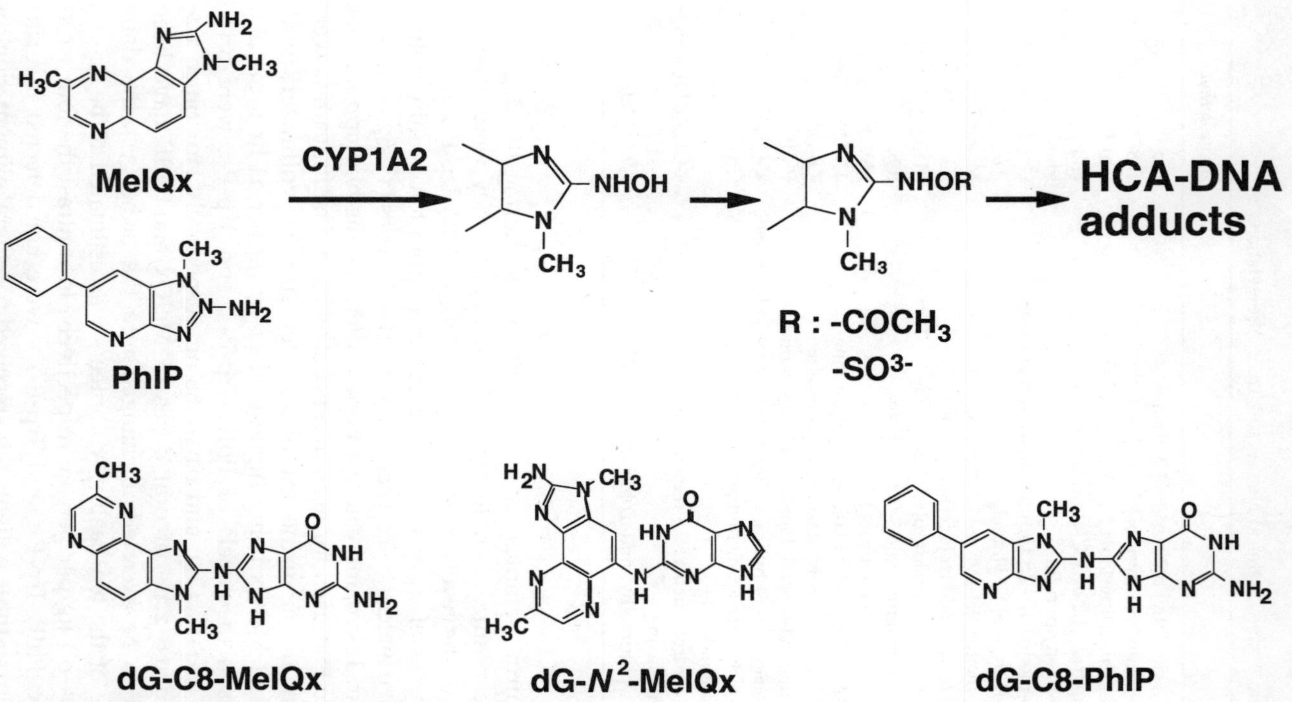

Figure 2. Metabolic activation pathways of MeIQx and PhIP.

Table 1
Heterocyclic Amine Chemical Names and Their Abbreviations

Chemical name	Abbreviation
3-Amino-1,4-dimethyl-5H-pyrido[4,3-b]indole	Trp-P-1
3-Amino-1-methyl-5H-pyrido[4,3-b]indole	Trp-P-2
2-Amino-6-methyldipyrido[1,2-a: 3′,2′-d]imidazole	Glu-P-1
2-Aminodipyrido]1,2-a: 3′,2′-d]imidazole	Glu-P-2
2-Amino-5-phenylpyridine	Phe-P-1
4-Amino-6-methyl-1H-2,5,10,10b-tetraazafluoranthene	Orn-P-1
2-Amino-9H-pyrido[2,3-b]indole	AαC
2-Amino-3-methyl-9H-pyrido[2,3-b]indole	MeAαC
2-Amino-3-methylimidazo[4,5-f]quinoline	IQ
2-Amino-3,4-dimethylimidazo[4,5-f]quinoline	MeIQ
2-Amino-3-methylimidazo[4,5-f]quinoxaline	IQx
2-Amino-3,8-dimethylimidazo[4,5-f]quinoxaline	MeIQx
2-Amino-3,4,8-trimethylimidazo[4,5-f]quinoxaline	4,8-DiMeIQx
2-Amino-3,7,8-trimethylimidazo[4,5-f]quinoxaline	7,8-DiMeIQx
2-Amino-1-methyl-6-phenylimidazo[4,5-b]pyridine	PhIP
2-Amino-1-methyl-6-(4-hydroxyphenyl)imidazo[4,5-b]pyridine	4′-OH-PhIP
4-Amino-1,6-dimethyl-2-methylamino-1H,6H-pyrrolo-[3,4-f]benzimidazole-5,7-dione	Cre-P-1
2-Amino-4-hydroxymethyl-3,8-dimethylimidazo-[4,5-f]quinolaxine	4-CH$_2$OH-8-MeIQx
2-Amino-1,7,9-trimethylimidazo[4,5-g]quinoxaline	7,9-DiMeIgQx

Since urine samples are convenient for monitoring the degree of human exposure to environmental carcinogens, they were used for analysis of the levels of four HCAs – MeIQx, PhIP, Trp-P-1 and Trp-P-2. Samples of 24-hr urine were obtained from ten healthy volunteers – five males (33–80 years old) and five females (13–67 years old) – living in Tokyo and eating a normal diet. The method applied was similar to that used for examining cooked food. The four HCAs were found in all the urine samples of ten healthy volunteers with amounts of MeIQx being highest, at 11–47 ng per 24-hr urine. For comparison the levels of PhIP, Trp-P-1, and Trp-P-2 were 0.12–1.97 ng, 0.04–1.43 ng, and 0.03–0.68 ng, respectively (30). Since 1.2–4.3% and 0.6–2.3% of oral doses of MeIQx and PhIP have been reported to be excreted unchanged into the urine (31), the daily exposure of the ten healthy volunteers was estimated to be 0.3–3.9 and 0.005–0.3 μg per person, respectively. In contrast the four HCAs – MeIQx, PhIP, Trp-P-1 and Trp-P-2 – were not detected in urine samples from three patients who received parenteral alimentation for

Table 2
Carcinogenicities of Heterocyclic Amines in Rats and Mice

Chemical	Species	Concentration (%)	Target organs
IQ	Rats	0.03	Liver, small & large intestines, Zymbal gland, clitoral gland, skin
	Mice	0.03	Liver, forestomach, lung
MeIQ	Rats	0.03	Large intestine, Zymbal gland, skin, oral cavity, mammary gland
	Mice	0.04, 0.01	Liver, forestomach
MeIQx	Rats	0.04	Liver, Zymbal gland, clitoral gland, skin
	Mice	0.06	Liver, lung, hematopoietic system
PhIP	Rats	0.04	Large intestine, mammary gland, prostate
	Mice	0.04	Lymphoid tissue
Trp-P-1	Rats	0.015	Liver
	Mice	0.02	Liver
Trp-P-2	Rats	0.01	Urinary bladder, clitoral gland
	Mice	0.02	Liver
Glu-P-1	Rats	0.05	Liver, small & large intestines, Zymbal gland, clitoral gland
	Mice	0.05	Liver, blood vessels
Glu-P-2	Rats	0.05	Liver, small & large intestines, Zymbal gland, clitoral gland
	Mice	0.05	Liver, blood vessels
AαC	Mice	0.08	Liver, blood vessels
MeAαC	Rats	0.02, 0.01	Liver
	Mice	0.08	Liver, blood vessels

one day before and two to four days after surgery (30). It has in fact been reported that urinary levels of MeIQx in residents of Los Angeles are positively associated with intake of cooked meat (32). From the available observations it is evident that humans are continuously exposed to low levels of HCAs derived from diet in our daily life.

Because the level of MeIQx in human urine was highest among the four HCAs analyzed, we next analyzed MeIQx-DNA adducts in human surgical and autopsy tissue samples by the ^{32}P-postlabeling method, under adduct intensification conditions with additional nuclease P1 and phosphodiesterase I digestion after kination at the 5'-hydroxyl termini.

Surgical specimens were obtained from eight Japanese patients (subjects I–VIII), undergoing operations for colorectal, liver, or renal cancers. DNA samples were prepared from apparently non-tumourous tissue surrounding the tumours. Autopsy specimens of liver, kidney, colon, pancreas, lung, and heart were also obtained from each of five

Table 3
Levels of dG-C8-MeIQx in Surgical and Autopsy Specimens

Subject	Age (years)	Sex	Disease	Test organ	
SURGICAL SPECIMENS					
I	46	M	Colon cancer	Transverse colon	N.D.[c]
II	63	M	Rectum cancer	Sigmoid colon	14 / 10^{10}
III	67	F	Colon cancer	Rectum	18 / 10^{10}
IV	68	M	Colon cancer	Transverse colon	N.D.
V	58	F	Liver cancer	Liver	N.D.
VI	65	M	Liver cancer	Liver	N.D.
VII	68	M	Renal cancer	Kidney	N.D.
VIII	69	M	Renal cancer	Kidney	N.D.
AUTOPY SPECIMENS					
IX	54	M	Cerebral hemorrhage	Six organs[a]	N.D.
X	71	M	Heart failure	Six organs[a]	N.D.
XI	74	M	Respiratory failure	Six organs[a]	N.D.
XII	81	M	Acute myocardial infarction	Six organs[a]	1.8 / 10^{10} (kidney)
XIII	81	M	Cerebral hemorrhage	Six organs[a]	N.D.

[a] DNA was isolated from six organs – the liver, kidney, colon, pancreas, lung, and heart.
[b] All DNA samples were analyzed twice, and the values are the means of the two assay results.
[c] N.D.: Not detectable ($< 1/10^{10}$ nucleotides).

Japanese patients (subjects IX–XIII) within two hours of death from diseases other than cancers (see table 3 for details).

Among 38 DNA samples obtained from 8 surgical and 30 autopsy specimens, 3 were found to contain an adduct spot corresponding to the standard 5'-pdG-C8-MeIQx. Two were surgical specimens of colon (subject II) and rectum (subject III) and one was an autopsy specimen of kidney (subject XII), and values for their relative adduct labeling (RAL) were 14, 18, and 1.8/10^{10} nucleotides, respectively (table 3) (33). Each adduct spot was extracted from TLC and identified to be 5'-pdG-C8-MeIQx by HPLC. The RAL of 5'-pdG-C8-MeIQx for other DNA samples was less than 1/10^{10} nucleotides, if present. Differences in MeIQx-DNA adduct levels from person to person are most likely due to variation in intake of MeIQx, capacity for metabolic activation and detoxification, and DNA adduct repair efficiency.

Several epidemiological studies have now been published indicating a positive association between consumption of cooked meat and development of such neoplasms as colorectal, pancreatic, and urothelial cancers (34–37). In addition it has also been demonstrated that the highest risk phenotype (rapid CYP1A2 and rapid NAT-2) combined with a dietary preference for well-done red meat has a relative odds ratio of 6.45 for colorectal cancer risk (38). The findings thus suggest that even if human exposure to HCAs is at microgram levels per day per person, DNA adducts are nevertheless formed in human organs and that these could be involved in cancer development in humans. This situation may also be true for other environmental carcinogens. Therefore it is important that exposure to known carcinogenic agents, including HCAs, should be reduced as far as possible with any available measures that are realistic and not so inconvenient as to cause an adverse impact.

REFERENCES

1 Doll R, Peto R. The causes of cancer: quantitative estimates of avoidable risks of cancer in the United States today. *J Natl Cancer Inst* 1981;66:1191–1308.

2 Sugimura T. Studies on environmental chemical carcinogenesis in Japan. *Science* 1986;233:312–318.

3 Sugimura T. Multistep carcinogenesis: a 1992 perspective. *Science* 1992;258:603–607.

4 Wakabayashi K, Nagao M, Esumi H, Sugimura T. Food-derived mutagens and carcinogens. *Cancer Res* 1992;52:2092s–2098s.

5 Felton JS, Knize MG, Shen NH, Lewis PR, Andresen BD, Happe J, Hatch FT. The isolation and identification of a new mutagen from fried ground beef: 2-amino-1-methyl-6-phenylimidazo[4,5-*b*]pyridine (PhIP). *Carcinogenesis* 1986;7:1081–1086.

6 Becher G, Knize MG, Nes IF, Felton JS. Isolation and identification of mutagens from a fried Norwegian meat product. *Carcinogenesis* 1988;9:247–253.

7 Watanabe M, Ishidate M, Jr, Nohmi T. Sensitive method for the detection of mutagenic nitroarenes and aromatic amines: new derivatives of *Salmonella typhimurium* tester strains possessing elevated *O*-acetyltransferase levels. *Mutat Res* 1990;234:337–348.

8 Nakayasu M, Nakasato F, Sakamoto H, Terada M, Sugimura T. Mutagenic activity of heterocyclic amines in Chinese hamster lung cells with diphtheria toxin resistance as a marker. *Mutat Res* 1983;118:91–102.

9 Ishidate M, Jr, Sofuni T, Yoshikawa K. Chromosomal aberration tests *in vitro* as a primary screening tool for environmental mutagens and/ or carcinogens. In: Inui N, Kuroki T, Yamada M, Heidelberger C, eds. *Mutation, promotion and transformation in vitro, GANN monograph on cancer research* no. 27. Tokyo: Japan Sci. Soc. Press 1981:95–108.

10 Tohda H, Oikawa A, Kawachi T, Sugimura T. Induction of sister-chromatid exchanges by mutagens from amino acid and protein pyrolysates. *Mutat Res* 1980;77:65–69.

11 Holme JA, Wallin H, Brunborg G, Soderlund EJ, Hongslo JK, Alexander J. Genotoxicity of the food mutagen 2-amino-1-methyl-6-phenylimidazo[4,5-*b*]pyridine (PhIP): formation of 2-hydroxyamino-PhIP, a directly acting genotoxic metabolite. *Carcinogenesis* 1989;10: 1389–1396.

12 Aeschbacher HU, Ruch E. Effect of heterocyclic amines and beef extract on chromosome aberrations and sister chromatid exchanges in cultured human lymphocytes. *Carcinogenesis* 1989;10:429–433.

13 Ohgaki H, Takayama S, Sugimura T. Carcinogenicities of heterocyclic amines in cooked food. *Mutat Res* 1991;259:399–410.

14 Esumi H, Ohgaki H, Kohzen E, Takayama S, Sugimura T. Induction of lymphoma in CDF₁ mice by the food mutagen, 2-amino-1-methyl-6-phenylimidazo[4,5-*b*]pyridine. *Jpn J Cancer Res* 1989;80:1176–1178.

15 Ito N, Hasegawa R, Sano M, Tamano S, Esumi H, Takayama S, Sugimura T. A new colon and mammary carcinogen in cooked food, 2-amino-1-methyl-6-phenylimidazo[4,5-*b*]pyridine (PhIP). *Carcinogenesis* 1991;12:1503–1506.

16 Shirai T, Sano M, Tamano S, Takahashi S, Hirose M, Futakuchi M, Hasegawa R, Imaida K, Matsumoto K, Wakabayashi K, Sugimura T, Ito N. The prostate: a target for carcinogenicity of 2-amino-1-methyl-6-phenylimidazo[4,5-*b*]pyridine (PhIP) derived from cooked foods. *Cancer Res*, 1997;195–198.

17 Adamson RH, Thorgeirsson UP, Snyderwine EG, Thorgeirsson SS, Reeves J, Dalgard DW, Takayama S, Sugimura T. Carcinogenicity of 2-amino-3-methylimidazo[4,5-*f*]quinoline in nonhuman primates: induction of tumors in three macaques. *Jpn J Cancer Res* 1990;81:10–14.

18 Kato R, Yamazoe Y. Metabolic activation and covalent binding to nucleic acids of carcinogenic heterocyclic amines from cooked foods and amino acid pyrolysates. *Gann* 1987;78:297–311.

19 Aoyama T, Gonzalez FJ, Gelboin HV. Mutagen activation by cDNA-expressed P1450, P3450, and P450a. *Mol Carcinog* 1989;1:253–259.

20 Ochiai M, Nagaoka H, Wakabayashi K, Tanaka Y, Kim SB, Tada A, Nukaya H, Sugimura T, Nagao M. Identification of N²-(deoxyguanosin-8-yl)-2-amino-3,8-dimethylimidazo[4,5-*f*]quinoxaline 3',5'-diphosphate,

a major DNA adduct, detected by nuclease P1 modification of the
^{32}P-postlabeling method, in the liver of rats fed MeIQx. *Carcinogenesis*
1993;14:2165–2170.
21 Turesky RJ, Rossi SC, Welti DH, Lay JO, Jr, Kadlubar FF. Characterization of DNA adducts formed *in vitro* by reaction of N-hydroxy-2-amino-3-methylimidazo[4,5-*f*]quinoline and N-hydroxy-2-amino-3,8-dimethylimidazo[4,5-*f*]quinoxaline at the C-8 and N^2 atoms of guanine. *Chem Res Toxicol* 1992;5:479–490.
22 Frandsen H, Grivas S, Andersson R, Dragsted L, Larsen JC. Reaction of the N^2-acetoxy derivative of 2-amino-1-methyl-6-phenylimidazo[4,5-*b*]pyridine (PhIP) with 2'-deoxyguanosine and DNA. Synthesis and identification of N^2-(2'-deoxyguanosin-8-yl)-PhIP. *Carcinogenesis* 1992;13:629–635.
23 Lin D, Kaderlik KR, Turesky RJ, Miller DW, Lay JO, Jr, Kadlubar FF. Identification of N-(deoxyguanosin-8-yl)-2-amino-1-methyl-6-phenylimidazo[4,5-*b*]pyridine as the major adduct formed by the food-borne carcinogen, 2-amino-1-methyl-6-phenylimidazo[4,5-*b*]pyridine, with DNA. *Chem Res Toxicol* 1992;5:691–697.
24 Fukutome K, Ochiai M, Wakabayashi K, Watanabe S, Sugimura T, Nagao M. Detection of guanine-C8-2-amino-1-methyl-6-phenylimidazo[4,5-*b*]pyridine adduct as a single spot on thin-layer chromatography by modification of the ^{32}P-postlabeling method. *Jpn J Cancer Res* 1994;85:113–117.
25 Kudo M, Ogura T, Esumi H, Sugimura T. Mutational activation of c-Ha-*ras* gene in squamous cell carcinomas of rat zymbal gland induced by carcinogenic heterocyclic amines. *Mol Carcinog* 1991;4:36–42.
26 Ushijima T, Makino H, Kakiuchi H, Inoue R, Sugimura T, Nagao M. Genetic alterations in HCA-induced tumors. In: Adamson RH, Gustafsson J, Ito N, Nagao M, Sugimura T, Wakabayashi K, Yamazoe Y, eds. *Heterocyclic amines in cooked foods: possible human cancer.* Princeton: Princeton Sci Publ, 1995:281–291.
27 Ushijima T, Kakiuchi H, Makino H, Hasegawa R, Ishizaka Y, Hirai H, Yazaki Y, Ito N, Sugimura T, Nagao M. Infrequent mutation of Ha-*ras* and *p53* in rat mammary carcinomas induced by 2-amino-1-methyl-6-phenylimidazo[4,5-*b*]pyridine. *Mol Carcinog* 1994;10:38–44.
28 Kakiuchi H, Watanabe M, Ushijima T, Toyota M, Imai K, Weisburger JH, Sugimura T, Nagao M. Specific 5'-GGGA-3' 5'-GGA-3' mutation of the *Apc* gene in rat colon tumors induced by 2-amino-1-methyl-6-phenylimidazo[4,5-*b*]pyridine. *Proc Natl Acad Sci USA* 1995;92:910–914.
29 Wakabayashi K, Ushiyama H, Takahashi M, Nukaya H, Kim SB, Hirose M, Ochiai M, Sugimura T, Nagao M. Exposure to heterocyclic amines. *Environ Health Perspect* 1993;99:129–133.

30 Ushiyama H, Wakabayashi K, Hirose M, Itoh H, Sugimura T, Nagao M. Presence of carcinogenic heterocyclic amines in urine of healthy volunteers eating normal diet, but not of inpatients receiving parenteral alimentation. *Carcinogenesis* 1991;12:1417–1422.

31 Lynch AM, Kninze MG, Boobis AR, Gooderham NJ, Davies DS, Murray S. Intra- and interindividual variability in systemic exposure in humans to 2-amino-3,8-dimethylimidazo[4,5-f]quinoxaline and 2-amino-1-methyl-6-phenylimidazo[4,5-b]pyridine, carcinogens present in cooked beef. *Cancer Res* 1992;52:6216–6223.

32 Ji H, Yu MC, Stillwell WG, Skipper PL, Ross RK, Henderson BE, Tannenbaum SR. Urinary excretion of 2-amino-3,8-dimethylimidazo [4,5-f]quinoxaline in white, black and Asian men in Los Angeles County. *Cancer Epidemiol Biomarkers Prev* 1994;3:407–411.

33 Totsuka Y, Fukutome K, Takahashi M, Takahashi S, Tada A, Sugimura T, Wakabayashi K. Presence of N^2-(deoxyguanosin-8-yl)-2-amino-3,8-dimethylimidazo[4,5-f]quinoxaline (dG-C8-MeIQx) in human tissues. *Carcinogenesis* 1996;17:1029–1034.

34 Norell SE, Ahlbom A, Erwald R, Jacobson G, Lindberg-Navier I, Olin R, Tornberg B, Wiechel KL. Diet and pancreatic cancer: a case-control study. *Am J Epidemiol* 1986;124:894–902.

35 Steineck G, Hagman U, Gerhardsson M, Norell SE. Vitamin A supplements, fried foods, fat and urothelial cancer: a case-referent study in Stockholm in 1985–87. *Int J Cancer* 1990;45:1006–1011.

36 Schiffman MH, Felton JS. Fried foods and the risk of colon cancer. *Am J Epidemiol* 1990;131:376–378.

37 Gerhardsson de Verdier M, Hagman U, Peters RK, Steineck G, Overvik E. Meat, cooking methods and colorectal cancer: a case-referent study in Stockholm. *Int J Cancer* 1991;49:520–525.

38 Lang NP, Butler MA, Massengill J, Lawson M, Stotts RC, Hauer-Jensen M, Kadlubar FF. Rapid metabolic phenotypes for acetyltransferase and cytochrome P4501A2 and putative exposure to food-borne heterocyclic amines increase the risk for colorectal cancer or polyps. *Cancer Epidemiol Biomarkers Prev* 1994;3:675–682.

JOZEF VICTOR JOOSSENS and HUGO KESTELOOT

Nutrition in Relation to Stomach Cancer and Stroke Mortality

Stomach cancer and stroke mortality were found to be strongly correlated among 18 countries in 1964 (1). From the start it was shown that this association persisted, using populations of different or identical age groups for stomach cancer and stroke, indicating that it was a population and not an individual association. Therefore it was undetectable by clinical investigation. This relationship still persists (figure 1, r = 0.71)).

Already in 1968 a quantitatively similar relation was found within countries that was confirmed later on (2,3). The regression equation from Canada, 1950 to 1992 (figure 2, r = 0.99), using the average of both sexes, confirms those findings and is not significantly different from the one obtained in figure 1. The same was true in Canada for men and women separately (r = 0.97 and 0.99, respectively) when compared with data from 34 countries. The similarity of the regression equations obtained between and within countries makes a spurious association unlikely, and favours the existence of a major factor linking both diseases.

Salt and Stomach Cancer and Stroke Mortality

Already in 1964 dietary salt intake was hypothesized to be the linking factor (1). This was confirmed for gastric cancer by several methods of investigation (ecological, case-control, prospective, and salt-preference

This research was funded by the Belgian Association Against Cancer.

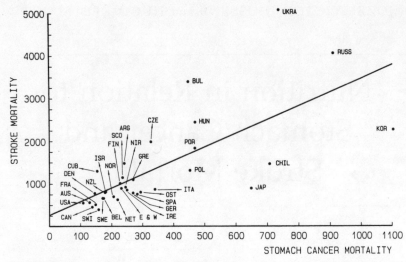

Figure 1. Positive correlation between stroke and stomach cancer mortality, using the average of both sexes in 34 countries worldwide. The values are the mean of the last three available years between 1989 and 1994, and are age-adjusted per million inhabitants 45–74 years to the age structure of the Standard European population. The regression equation of this correlation was y = 258 + 3.16x, with r = 0.71, p < 0.0001 and n = 34.

studies) (4,5) and also in a large cohort study (6). The conclusion was that a high salt intake is a risk factor for stomach cancer through the production of atrophic gastritis.

Experimental research, mostly in rats, showed that hypertonic salt solutions were co-carcinogenic when given with the carcinogen and stomach cancer–promoting when given after the carcinogen (7). The underlying molecular mechanism proposed is through induction of ornithine decarboxylase and increased mitotic activity. Inhibitors of ornithine decarboxylase inhibit the co-carcinogenic action of salt (8). A high salt intake also produces atrophic gastritis in mice (9).

The relation between salt and blood pressure and between blood pressure and stroke is well documented, but the association of salt intake and stroke is only provided by ecological studies (10). A possible confounding factor is fat intake, especially saturated fat, which promotes cerebral thrombosis, and polyunsaturated fat, which may play a protective role. Fat intake by its inverse relationship to salt intake could spuriously seem to protect against stomach cancer.

It is widely accepted that fruits and vegetables protect against stomach cancer (4,5,11), and they may also be protective against

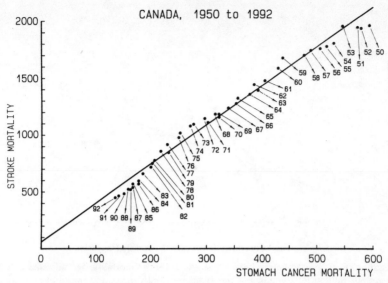

Figure 2. Positive correlation between stroke and stomach cancer mortality. The values are age-adjusted 45–74 years per million inhabitants and the average of both sexes, using data of singular years from 1950 to 1992 in Canada. The regression equation of this correlation is y = 46 + 3.46x, with r = 0.991, p < 0.00001 and n = 43. There is no significant difference between the regression equations obtained among countries (figure 1) and within a country (figure 2), making a spurious association unlikely. Both diseases decreased more than fourfold over time.

stroke. However fruits and vegetables are only useful in the presence of harmful factors and do not confound the relation between stroke and stomach cancer mortality, since they are presumed to be protective for both diseases. The within-country relationship of stomach cancer and stroke is consistent with the decline in salt intake observed in Belgium, Switzerland, and Finland and best documented in Japan where the salt intake measured by 24-hr urine excretion in the fifties was halved in the eighties (12). The decline in salt intake at the population level is mainly due to the massive introduction of refrigerators (from 1930 onwards in the U.S. and from 1965 in Japan), and since the seventies to health education, at least in certain countries (12).

Nitrate, Salt, and Stomach Cancer Mortality

The role of nitrate in stomach cancer mortality is still controversial. Nitrate in drinking water in France and the U.K. was negatively

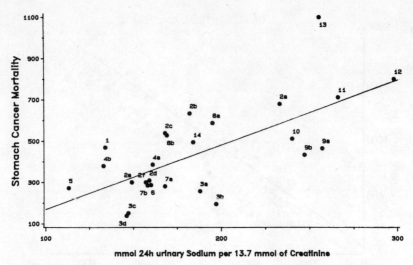

Figure 3. Positive correlation between stomach cancer mortality, age adjusted 45–74 years per million inhabitants and the average of both sexes, and mmol of 24-hr urinary sodium excretion standardized to 13.7 mmol of creatinine. The latter was done in order to correct for errors in urine collection and differences in weight among the countries. The data for sodium and creatinine are from 26 references from 14 countries (1961–1983). Those data are unstandardized and uncontrolled (3). The obtained regression equation was y = −144 + 3.14x, with r = 0.68, p < 0.001 and n = 26. 1 = Netherlands, 1978; 2 = North of Belgium, 1966–1983; 3 = U.S., 1961–1977; 4 = E&W, 1978–1978; 5 = France, 1977; 6 = New Zealand, 1975; 7 = Australia, 1973–1974; 8 = FRG, 1973–1976; 9 = Finland, 1977–1979; 10 = Scotland, 1972; 11 = Portugal, 1978; 12 = Bulgaria, 1970; 13 = Japan, 1979; 14 = Italy, 1979.

associated with stomach cancer, whereas in Colombia it was positively associated (references in 12). The ECP-Intersalt study on salt and nitrate in 24 countries all over the world made the issue less controversial (12). The data for the ECP-Intersalt study were obtained in two quality-controlled laboratories (one for salt in Leuven, Belgium, and one for nitrate in Porton Down, Salisbury, England) using deep-frozen urine specimens obtained from randomized, age-stratified populations worldwide, from the previous Intersalt study (13).

When comparing the ECP-Intersalt results with previously published data obtained with unstandardized techniques and from different laboratories, the relations with stomach cancer were not significantly different (figures 3 and 4 for salt, figures 5 and 6 for nitrate). Both salt and nitrate were associated with stomach cancer, but the relationship with salt was always stronger (12). There are no

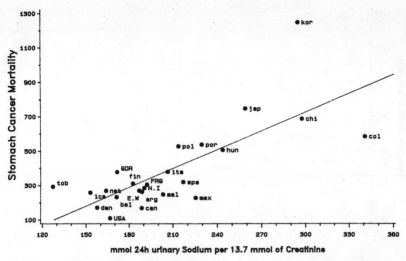

Figure 4. Positive correlation between stomach cancer mortality, age adjusted 45–74 years per million inhabitants and the average of both sexes, and mmol of 24-hr urinary sodium excretion standardized to 13.7 mmol of creatinine (average of both sexes). The data for sodium and creatinine are from the standardized and controlled ECP-Intersalt study, collected from 1986 to 1988 (13). The obtained regression equation $y = -366 + 3.65x$, $r = 0.74$, $p < 0.001$ and $n = 24$, is not significantly different from the one in figure 3, increasing thereby the reliability of the results. Chi = People's Republic of China; GDR = East Germany; FRG = West Germany.

indications that nitrate increases stroke mortality. In a multiple regression analysis nitrate in men contributed less to the level of stomach cancer mortality than salt, whereas in women the role of nitrate was not significant. However there was a possibility that nitrate enhanced the role of salt and therefore a multiple regression was performed including an interaction term: sodium*nitrate. The correlation increased to an R^2 of 0.74 ($p < 0.0001$).

When visualizing the role of salt at different levels of nitrate intake, it became clear that at lower levels of salt intake (hypotonic salt levels in the stomach) nitrate was negatively associated with stomach cancer mortality (figure 7). This relationship is probably spurious and due to an increased intake of vegetables, which are a major source of nitrates in populations with low salt intakes. On the other hand nitrate increases the risk of stomach cancer when the high salt intake produces a hypertonic stomach content (figure 7). Using the equation from nitrate and sodium*nitrate obtained in the ECP-

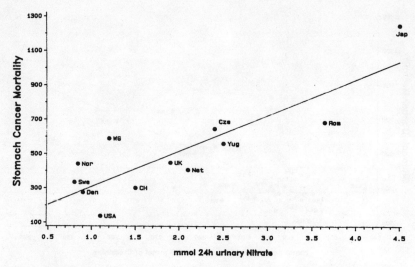

Figure 5. Positive relation between stomach cancer mortality, age adjusted 45–74 years per million inhabitants and the average of both sexes, and mmol of 24-hr urinary nitrate. The unstandardized and uncontrolled nitrate data are from reference 18. The obtained regression equation is $y = 100 + 208x$, with $r = 0.85$, $p < 0.001$ and $n = 12$. The urines were collected in the seventies and early eighties. WG = West Germany; Rom = Romania; CH = Switzerland.

Intersalt study, it is possible to calculate the stomach cancer mortality levels in 24 countries and to compare them with the observed values (figure 8).

All data were shown for the combined average of men and women in figures 1–8, but the relations obtained in men and women separately were similar.

Helicobacter pylori Infections of the Stomach and Stomach Cancer

The discovery that *Helicobacter pylori* (HP) infection of the stomach could be related to stomach cancer was hailed with great enthusiasm and a multitude of articles. The Eurogast Study (14) showed a between-countries relationship for HP infection and stomach cancer. However the Eurogast HP data also correlated significantly with salt intake (12) and this was confirmed by Japanese data (15). In certain African regions 70–80% of the inhabitants, generally with a lower salt intake (12), were infected with HP from an early age on, but stomach cancer and intestinal metaplasia were rare in those areas (16).

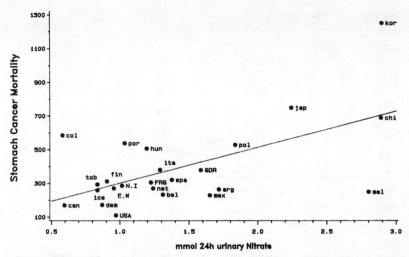

Figure 6. Positive relation between stomach cancer mortality, age adjusted 45–74 years per million inhabitants and the average of both sexes, and mmol 24h urinary nitrate. The urines were collected from 1986 to 1988. The data on nitrate excretions are derived from the standardized and controlled ECP-Intersalt study (12). The obtained regression equation y = 88 + 214x, with r = 0.59, p < 0.003 and n = 24, is not significantly different from the one in figure 5. Chi = People's Republic of China; WG = West Germany; Tob = Tobago and Trinidad; N.I = Northern Ireland.

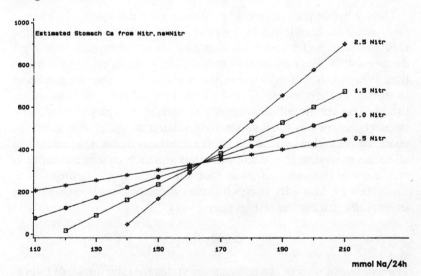

Figure 7. Multiple regression between stomach cancer mortality and 24-hr urinary nitrate and the interaction factor nitrate*sodium. The lines have a crossing point around 164 mmol sodium excretion, near to the isotonicity level of NaCl solutions (12). R^2 = 0.74, p < 0.00001 and n = 24.

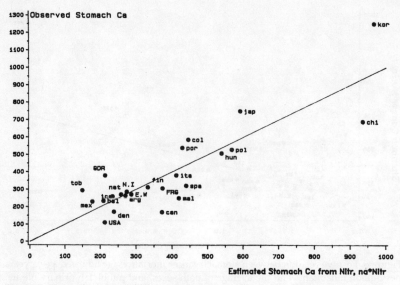

Figure 8. Using the same multiple regression equations as in figure 7 it is possible to compare the estimated with the observed stomach cancer mortality levels, using 24-hr nitrate and nitrate*sodium as independent variables. Total R^2 is now 0.74.

The HP hypothesis has never explained why the levels of HP infection are so high in Japan (15) and in China (17), and so low in the U.S. (3). The salt hypothesis explains those differences. A high dietary salt intake predisposes to atrophic gastritis and to HP infection. Whether HP infection contributes to the causation or promotion of stomach cancer mortality and to what extent remains to be established. The HP hypothesis cannot at any rate explain either why stomach cancer has been so strongly related to stroke for nearly 40 years, or why stomach cancer in 34 countries (figure 1) is related to all-cause mortality (r = 0.58), although stomach cancer mortality is only 2.6% of the mean all-cause mortality in those 34 countries. Neither can it explain why stomach cancer mortality has been declining universally during the last 40 years.

Conclusion

The salt hypothesis of stomach cancer states that the intake of hypertonic salt solutions, through their caustic properties, is the main cause of atrophic gastritis. At that stage the carcinogenic properties of nitroderivatives, synthesized from nitrate/nitrite and possibly enhanced by HP infections, can lead to stomach cancer. The present data suggest that nitrate from foods is only harmful at salt intake levels above 10 g/d. On the other hand salt intake increases blood pressure over the years, and as a consequence the risk of stroke. Antioxidants from fruits and vegetables inhibit those harmful mechanisms.

The data presented are consistent with this hypothesis. Dietary salt intake is likely the rate-limiting factor for stomach cancer and stroke mortality. A preventive strategy of consuming less salt, more fruits and vegetables, and less fat (stroke only) can be derived from those findings.

Technical Note

The data on salt and nitrate in 24 populations from the ECP-Intersalt study were median values. In this report mean values were used. However the results are very similar as already stated in reference 12.

REFERENCES

1 Joossens JV. The riddle of cancer mortality (Dutch). *Verh K Vl Acad Geneeskd Belg* 1965;27:489–545.

2 Joossens JV. La relation entre l'épidémiologie des accidents cérébro-vasculaires et du cancer de l'estomac. *L'Évolution Médicale* 1968;12:381–385.

3 Joossens JV, Kesteloot H. Salt and stomach cancer. In: Reed PI, Hill MJ, eds. *Gastric carcinogenesis*. Amsterdam: Excerpta Medica, 1988:105–126.

4 Forman D. The etiology of gastric cancer. In: O'Neill IK, Chen J, Bartsch H, eds. *Relevance to human cancer of N-nitroso compounds, tobacco smoke and mycotoxins*. Lyon: International Agency for Research on Cancer, 1991:22–31.

5 Kono S, Hirohata T. Nutrition and stomach cancer. *Cancer Causes Control* 1996;7:41–55.

6 Hirayama T. Life-style and cancer: from epidemiological evidence to public behavior change to mortality reduction to target cancers. *JNCI Monograph* 1992;12:65–74.

7 Takahashi M, Hasegawa R. Enhancing effects of dietary salt on both initiation and promotion stages of rat gastric carcinogenesis. In: Hayashi Y, Nagao M, Sugimura T et al., eds. *Diet, nutrition and cancer*. Tokyo: Japan Scientific Societies Press, 1986:169–182.

8 Tatsuta M, Iishi H, Baba M et al. Ornithine decarboxylase inhibitor
   attenuates NaCl enhancement of gastric carcinogenesis induced by N-
   methyl-N'-nitro-N-nitrosoguanidine. *Carcinogenesis* 1995;16:2107–2110.

9 Kodama M, Kodama T, Suzuki H, Kondo K. Effect of rice and salty
   rice diets on the structure of mouse stomach. *Nutr Cancer* 1984;6:135–
   147.

10 Xie J, Sasaki S, Joossens JV, Kesteloot H. The relationship between urinary cations obtained from the Intersalt study and cerebrovascular
   mortality. *J Human Hypertens* 1992;6:17–21.

11 Weisburger JH. Causes of gastric and esophageal cancer. Possible
   approach to prevention by vitamin C. *Int J Vit Nutr Res* 1985;27:381–
   402.

12 Joossens JV, Hill MJ, Elliott P et al. Dietary salt, nitrate and stomach
   cancer mortality in 24 countries. *Int J Epidemiol* 1996;25(3):494–504.

13 Intersalt Cooperative Research Group. Intersalt: an international study
   of electrolyte excretion and blood pressure. Results for 24 hour urinary
   sodium and potassium excretion. *Br Med J* 1988;297:319–328.

14 The Eurogast Study Group. An international association between *Helicobacter pylori* infection and gastric cancer. *Lancet* 1993;341:1359–1362.

15 Tsugane S, Tei Y, Takahashi T et al. Salty food intake and risk of *Helicobacter pylori* infection. *Jpn J Cancer Res* 1994;85:474–478.

16 Holcombe C. *Helicobacter pylori*: the African enigma. *Gut* 1992;33:429–
   431.

17 Chang-Claude J, Raedsch R, Waldherr R et al. Prevalence of *Helicobacter pylori* infection and gastritis among young adults in China. *Eur J
   Cancer Prev* 1995;4:73–79.

18 Hartman PE. Review: putative mutagens and carcinogens in foods. I.
   Nitrate/nitrite ingestion and gastric cancer mortality. *Environ Mutagen*
   1983;5:111–121.

GAIL McKEOWN-EYSSEN
and M. ELISABETH DEL GUIDICE

Epidemiology of Breast and Colon Cancers: Old Risk Factors, New Mechanisms?

Cancers of the breast and colon have considerable similarities in their patterns of occurrence and in dietary and lifestyle risk factors. This paper will describe these epidemiological factors and will consider the possibility that similar biological mechanisms may be involved in the development of both types of tumour.

Among Canadian women the breast is the site of cancer with the highest incidence rate and second highest mortality rate, exceeded only by that of lung cancer. The colon is the site of cancer with the third highest incidence and mortality rates, its rates being exceeded only by those of breast and lung cancers among women, and of the lung and prostate cancers among men (1). Similarly high rates of breast and colon cancers are observed elsewhere in North America and Western Europe, but rates are substantially lower in Japan and other parts of Asia (2), with incidence rates varying more than five-fold around the world. Migrants who move from low-risk to high-risk areas acquire disease rates of their new country within one or two generations (3–6). These observations strongly suggest that environmental factors play a major role in the etiology of these diseases.

That diet may be one such environmental factor was suggested over 20 years ago by the observation that indices of national per capita fat consumption were highly correlated with the incidence and mortality of breast and colon cancers (7), with correlations ranging from 0.74 (for male colon cancer incidence) to 0.89 (for female breast cancer mortality). These observations led to epidemiological studies that have explored the possibility that dietary fat and foods

that contain fat, such as meats and dairy products, may be associated
with the risk of cancer at both sites. Early international studies also
provided evidence of strong inverse correlations between sources of
dietary fibre, such as cereals, and the risk of breast and colon cancers
(7). This led to many studies examining the association between
colon cancer and dietary fibre or consumption of plant foods, but it
is only recently that associations involving plant foods or their components have been examined for breast cancer.

Dietary Fat and Fat-Containing Foods

The relationship between dietary fat intake and breast cancer has
been more extensively studied than any other dietary factor. The
findings of case-control studies of breast cancer have been assembled
in two meta-analyses (8,9). Howe and colleagues (8) estimated odds
ratios using raw data from 12 case-control studies, including 4,427
cases and 6,095 controls. They observed a significant positive association between total fat consumption (RR = 1.48, p < 0.0001) among
postmenopausal women, but found no significant association among
premenopausal women (RR = 1.13, p = 0.21). Boyd and colleagues (9)
assembled published relative risks from 16 case-control studies comprising 6,831 cases and 7,105 controls. Ten of these studies showed
positive, though not necessarily significant, associations between fat
intake and breast cancer, and 5 studies showed negative associations.
These investigations produced a pooled relative risk of 1.21 (95%
confidence limits [CL]: 1.10–1.34), indicating a significant positive
association between total dietary fat and breast cancer risk.

Case-control studies also provided evidence of positive associations between breast cancer and fat-containing foods. Boyd et al. (9)
reported results from 13 analyses describing the association between
breast cancer and meat intake; of these, 10 odds ratios were positive
and 3 were negative, with a pooled odds ratio of 1.14 (95% CL: 1.02–
1.29). Milk consumption was positively related to breast cancer in
five of seven case-control studies and cheese consumption was positively associated with risk in 5 of 6 case-control studies. Pooled estimates of relative risk were 1.17 (95% CL: 1.04–1.31) for milk and 1.17
(95% CL: 1.02–1.36) for cheese.

Weaker associations with dietary fat have, however, been observed
in cohort studies. Boyd et al. (9) assembled published estimates of
relative risk from seven cohort studies, comprising 3,007 cases in a
total population of 252,765, and obtained a pooled estimate of relative

risk of 1.01 (95% CL: 0.90–1.13), comparing highest and lowest fat consumption categories. Hunter et al. (10) estimated relative risks using raw data from 7 cohort studies comprising an analysis of 4,980 cases in a total population of 337,819; this analysis included 5 studies in common with those in the analysis by Boyd et al. (9). Comparing the highest to the lowest quintiles of consumption, the energy-adjusted relative risk for fat intake was 1.05 (95% CL: 0.94–1.16). Cohort studies have, however, shown positive associations with some fat-containing foods. Five studies showed positive associations with meat intake, with a pooled estimate of relative risk of 1.37 (95% CL: 1.07–1.76) and one study showed a positive association with consumption of milk and cheese.

Several methodological issues have been suggested as explanations of the failure of cohort studies to confirm the positive associations between breast cancer and dietary fat intake observed in case-control studies. First, in case-control studies, it is possible that recall bias, in which cases over-reported their fat consumption, led to over-estimation of the strength of the dietary fat association. Two investigations have examined this possibility by comparing results from data collected prospectively and retrospectively within prospective cohorts (11,12). Both investigations failed to find evidence of significant recall bias, although small differences in relative risks obtained using prospectively and retrospectively collected data were in the direction expected for recall bias. Second, in cohort studies, it is possible that random error in estimates of nutrient intake may have led to underestimation of the true association. Hunter et al. (10) attempted in their meta-analysis to evaluate this possibility by adjusting the relative risk for measurement error. They obtained a relative risk of 1.07 per 25 g fat consumption, higher than that obtained without adjustment, 1.02 per 25 g, though neither estimate was statistically significant. Third, all cohort studies reported by Boyd et al. (9) and by Hunter et al. (10) were conducted in North America and Europe and it is possible that the range of fat consumption among participants was too narrow to allow strong associations with risk to be detected. The lowest deciles of consumption in studies included in Hunter's meta-analysis (10) corresponded to 25–30% of calories as fat, substantially above the 15% energy from fat consumed by some women in Asian countries with low breast cancer rates. As case-control studies also suffer from the problem that the range of fat consumption within countries is substantially lower than is seen internationally, it is possible that both case-control and cohort studies may underestimate the association between dietary fat and breast cancer.

As with breast cancer, many investigations have been carried out to examine the relationship between fat and fat-containing foods and the risk of colon cancer. Thirteen of 16 studies reviewed by Potter et al. (13) showed a positive association of fat intake with risk. A total of 8 of 10 well-conducted investigations found a positive association with meat consumption, and 5 studies reported a positive association with egg consumption. However when the results of 13 case-control studies were assembled in a meta-analysis, Howe et al. (14) investigated whether associations between colorectal cancer and total fat were accounted for by the energy received from fat or from other characteristics of the fat consumed. They concluded that total energy intake was associated with risk (RR = 1.63, p < 0.0001 comparing the highest and lowest quintiles of consumption) and that there was no association with intake of fat that was independent of energy (RR = 0.92, p = 0.67, comparing lowest and highest quintiles). Cholesterol was the only type of fat found to be associated with risk after adjustment for energy and the authors concluded that this could be indicative of the intake of specific foods, such as meat or eggs. Three cohort studies have examined dietary fat with adjustment for energy intake. Results from a cohort of American nurses (15) provided evidence of an association with animal fat (RR = 1.89, 95% CL: 1.13–3.15) and observed an even stronger association with an index of intake of meat compared with chicken (RR = 2.49, 95% CL: 1.50–4.13). However 2 additional cohort studies, one of women from Iowa (16), and one of men and women from the Netherlands (17), both failed to find associations with fat intake or with fat-containing foods. Thus while colon cancer has been associated with the intake of fat and fat-containing foods, the role of energy and other mechanisms by which these eating patterns contribute to disease remains to be fully understood.

Plant Foods and Their Components

The possibility that dietary fibre may be related to the risk of breast cancer has been examined much less extensively than the association with dietary fat. Howe et al. (8) reported a negative association between fibre intake and the risk of breast cancer in their meta-analysis of 12 case-control studies from which fibre intake could be calculated. Relative risks were 0.83 (p = 0.002) for postmenopausal and 0.89 (p = 0.15) for premenopausal women. In an analysis of dietary data from the prospective Canadian National Breast Cancer Screening Study, Rohan et al. (18) reported a 30% reduction in risk associated with the highest quintile of fibre intake, with an odds ratio of 0.68 (95% CL: 0.46–1.0) after adjustment for a number of breast cancer risk factors. A reduction of risk of similar size was associated with intake of cereals, pasta, and vegetables rich in vitamins A and C (18). In contrast 2 cohort studies (19,20) showed no association between dietary fibre intake and breast cancer risk.

Unlike with breast cancer, the relationship between colon cancer and plant foods or their components has been extensively studied. Vegetable consumption has been consistently inversely associated with risk in 23 of 28 studies reviewed by Potter et al. (13). Inverse associations with fruit have been reported somewhat less frequently. Ten of 16 studies showed that foods high in fibre were protective (13) and a meta-analysis of 13 case-control studies (21) showed a relative risk of 0.53 comparing the highest and lowest quintiles of consumption, together with a significant dose-response relationship (p < 0.0001).

Other Lifestyle Factors

In addition to diet a number of lifestyle factors – alcohol intake, physical activity, and body size – have been implicated in the etiology of both breast and colon cancers.

ALCOHOL

The relationship between intake of alcohol and the risk of breast cancer has been the subject of two meta-analyses (8,22). Reviewing 28 case-control and 10 cohort studies in 1992, Longnecker (22) reported a positive association, with a relative risk of 1.38 (95% CL: 1.23–1.55) for an intake of three drinks per day. The analysis by Howe et al. (8) of 6 case-control studies in 1991 also produced evidence of a positive association, with relative risks per 10 g of alcohol per day of 1.10 (95% CL: 1.1–1.19) for premenopausal women and 1.06 (95% CL: 0.99–1.12) for postmenopausal women. They observed a significant relative risk (RR = 1.69, 95% CL: 1.19–2.40) when consumption reached 40 g (three drinks) per day.

A positive association between the risk of colon cancer and consumption of alcohol, especially beer, has been observed in geographic correlation studies, with investigations of international patterns of alcohol consumption leading to correlations with colon cancer in the range 0.58–0.76 (13). However 8 cohort studies of alcoholics or of male brewery workers failed to show associations, possibly because 5 of the studies contained under 20 cases of colon cancer and no study had more than 85 cases (13). Significant positive associations were reported in 7 of 14 case-control studies and 2 of 4 population cohort studies (13). The strongest associations were reported in a Japanese cohort in which daily users of alcohol had a relative risk of 5.4 compared to abstainers; other studies showed that alcohol consumption was associated with up to a twofold increase in risk (13).

PHYSICAL ACTIVITY

Physical activity has been associated with a decrease of 10–60% in the risk of breast cancer in 8 of 11 studies in which this was examined (23). In contrast 2 prospective cohort studies showed a 23–60% increase in risk associated with increased activity and a third showed no association (23). Only 2 of the investigations that examined physical activity were adjusted for body size, so further research is needed to separate the effects of physical activity from those of body size.

A negative association has been observed consistently between exercise and the risk of colon cancer (13). Ten case-control and 7 cohort studies have shown up to a twofold increase in risk associated with sedentary occupations or lifestyle. While findings have been consistent for colon cancer, results have been somewhat less consistent for rectal cancer or when cancers of the colon and rectum have been combined (13).

BODY SIZE

Associations between breast cancer and body size have been examined using three indicators of body size: body mass index (BMI), waist-to-hip ratio, and height. Findings for BMI appear to be different for premenopausal and postmenopausal women. Among postmenopausal women increased body size has been consistently associated with increased breast cancer risk in case-control studies (24). Twelve of 13 case-control studies of postmenopausal women reviewed by Hunter and Willett (25) showed a positive association, with relative risks comparing the highest to lowest categories of body mass ranging from 1.1 to 2.7. Prospective studies also showed predominantly positive, though somewhat weaker, associations, with relative risks from 0.7 to 1.2 in 6 cohort studies (25). In contrast the balance of evidence suggests a negative association among pre-menopausal women. Among 13 case-control studies of premeno-pausal women (25), 4 showed negative associations, with relative risks from 0.5 to 0.8, 3 showed no association (RR = 1.0), and 6 showed positive associations, with relative risks from 1.2 to 1.3. Four of 5 cohort studies showed a negative association, with relative risks from 0.4 to 0.8; one study showed no association (RR = 1.0). A formal meta-analysis of studies of premenopausal breast cancer (26) showed a relative risk of 0.88 (95% CL: 0.76–1.02) for each 8 kg/m² of BMI, based on 19 case-control studies, and a similar relative risk, 0.70 (95% CL: 0.54–0.91), based on 4 cohort studies.

Waist-to-hip ratio has been consistently positively related to breast cancer risk in postmenopausal women in both case-control and cohort studies (27–29), with relative risks observed between 2 and 5, after adjustment for other risk factors.

Height has also been consistently positively related to breast cancer risk in seven prospective studies of both pre- and postmeno-pausal women, with relative risks ranging from 1.1 to 2.6 (25). This is consistent with findings from the majority of case-control studies on postmenopausal women, as 2 of 3 reported relative risks above 1 (1.1–1.3). However among premenopausal women 2 of 3 case-control studies reported relative risks below 1 (0.7–0.8). Because height is influenced by early nutrition, a positive association between height and breast cancer risk may suggest a role for early nutrition in the etiology of breast cancer.

For colon cancer a positive association with BMI has been sug-gested by the findings of 7 of 11 case-control studies reviewed by Potter et al. (13), with people in the highest quintile of body size having as much as a twofold increase in risk. Two prospective stud-ies (16,30) also observed positive associations. The distribution of body fat was examined in one investigation (16), with an increase in risk observed in the highest quintile of measured waist-to-hip ratio. Height, independent of weight, has also been associated with increased risk, with relative risks from 1.6 to 2.1 (16,31,32). In addi-tion colorectal cancer recurrence (33) has been positively associated with body mass, height, and weight.

Biological Mechanisms

Explanations for associations between breast cancer and lifestyle risk factors are often based on the role of hormones, especially estrogens.

Dietary fat can alter the metabolic disposition of endogenous steroids (34), fibre-rich foods can alter the enterohepatic cycling of estrogen (18), alcohol may influence metabolism and clearance of estrogen by the liver and may act on pituitary prolactin secretion (35), physical activity reduces resting levels of estrogen, progesterone, prolactin, and other hormones (13), and obesity influences the production, metabolism, and disposition of estrogens (34).

Associations between colorectal cancer and the same epidemiological risk factors are usually explained by other mechanisms involving the contents of the colonic lumen. Fat increases bile acid metabolism and is thus thought to increase exposure of the colon to the toxic, trophic, and promoting effects of bile acids (13). Fibre binds bile acids, reduces exposure to bile acids by reducing transit time, dilutes bile acids by increasing stool bulk, and ferments to volatile fatty acids that may reduce the conversion of primary to secondary bile acids by lowering colonic pH. In addition vegetables contain micronutrients and phytochemicals that may influence the steps in carcinogenesis from activation of procarcinogens to DNA damage, DNA synthesis and replication, cell replication with abnormal DNA, and abnormal protein synthesis (13). Physical activity stimulates colon peristalsis and thereby decreases the time that bile acids and carcinogens are in contact with colonic tissue. It also has potentially beneficial effects on the immune system (13). Body size may reflect early development and this may influence cell numbers and organ size or may effect some early tumour event (13).

Evidence is, however, accumulating that dietary and lifestyle risk factors for breast and colon cancer may act through a common mechanism involving insulin resistance (36–38), a syndrome characterized by increased insulin, glucose, and triglycerides. The similarity of epidemiological risk factors for insulin resistance, breast cancer, and colon cancer, discussed below, provides indirect evidence for this hypothesis and biological mechanisms exist that could account for these associations.

Insulin, glucose, and triglycerides could all increase growth of neoplastic cells. Insulin is considered to be a growth factor (39–41). Receptors for insulin and for insulin-like growth factors are observed in both normal and malignant breast (40–44) and colorectal (45,46) tissue. Cross reactions can occur between these receptors and their hormones (40,41,46). Thus insulin may stimulate growth directly or indirectly, by mimicking growth-promoting actions of insulin-like growth factors, or by influencing circulating levels of insulin-like growth factor (47,48) and/or its binding proteins (49). An effect of insulin in carcinogenesis is further suggested by the finding that insulin is capable of damaging DNA in endothelial cells (50) and an insulin analogue, BioAsp, has been shown to cause a dose-dependent increase in the incidence of spontaneous adenocarcinomas and fibroepithelial mammary tumours in female rats (51). In culture insulin has been shown to induce morphological changes in the epithelium of normal, dysplastic, and fibroadenoma breast tissue (52–54). Insulin has been shown to induce phenotypic changes in human and animal fibroblast cells in culture with over-expressed insulin (55) and insulin-like growth factor I receptor (56). Further insulin is negatively associated with somatostatin (57), a hormone with atrophic effects (58) that has been shown to inhibit mouse colon adenocarcinoma (59).

Plasma glucose and/or serum triglycerides may be indicators of energy available for neoplastic cells. Plasma glucose is a major source of energy for neoplastic cells (60). Fasting serum triglycerides may be a general marker of energy availability because VLDL triglycerides (the major component of serum triglycerides) represent the triglycerides that are sent from liver to adipose tissues for long-term storage and to peripheral tissues for energy. In addition high glucose and triglycerides may be indicators of enhanced production and/or transport of lipid peroxidation products. Lipid peroxidation is a potential source of endogenous DNA adducts (61,62), and such damage to DNA may be a contributor to cancer (63). Studies of diabetics and people with impaired glucose tolerance have suggested that levels of glucose and triglycerides are positively correlated with indicators of lipid peroxidation (64,65). Finally serum triglycerides have been observed to be correlated with fecal bile acids (36), which have been positively related to the risk of colorectal cancer in a number of epidemiological studies (66–72). Thus several biological mechanisms involving either circulatory or luminal paths could account for associations between insulin, glucose, and triglycerides and the risk of breast and colon cancers.

Epidemiological Evidence of Association between Insulin Resistance and Breast and Colon Cancers

Recent studies have provided direct evidence of an association between biological factors related to insulin resistance and the risks of both breast and colon cancers. Bruning et al. (73) reported significantly higher levels of C-peptide, an indicator of insulin secretion, in breast cancer cases than in controls for both pre- and postmenopausal women. Del Guidice (38) reported higher fasting plasma insulin among premenopausal breast cancer patients than in controls, after adjustment for age and body size. In the same study Goodwin et al. (74) observed a positive association between triglycerides and breast cancer. In addition a positive association between triglycerides and breast cancer has been supported in 3 (75–77) of 5 other studies (75–79) and an association with colorectal cancer has been reported in 3 studies (62,80,81).

Studies that have included direct measures of glucose levels or glucose tolerance tests have shown positive associations with breast cancer (82–87) and with colon cancer (83,88,89), though some are based on small numbers of cases and do not provide adequate statistical evaluation. Indirect evidence of an association between cancer and insulin, glucose, and/or triglycerides comes from studies of diabetics. Positive associations with breast cancer have been reported in 3 (90–92) of 5 (90–94) studies and positive associations with colon cancer have been reported in 5 (95–99) of 6 (83,95–99) investigations.

These findings are supported by the observation that epidemiological risk factors for breast and colon cancers are also associated with insulin, glucose, and/or triglycerides. Diets high in fat and energy density are associated with decreased insulin sensitivity (100) and feeding trials have shown that such diets increase triglycerides when compared with low-fat, low-energy-dense diets (101–103). Diets that are high in fibre-rich carbohydrates are associated with reduced fasting insulin levels (104), increased insulin sensitivity (100), and reduced serum triglycerides (105–114). Plant foods, a source of dietary fibre, produce a low postprandial glycemic response (105–107,115,116). Alcohol, like carbohydrate, has long been recognized as increasing serum triglycerides (117) and beer is a source of both alcohol and carbohydrate (about 30g/l) (117). Alcohol intake has also been positively associated with hyperglycemia and reduced insulin sensitivity (118). However the relationship may be complex because alcohol can result in hyperglycemia when taken after meals, but not in a fasting state (117), and low to moderate intake has been associated with reduced insulin levels (119–121). Thus alcohol can affect serum triglycerides, plasma glucose, and insulin sensitivity, but patterns of consumption may be important and need to be considered in detail in epidemiological studies of the relationship between alcohol intake and the risk of breast and colon cancers. Positive associations between obesity, serum triglycerides, and blood glucose are well established (122–124). Clinical studies have shown that the degree of obesity is associated with production of VLDL triglycerides, and with elevated levels of blood glucose and that increases in weight are associated with increases in triglycerides and glucose (124). Further the regional distribution of body fat can influence both serum triglycerides and blood glucose (122–128). Obesity and high waist-to-hip ratio have been associated with impaired glucose tolerance and high insulin levels (129). Exercise reduces serum triglycerides and insulin levels and improves glucose tolerance and insulin sensitivity (130–134). Studies comparing lipids in persons with different levels of physical activity have shown higher serum triglycerides in inactive people (135–140). Studies of physical training have shown reductions in triglycerides (141–143), together with increases in glucose tolerance (132); even a single exercise session can improve insulin responsiveness (144).

Conclusion

Evidence is accumulating to suggest that cancers of the breast and colon may arise through common mechanisms involving insulin, glucose, and/or triglycerides. Such mechanisms could explain the similarity of epidemiological risk factors that have been suggested for these two cancers. Future research will require collaboration between basic scientists and epidemiologists in order to develop an understanding of the effects of dietary and lifestyle risk factors on the relevant biological and metabolic processes, and to link these models with an understanding of the genetics of neoplastic cells. Such studies may also lead to an understanding of biological processes involved in cancers of the endometrium, ovary, and prostate, as these sites share risk factors with breast and colon cancers (1,2).

REFERENCES

1 National Cancer Institute of Canada. *Canadian cancer statistics 1996*. Toronto: 1996.
2 Muir C, Waterhouse J, Mack T et al. *Cancer incidence in five continents*, vol. 5, IARC scientific publication 88. Lyon, France: International Agency for Research on Cancer, 1987.

3 Haenszel W. Cancer mortality among foreign-born in the United States. *J Natl Cancer Inst* 1961;26:37–132.
4 McMichael AJ, McCall MG, Hartshorne JM et al. Patterns of gastro-intestinal cancer in European migrants to Australia: the role of dietary change. *Int J Cancer* 1980;25:431–437.
5 McMichael AJ, Giles GG. Cancer in migrants to Australia: extending the descriptive epidemiological data. *Cancer Res* 1988;48:751–756.
6 Steinitz R. Cancer risks in immigrant populations in Israel. In: Aoki K, ed. *Proceedings of the first UICC conference on cancer prevention in developing countries*. Nagoya: University of Nagoya Press, 1982:363–381.
7 Armstrong B, Doll R. Environmental factors and cancer incidence and mortality in different countries, with special reference to dietary practices. *Int J Cancer* 1975;15:617–631.
8 Howe GR, Hirohata T, Hislop TG et al. Dietary factors and risk of breast cancer: combined analysis of 12 case-control studies. *J Natl Cancer Inst* 1990;82:561–569.
9 Boyd NF, Martin LJ, Noffel M et al. A meta-analysis of studies of dietary fat and breast cancer risk. *Br J Cancer* 1993;68:627–636.
10 Hunter DJ, Spiegelman D, Adani HO et al. Cohort studies of fat intake and risk of breast cancer: a pooled analysis. *N Engl J Med* 1996;334:356–361.
11 Freidenreich CM, Howe GR, Miller AB. The effect of recall bias on the association of calorie-providing nutrients and breast cancer. *Epidemiology* 1991;2:424–429.
12 Giovannucci E, Stampfer MJ, Colditz GA et al. A comparison of prospective and retrospective assessments of diet in the study of breast cancer. *Am J Epidemiol* 1993;133:502–511.
13 Potter JD, Slattery ML, Bostick RM, Gapstur SM. Colon cancer: a review of the epidemiology. *Epidemiol Rev* 1993;15:499–545.
14 Howe GR, Aronson KJ, Benito E et al. The relationship between dietary fat intake and risk of colorectal cancer: evidence from the combined analysis of 13 case-control studies. *Cancer Causes Control* 1997;8:215–228.
15 Willett WG, Stampfer MJ, Colditz GA et al. Relation of meat, fat and fiber intake to the risk of colon cancer in a prospective study among women. *N Engl J Med* 1990;323:1664–1672.
16 Bostick RM, Potter JD, Kushi LH et al. Sugar, meat and fat intake and non-dietary risk factors for colon cancer incidence in Iowa women (United States). *Cancer Causes Control* 1994;5:38–52.
17 Goldbohm RA, Van den Brandt PA, Van't Veer P et al. A prospective cohort study of the relation between meat consumption and the risk of colon cancer. *Cancer Res* 1994; 54:718–723.

18 Rohan TE, Howe GR, Friedenreich CM et al. Dietary fibre, vitamins A, C and E and risk of breast cancer: a cohort study. *Cancer Causes Control* 1993;4:29–37.

19 Graham S, Zielezny M, Marshall J et al. Diet in the epidemiology of postmenopausal breast cancer in the New York State cohort. *Am J Epidemiol* 1992;136:1327–1337.

20 Willett WC, Hunter DJ, Stampfer MJ et al. Dietary fat and fiber in relation to the risk of breast cancer: an 8 year follow-up. *JAMA* 1992;268:2037–2044.

21 Howe GR, Benito E, Castelleto R et al. Dietary intake of fiber and decreased risk of cancers of the colon and rectum: evidence from the combined analysis of 13 case-control studies. *J Natl Cancer Inst* 1992;84:1887–1896.

22 Longnecker MP. Alcoholic beverage consumption in relation to risk of breast cancer: meta-analysis and review. *Cancer Causes Control* 1994;5:73–82.

23 Friedenreich CM, Rohan TE. A review of physical activity and breast cancer. *Epidemiology* 1995;6:311–317.

24 Kelsey JL. Breast cancer epidemiology: summary and future directions. *Epidemiol Rev* 1993;15:255–263.

25 Hunter DJ, Willett WC. Diet, body size and breast cancer. *Epidemiol Rev* 1993;15:110–132.

26 Ursin G, Longnecker MP, Hacle RW et al. A meta-analysis of body mass index and risk of premenopausal breast cancer. *Epidemiology* 1995;6:137–141.

27 Ballard-Barbash R, Schatzkin A, Carter CL et al. Body fat distribution and breast cancer in the Framingham study. *J Natl Cancer Inst* 1990;82:286–290.

28 Folsom AR, Kage SA, Prineas RJ et al. Increased incidence of carcinoma of the breast associated with abdominal adiposity in postmenopausal women. *Am J Epidemiol* 1990;131:794–803.

29 Schapira DV, Kumar NB, Lyman GH, Cox CE. Abdominal obesity and breast cancer risk. *Ann Int Med* 1990;112:182–186.

30 Lew EA, Garfinkel L. Variations in mortality by weight among 750,000 men and women. *J Chron Dis* 1979;32:563–576.

31 Albanes D, Jones DY, Schatzkin A, Micozzi MS. Adult stature and risk of cancer. *Cancer Res* 1988;48:1658–1662.

32 Albanes D, Taylor PR. International differences in body height and weight and their relationship to cancer incidence. *Nutr Cancer* 1990;14:69–77.

33 Tartter PI, Slater C, Paptestas G, Aufses AH. Cholesterol, weight, height, Quetelet's index and colon cancer recurrence. *J Surg Oncol* 1984;27:232–235.

34 Herschcopt RJ, Bradlow HL. Obesity, diet, endogenous estrogens and the risk of hormone-sensitive cancer. *Am J Clin Nutr* 1987;47:283–289.
35 Rosenberg L, Metzger LS, Palmer JR. Alcohol consumption and risk of breast cancer: a review of the epidemiological evidence. *Epidemiol Rev* 1993;15:133–144.
36 McKeown-Eyssen GE. The epidemiology of colorectal cancer revisited: are plasma glucose and serum triglycerides associated with risk? *Cancer Epidemiol Biomarkers Prevent* 1994;3:687–695.
37 Kazer RR. Insulin resistance, insulin-like growth factor I and breast cancer: a hypothesis. *Int J Cancer* 1995;63:403- 406.
38 Del Guidice ME, Fantus IG, Ezzat S et al. Insulin and related factors in premenopausal breast cancer risk. *Breast Cancer Rest Treat.* In press.
39 Korc M. Growth factors and oncogenes. *Regl Pept Lett* 1990;2:7–11.
40 Hill DJ, Millner RDG. Insulin as a growth factor. *Pediatr Res* 1985;19:879–886.
41 Straus DS. Growth-stimulatory actions of insulin in vitro and in vivo. *Endocr Rev* 1984;5:356–369.
42 Benson EA, Holdaway IM. Regulation of insulin binding to human mammary carcinoma. *Cancer Res* 1982;42:1137–1141.
43 Holdaway IM, Friesen HG. Hormone binding by human mammary carcinoma. *Cancer Res* 1977;37:1946–1952.
44 Papa V, Pezzino V, Costantino A et al. Elevated insulin receptor content in human breast cancer. *J Clin Invest* 1990;86:1503–1510.
45 Wong M, Holdaway IM. Insulin binding by normal and neoplastic colonic tissues. *Int J Cancer* 1985;35:335–341.
46 Cullen KJ, Yee D, Rosen N. Insulin-like growth factors in human malignancy. *Cancer Invest* 1991;9:443–454.
47 Salamon EA, Luo J, Murphy LJ. The effect of acute and chronic insulin administration on insulin-like growth factor-I expression in the pituitary-intact and hypophysectomised rat. *Diabetologia* 1989;32:348–353.
48 Daughaday WH, Phillips LS, Mueller MC. The effects of insulin and growth hormone on the release of somatomedin by isolated rat liver. *Endocrinology* 1976;98:1214–1219.
49 Holly JMP, Wass JAH. Insulin-like growth factors: autocrine, paracrine or endocrine? New perspectives of the somatomedin hypothesis in the light of recent developments. *J Endocrinol* 1989;122:611–618.
50 Lorenzi M, Montisano DF, Toledo S, Barvieux A. High glucose induces DNA damage in cultured human endothelial cells. *J Clin Invest* 1986;77:322–325.
51 Dideriksen LH, Jorgensen LN, Drejer K. Carcinogenic effect on female rats after 12 months administration of the insulin analogue B10 Asp. *Diabetes* 1992;41(suppl 1):143A.

52 Barker BE, Fanger H, Farnes P. Human mammary slices in organ cul-
    ture. I. Methods of culture and preliminary observations on the effects
    of insulin. *Exp Cell Res* 1964;35:437–448.
53 Ceriani RL, Contesso GP, Nataf BM. Hormone requirements for
    growth and differentiation of the human mammary gland in organ cul-
    ture. *Cancer Res* 1972;32:2190–2196.
54 Elias JJ, Armstrong RC. Hyperplastic and metaplastic responses of
    human mammary fibroadenomas and dysplasias in organ culture.
    J Natl Cancer Inst 1973;51:1341–1343.
55 Giorgino F, Belfiore A, Milazzo G et al. Overexpression of insulin
    receptors in fibroblast and ovary cells induces a ligand-mediated trans-
    formed phenotype. *Mol Endocrinol* 1991; 5:452–459.
56 Kaleko M, Rutter WJ, Miller AD. Overexpression of the human insulin-
    like growth factor I receptor promotes ligand-dependent neoplastic
    transformation. *Mol Cell Biol* 1990;10:464–473.
57 Schade DS, Santigao JV, Skyler JS, Rizza RA. *Intensive insulin therapy.*
    Amsterdam: Excerpta Medica, 1983:23–25.
58 Bristol JB, Williamson RCN. Large bowel growth. In: Pollak JM, Bloom
    SR, Wright NA, Butler AG, eds. *Basic science in gastroenterology.* Ware,
    Herts, U.K.: Glaxo Group Research Ltd, 1984:307–316.
59 Townsend, CM. Peptides and gastrointestinal cancer growth. *Regl Pept
    Lett* 1990;2:12–15.
60 Newsholme EA, Board M. Application of metabolic-control logic to
    fuel utilization and its significance in tumour cells. *Adv Enz Reg*
    1991;31:225–246.
61 Welsch CW. Review of the effects of dietary fat on experimental mam-
    mary gland tumorigenesis: role of lipid peroxidation. *Free Radical Biol
    Med* 1995;18:757–773.
62 Chaudhary AK, Nokubo M, Reddy GR et al. Detection of endogenous
    malondialdehyde-deoxyguanosine adducts in human liver. *Science*
    1994;265:1580–1582.
63 Ames BN, Gold LS, Willett WC. The causes and prevention of cancer.
    Proc Natl Acad Sci 1995;92:5258–5265.
64 Aktomore E, Venemcale G, Chicco D et al. Increased lipid peroxidation
    in type 2 poorly controlled diabetic patients. *Diabetes Metab*
    1992;18:264–271.
65 Haffner SM, Stern MP, Agil A et al. Plasma oxidizability in subjects
    with normal glucose tolerance, impaired glucose tolerance and NIDDM.
    Diabetes Care 1995;18:646–653.
66 Committee on Diet and Health. *Diet and health: implications for reducing
    chronic disease risk.* Washington: National Academy Press, 1989:159–
    258.

67 Stadler J, Yeung KS, Furrer R et al. Proliferative activity of rectal
    mucosa and soluble fecal bile acids in patients with normal colons
    and in patients with colonic polyps or cancer. *Cancer Lett* 1988;38:315–
    320.

68 Yeung KS, McKeown-Eyssen GE, Li GF et al. Comparisons of diet and
    biochemical characteristics of stool and urine between Chinese popula-
    tions with low and high colorectal cancer rates. *J Natl Cancer Inst*
    1991;83:46–50.

69 Rafter JJ, Child P, Anderson AM et al. Cellular toxicity of fecal water
    depends on diet. *Am J Clin Nutr* 1987;45:559–563.

70 Rafter JJ, Eng VWS, Furrer R et al. Effect of calcium and pH on the
    mucosal damage produced by deoxycholic acid in the rat colon. *Gut*
    1986;27:1320–1329.

71 Narisawa T, Magadia NE, Weisburger JH, Wynder EL. Promoting
    effects of bile acids on colon carcinogenesis after intra-rectal instilla-
    tion of N-methyl-N-nitrosoguanine in rats. *J Natl Cancer Inst*
    1974;53:1093–1095.

72 Sarwal AN, Cohen BI, Raicht RF et al. Effects of dietary administra-
    tion of chenodeoxycholate on N-methyl-N-nitrosourea induced colon
    cancer in rats. *Biochim Biophys Acta* 1979;574:423–432.

73 Bruning PF, Bonfrer JMG, Van Noord PAH et al. Insulin resistance and
    breast cancer risk. *Int J Cancer* 1992;52:511–516.

74 Goodwin PJ, Boyd NF, Hanna W et al. Elevated levels of plasma trig-
    lycerides are associated with histologically defined premenopausal
    breast cancer. *Nutr Cancer* 1997;27:284–292.

75 Dilman VM, Berstein LM, Ostroumova MN et al. Peculiarities of hyper-
    lipidemia in tumour patients. *Br J Cancer* 1981;43:637–643.

76 Bani IA, Williams CM, Boulter PS, Dickerson JWT. Plasma lipids and
    prolactin in patients with breast cancer. *Br J Cancer* 1986;54:439–446.

77 Kumar K, Sachdanandam P, Arivazhagan R. Studies on the changes in
    plasma lipids and lipoproteins in patients with benign and malignant
    breast cancer. *Biochem Intern* 1991;23:581–589.

78 Gerber M, Cavallo F, Marubini E et al. Lipsoluble vitamins and lipid
    parameters in breast cancer. A joint study in northern Italy and south-
    ern France. *Int J Cancer* 1988;421: 489–494.

79 Vatten LJ, Foss OP. Total serum cholesterol and triglycerides and risk
    of breast cancer: a prospective study of 24,329 Norwegian women.
    Cancer Res 1990;50:2341–2346.

80 Kono S, Ikeda N, Yani F et al. Serum lipids and colorectal adenoma
    among male self-defense officials in northern Kyushu, Japan. *Intern J
    Epidemiol* 1990;19:274–278.

81 Kovalenko IG, Bershtein LM, Ostrouvova MN, Dil'man UM. Body weight, blood lipids, blood cortisol and prognosis of patients with cancer of the large intestine and breast. *Voprosy Onkologii* 1989;35:816–822.

82 Glicksman AS, Myers WPL, Rawson RW. Diabetes mellitus and carbohydrate metabolism in patients with cancer. *Med Clin N Am* 1956;40:887–900.

83 Glicksman AS, Rawson RW. Diabetes and altered carbohydrate metabolism in patients with cancer. *Cancer* 1956;9:1127–1134.

84 Pearson OH, Llerena O, Samaan N et al. Serum growth hormone and insulin levels in patients with breast cancer. In: Forrest APM, Kunkler PB, eds. *Prognostic factors in breast cancer, proc. of 1st Tenovus symposium.* Cardiff: E and S Livingstone, 1968:421–430.

85 Carter AC, Lefkon BW, Farlin M et al. Metabolic parameters in women with metastatic breast cancer. *J Clin Endocrin Metab* 1975;40:260–264.

86 Muck BR, Trotnow S, Hommel G. Cancer of the breast, diabetes and pathological glucose tolerance. *Arch Gynak* 1975;220: 73–81.

87 Muck BR, Trotnow S, Egger H et al. Altered carbohydrate metabolism in breast cancer and benign breast affections. *Arch Gynak* 1976;221:83–91.

88 Levine W, Dryer AR, Shekelle RB et al. Post-load glucose and cancer mortality in middle-aged men and women. *Am J Epidemiol* 1990;131:254–262.

89 Smith GD, Egger M, Shipley MJ, Marmot MG. Post-challenge glucose concentration, impaired glucose tolerance, diabetes and cancer mortality in men. *Am J Epidemiol* 1992;136:1110–1114.

90 Repert RW. Breast cancer: relation to thyroid disease and diabetes. *J Michigan State Med Soc* 1952;52:1315–1320.

91 Lancaster HO, Maddox JK. Diabetic mortality in Australia. *Australas Ann Med* 1958;7:145–151.

92 Unger C, Rageth JC, Wyss P et al. Risk factors in breast carcinoma. *J Suisse de Médecine* 1991;121:30–36.

93 Kopp S. Current evidence about association between diabetes mellitus and breast cancer. *Arch Geschwulstforsch* 1989;59:367–373.

94 Franceschi S, La Vecchia C, Negri E et al. Breast cancer risk and history of selected medical conditions linked with female hormones. *Eur J Cancer* 1990;26:781–785.

95 Wilson EB, Maher HC. Cancer and tuberculosis with some comments on cancer and other diseases. *Am J Cancer* 1932;16:227–250.

96 O'Mara BA, Byers T, Schoenfeld E. Diabetes mellitus and cancer risk: a multisite case-control study. *J Chron Dis* 1985;38:435–441.

97 Adami HO, McLaughlin J, Ekbom A et al. Cancer risk in patients with diabetes mellitus. *Cancer Causes Control* 1991; 2:307–314.

98 Ragozzino M, Melton LJ, Chu CP, Palumbo PJ. Subsequent cancer risk in the incidence cohort of Rochester, Minnesota, residents with diabetes mellitus. *J Chron Dis* 1982;35:13–19.

99 Kessler II. Cancer mortality among diabetics. *J Nat Cancer Inst* 1970;44:673–686.

100 Lovejoy J, Di Girolamo M. Habitual dietary intake and insulin sensitivity in lean and obese adults. *Am J Clin Nutr* 1992;55:1174–1179.

101 Antonis A, Bersohn I. Influence of diet on serum triglycerides. *Lancet* 1961;3–9.

102 Hatch JT, Abell LL, Kendall FE. Effects of restriction of fat and cholesterol upon serum lipids and lipoproteins in patients with hypertension. *Am J Med* 1955;19:48–60.

103 Grundy SM. Comparison of monounsaturated fatty acids and carbohydrates for lowering plasma cholesterol. *N Engl J Med* 1986;314:745–749.

104 Fukawaga NK, Anderson JW, Hageman G et al. High-carbohydrate, high-fibre diets increase peripheral insulin sensitivity in healthy young and old adults. *Am J Clin Nutr* 1990;52:524–528.

105 Jenkens DJ. Lente carbohydrate: a newer approach to dietary management of diabetes. *Diabetes Care* 1982;5:634–639.

106 Karlstrom B, Vessby B, Asp NG et al. Effects of an increased content of cereal fibre in the diet of type 2 (non-insulin dependent) diabetic patients. *Diabetologia* 1984;26:272–277.

107 Riccardi G, Rivellesa A, Pacioni D et al. Separate influence of dietary carbohydrate and fibre on the metabolic control in diabetes. *Diabetologia* 1984;26:116–121.

108 Anderson JW, Chen WJL, Sieling B. Hypolipidemic effects of high carbohydrate high fibre diets. *Metabolism* 1980;29:551–558.

109 Albrink MJ, Ullrich IH. Interaction of dietary sucrose and fiber on serum lipids in healthy young men fed high carbohydrate diets. *Am J Clin Nutr* 1986;43:419–428.

110 Anderson JW, Story L, Sieling RD et al. Hypocholesterolemic effects of oat bran or bean intake for hypercholesterolemic men. *Am J Clin Nutr* 1984;40:1146–1155.

111 Bosello O, Cominacini L, Zocca I et al. Effects of guar gum on plasma lipoproteins and apolipoproteins C-II and C-III in patients affected by familial hyperlipoproteinemia. *Am J Clin Nutr* 1984;40:1165–1174.

112 Angelico F, Clemente P, Menoti A et al. Bran and changes in serum lipids: observations during a project of primary prevention of coronary

heart disease. In: Carlson LA, ed. *International conference on atherosclerosis.* New York: Raven Press, 1978.

113 Hollenbeck CB, Coulston AM, Reaven GM. To what extent does increased dietary fibre improve glucose and lipid metabolism in patients with noninsulin-dependent diabetes mellitus (NIDDM)? *Am J Clin Nutr* 1986;43:16–24.

114 Salvioli G, Lugli R, Pradelli JM. Cholesterol absorption and sterol balance in normal subjects receiving dietary fibre or ursodeoxycholic acid. *Dig Dis Sci* 1985;30:301–307.

115 Wahlquist ML. Dietary fibre and carbohydrate metabolism. *Am J Clin Nutr* 1987;45:1232–1236.

116 Miettinen TA. Dietary fibre and lipids. *Am J Clin Nutr* 1987;45:1237–1242.

117 Committee on Diet and Health. *Diet and health: implications for reducing chronic disease risk.* Washington: National Academy Press, 1989:431–464.

118 Gerard MJ, Klatsky AL, Siegelaub AB et al. Serum glucose levels and alcohol-consumption habits in a large population. *Diabetes* 1977;26:780–785.

119 Razay G, Heaton KW, Bolton CH, Hughes AO. Alcohol consumption and its relation to cardiovascular risk factors. *Br Med J* 1992;304:80–83.

120 Facchini F, Chen YD, Reaven GM. Light-to-moderate alcohol intake is associated with enhanced insulin sensitivity. *Diabetes Care* 1994;17:115–119.

121 Mayer EJ, Newman B, Quesenberry CP. Alcohol consumption and insulin concentrations. Role of insulin in associations of alcohol intake with high-density lipoprotein cholesterol and triglycerides. *Circulation* 1993;88:2190–2197.

122 Ashley FW, Kannel WB. Relation of weight change to changes in atherogenic traits: the Framingham study. *J Chron Dis* 1974;27:103–104.

123 Committee on Diet and Health. *Diet and health: implications for reducing chronic disease risk.* Washington: National Academy Press, 1989:529–547.

124 Committee on Diet and Health. *Diet and health: implications for reducing chronic disease risk.* Washington: National Academy Press, 1989:563–592.

125 Lapidas L, Bengtsson C, Larsson B et al. Distribution of adipose tissue and risk of cardiovascular disease and death: a 12 year follow-up of participants in the population study of women in Gothenburg, Sweden. *Br Med J* 1984;289:1257–1261.

126 Bjorntorp P. Adipose tissue in obesity (Willendorf lecture). In: Hirsch J, Van Itallie TB, eds. *Recent advances in obesity research*, vol. 4. London: John Libbey, 1985:163–170.

127 Krotkiewski M, Bjorntorp P, Sjostrom L, Smith U. Impact of obesity on metabolism in men and women. Importance of regional adipose tissue distribution. *J Clin Invest* 1983;72:1150–1162.

128 Hartz RJ, Rupley DC, Rim AA. The association of girth measurements with disease in 32,856 women. *Am J Epidemiol* 1984;119:71–80.

129 Hauner H, Pfeiffer EF. Relation between body fat distribution, insulin levels and glucose tolerance in obese females. *Klin Wochenschr* 1988;66:216–222.

130 Huttunen JK, Lansimies E, Voutilainen E et al. Effect of moderate physical exercise on serum lipoproteins: a controlled clinical trial with special reference to serum high-density lipoproteins. *Circulation* 1979;60:1220–1229.

131 Committee on Diet and Health. *Diet and health: implications for reducing chronic disease risk*. Washington: National Academy Press, 1989:139–158.

132 Helmrich SP, Ragland DR, Leung RW et al. Physical activity and reduced occurrence of non-insulin-dependent diabetes mellitus. *N Engl J Med* 1991;325:147–152.

133 Reitman JS, Vasquez B, Klimes Z et al. Improvement of glucose homeostasis after exercise training in non-insulin dependent diabetes. *Diabetes Care* 1984;7:434–441.

134 Zimmet PZ, Collins VR, Dowse GK, Alberti KG. The relation of physical activity to cardiovascular disease risk factors in Mauritians. Mauritius Non-Communicable Disease Study Group. *Am J Epidemiol* 1991;134:862–875.

135 Cooper KH, Pollock ML, Martin RP et al. Physical fitness levels vs selected coronary risk factors. *JAMA* 1976;236:166–169.

136 Montoge HJ, Block WD, Metzner HL, Keller JB. Habitual physical activity and serum lipids: males age 16–64 in a total community. *J Chron Dis* 1976;29:697–709.

137 Nikkila EA, Kussi T, Myllynen P. High density lipoprotein and apoliprotein A-1 during physical inactivity. *Atherosclerosis* 1980;37:457–462.

138 Kussi T, Nikkila EA, Saarinen P et al. Plasma high density liproteins HDL_2, HLD_3 and postheparin plasma lipases in relation to parameters of physical fitness. *Atherosclerosis* 1982;41:209–219.

139 Hartung GH, Foreyt JP, Mitchell RE et al. Relation of diet to high-density-lipoprotein cholesterol in middle-aged marathon runners, joggers and inactive men. *N Engl J Med* 1980;302:357–361.

140 Wood PD, Haskell WL. The effect of exercise on plasma high density lipoproteins. *Lipids* 1979;14:417–427.
141 Huttunen JK, Lansimies E, Voutilainen E et al. Effect of moderate physical exercise on serum lipoproteins. *Circulation* 1979;60:1220–1229.
142 Blairs N, Copper KH, Gibbons LW et al. Changes in coronary heart disease risk factors associated with increased treadmill time in 753 men. *Am J Epidemiol* 1983;118:352–359.
143 Lipson LC, Bonow RO, Schafer EJ et al. Effect of exercise conditioning on plasma high density lipoproteins and other lipoproteins. *Atherosclerosis* 1980;37:529–538.
144 Zierath JR, Wallberg-Henriksson H. Exercise training in obese diabetic patients. Special considerations. *Sports Med* 1992;14:171–189.

DAVID KRITCHEVSKY

Cancer: Influences of
Fat and Calories

In primitive times, lack of food gave languishing bodies to death; now, on
the other hand, it is abundance that buries them.

Lucretius, "De Rerum Natura" V, 1097, ca 50 B.C.E.

More than 60 years ago Watson and Mellanby (1) showed that
tumour growth could be influenced by dietary fat when they added
12.5–25.0% butter to a diet containing 3% fat and increased the incidence of coaltar-induced skin tumours in mice by 68%. In the early
1940s Baumann's group at the University of Wisconsin demonstrated
that increasing levels of dietary fat increased the incidence of some
chemically-induced tumours in mice and found further that saturated fat was less co-carcinogenic than unsaturated fat (2–5). The
latter observation was confirmed by Carroll and his co-workers (6,7).
Ip et al. (8) demonstrated a positive requirement of linoleic acid for
tumourigenesis. Carroll and Khor (7) also showed a threshold level
for the fat effect. They increased levels of dietary corn oil in diets
of 7,12-dimethylbenz(a)anthracene (DMBA)-treated rats. A tenfold
increase in dietary fat, from 0.5 to 5% of the diet did not affect
tumour incidence or multiplicity. An increase of dietary fat to 10%
increased tumour incidence and multiplicity by 22 and 43%, respectively. Doubling fat content of the diet again, to 20%, had no further
effect (table 1). Tannenbaum (9) had concluded from his own work
that a sharp increase in tumourigenicity occurred when dietary fat
levels reached 8%.

In 1909 Moreschi (10) reported that the growth of a sarcoma transplanted into mice was inhibited when they were underfed. Rous (11)

Supported in part by a Research Career Award (HL-00734) from the National Institutes of Health.

Table 1
Influence of Dietary Fat Level on DMBA-Induced Mammary Tumours in Rats*

Corn oil (% in diet)	Incidence (%)	Tumour multiplicity**	Latency (days)
0.5	70	2.5 ± 0.4	78.4 ± 4.5
5.0	76	2.3 ± 0.4	77.4 ± 4.4
10.0	93	4.0 ± 0.5	68.0 ± 4.5
20.0	90	3.7 ± 0.6	68.2 ± 4.3

* After Carroll and Khor (7).
** Multiplicity = tumours/tumour-bearing rat.

Table 2
Institution of Caloric Restriction Related to Tumour Incidence*
(Benzo(a)pyrene-induced skin tumours in mice)

Regimen		Incidence (%)
Initiation	Promotion	
Ad libitum	Ad libitum	69
Ad libitum	Restricted	34
Restricted	Ad libitum	55
Restricted	Restricted	24

* After Tannenbaum (9).

showed that underfeeding inhibited growth of both spontaneous and transplanted tumours in mice. There was considerable interest in the underfeeding phenomenon for about 10 years and then it waned, possibly because investigators had gone about as far as the knowledge and techniques of the time could take them.

In the 1940s the laboratories of Baumann at the University of Wisconsin and of Tannenbaum at the Michael Reese Hospital in Chicago revived interest in undernutrition and cancer. Lavik and Baumann (12) compared the separate effects of fat and calories on the growth of methylcholanthrene (MC)-induced skin tumours in mice. When the diet was low in both fat and calories, no tumours were observed. A diet low in fat but high in calories led to a 54% incidence of tumours, whereas one high in fat but low in calories resulted in a tumour incidence of only 28%. Tumour incidence rose to 66% when the diet was high in both calories and fat. Tannenbaum showed that underfeeding was only effective when instituted during the promotion phase of tumourigenesis (13) (table 2). His work also demonstrated that underfeeding inhibited growth of spontaneous or chemically-induced tumours (14). In the course of his work Tannenbaum formulated a diet from which he could calculate caloric intake and thus he instituted studies of caloric (energy) restriction rather than only underfeeding. Boutwell et al. (15) carried out the first studies in which a scientifically prepared semi-purified diet was used in studies of caloric restriction and cancer and confirmed the earlier findings.

After about 1950 the work on caloric restriction languished until our laboratory began in-depth investigations in the 1980s. Our early studies were summarized in the earlier London symposium (16). Briefly we observed that when rats were treated with DMBA or 1,2-dimethylhydrazine (DMH) and fed 40% fewer calories than control rats they exhibited significantly fewer mammary (DMBA) or colon (DMH) tumours, even when their diets contained twice as much fat as the control diets (17). Tumour multiplicity and tumour burden, but not incidence, were reduced even by 10% restriction, and incidence of tumours was reduced at 20% restriction (18). Rats fed 26.7% corn oil but 25% fewer calories than controls fed *ad libitum* diets containing 5% corn oil had a significantly lower incidence of DMBA-induced mammary tumours and lower tumour multiplicity and tumour burden (19). Spontaneously obese LAN/cp rats showed a significant reduction in DMBA-induced mammary tumourigenesis when placed on 40% energy restriction (20).

Tannenbaum (9) showed that tumour growth was inhibited even when energy restriction was instituted in 9-month-old mice. Weindruch and Walford (21) restricted energy intake by 44% in 1-year-old mice of a strain prone to spontaneous tumourigenicity. Tumour incidence was reduced and life span increased. There is a positive relationship between feed efficiency and tumourigenesis (22).

Exercise will also increase caloric flux. Rusch and Kline (23) showed that exercise could decrease the weight of a transplanted tumour in mice by 30%. We (24) demonstrated that vigorous treadmill exercise could reduce the incidence of DMH-induced colon tumours in *ad libitum*–fed rats to the same extent as 25% caloric restriction. Cohen et al. (25) found that voluntary exercise reduced the incidence of N-nitrosomethylurea (NMU)-induced mammary tumours in rats.

Relevance to Humans

Seventy years ago Hoffman (26) proposed that energy excess was an important factor in cancer development. Twenty years ago Berg (27)

Table 3
Colon Cancer as Related to Lifetime Work Energy Output*

P	Age 30–65			Age 66–79		
	Cases	Controls	OR	Cases	Controls	OR
None	32	380	1.00	32	209	1.00
1–40%	49	365	1.59	20	85	1.54
41–100%	44	269	1.94[a]	33	123	1.75[b]

* After Vena et al. (31).
OR = odds ratio. P = Proportion of life spent in sedentary or light work.
[a] $p < 0.01$. [b] $p < 0.05$.

proposed that cancers prevalent in the United States might be related to high energy intake. Lew and Garfinkel (28) and Garfinkel (29) have shown a positive relationship between being overweight and cancer incidence and mortality in a cohort of over one million people.

The influence of lifelong energy expenditure has been assessed in a number of studies relating to the effects of vigorous occupational activity. Garabrant et al. (30), Vena et al. (31), and Gerhardsson et al. (32), among others, have shown that the risk of colon cancer is reduced significantly in men who have spent over 40% of their working careers at occupations that require high energy output (table 3). In 1921 Sivertsen and Dahlstrom (33) showed a negative relationship between occupational energy output and death from cancer but the group with lowest energy output and highest cancer mortality lived 10–15 years longer. A number of studies (34–36) have adduced a positive association between energy intake and colon cancer risk.

Mechanisms

We have now learned enough about the carcinogenic process and tumour biology to investigate the mechanisms by which energy restriction affects tumourigenesis.

Ruggeri (37) summarized the possible mechanisms (table 4) drawing on the available literature. Free radicals have been implicated as factors in tumourigenesis. Rao et al. (38) showed that energy restriction increased the activities of superoxide dismutase, catalase, and glutathione peroxidase in livers of ageing rats. The activities of superoxide anion, hydroxyl anion, and hydrogen peroxide fall by 27, 28, and 6%, respectively, in the livers of energy-restricted rats (39).

Table 4
Mechanisms by Which Caloric Restriction Might Inhibit Tumourigenesis*

1 Elevated glucocorticoid levels leading to growth inhibition
2 Reduction of mitotic activity and cell proliferation
3 Prolonged and/or increased immune response
4 "Starvation" of preneoplastic cells
5 Influence on specific hormones (mammotrophic hormones in the case of
  mammary tumours)
6 Influence on peptide growth factors or receptors
7 Modulation and repair of DNA damage

* After Ruggeri (37).

Table 5
Dietary Fat and Endogenous Oxidative DNA Damage in Rats*

Diet group	Calories (kcal/day)	DNA damage[a] Liver	Mammary
3% Fat	44.6 ± 0.3	2.30 ± 0.68	1.19 ± 0.40
5% Fat	46.0 ± 3.6	3.28 ± 1.32	1.76 ± 0.49
20% Fat	49.3 ± 2.0	2.59 ± 0.66	1.12 ± 0.26
CR (40%)[b]	26.8 ± 0.3	1.86 ± 0.36	1.10 ± 0.26

* After Djuric et al. (40).
Data ± SD, 12 rats/group.
[a] 5-hydroxymethyluracil/104 thymine residues.
[b] CR = caloric restriction.

Energy restriction significantly reduces oxidative DNA damage (40) (table 5). Energy restriction also enhances DNA repair (41) and increases formation of DNA adducts called I-compounds (42). Oncogenic expression in rats (43) and mice (44) is reduced by caloric restriction, as is expression of c-fos and c-ki-ras mRNA in mice (45). Heydari et al. (46) have summarized the effects of dietary restriction on expression of specific genes in mice and rats. A partial but representative list is given in table 6.

In 1949 Boutwell et al. (47) suggested that energy restriction of female rats resulted in "pseudohypohysectomy" reducing the size of the ovaries and uterus. They also observed adrenal hypertrophy. In 1992 Pashko and Schwartz (48) demonstrated that the influence of energy restriction on mouse skin tumour promotion could be reversed by adrenalectomy. More recently (49) they have shown the

Table 6
Effect of Dietary Restriction on Expression of Specific Genes in Rats and Mice*

Rat (male F344)		Mouse (female C3B10RF1)	
Gene	Change	Gene	Change
Catalase (L)	+	IGF-I (L)	+
c-myc (L)	0	c-jun	0
Cytochrome P450 (L)	+	Cytochrome P450 (L)	+
Androgen receptor (L)	+		
Calcitonin (T)	−		
Somatostatin (T)	−		

* After Heydari et al. (46).
L = liver; T = thyroid.
+ = increase; o = no change; − = decrease.

Table 7
Adrenalectomy Reverses Energy Restriction–Induced Inhibition of Lung
Tumourigenesis in Mice*

Group	No. of mice	Lung tumours/Mouse
Sham, AL	30	2.03 ± 0.29
Sham, ER	29	0.52 ± 0.10
Adrex, AL	28	4.46 ± 0.83
Adrex, ER	26	4.65 ± 0.97

* After Pashko and Schwartz (49).
DMBA-induced tumors. AL = ad libitum; ER = energy restricted.

same to be true of DMBA-induced lung tumourigenesis (table 7). In both cases, plasma corticosterone levels were increased significantly. Dietary restriction has been shown to increase serum corticosterone levels in normal mice when they were 7, 15, or 30 months of age (50). Energy restriction enhances production of glucocorticoid receptor mRNA in mice (51).

Insulin is a growth factor for tumours. Insulin deprivation inhibits tumour growth and cell division (52,53). When rats are subjected to caloric restriction, their plasma insulin levels fall (18,19) (table 8). The levels of plasma insulin fall immediately upon institution of energy restriction and remain low throughout the duration of restriction (54). Hepatic insulin receptors are increased in energy-restricted rats (55).

Table 8
Plasma Insulin Levels in DMBA-Treated Rats Fed *Ad libitum* (AL) or Energy Restricted (ER) Diets

Regimen	% Fat	Tumour incidence (%)	Insulin (µU/ml)
Study 1[a]			
AL	5	60	122 ± 16
10% ER	5	60	191 ± 10
20% ER	5	40	109 ± 13
30% ER	5	35	42 ± 5
40% ER	5	5	41 ± 8
		p < 0.005	p < 0.001
Study 2[b]			
AL	5	65	143 ± 16
AL	15	85	164 ± 15
AL	20	80	158 ± 11
25% ER	20	60	100 ± 2
25% ER	26.7	30	117 ± 13
		p < 0.005	p < 0.02

[a] Klurfeld et al. (18).
[b] Klurfeld et al. (19).

Table 9
Mammary Tumours in DMBA-Treated Female Sprague Dawley Rats Subjected to Energy Restriction (ER)*

Regimen	Tumour incidence (%)	Multiplicity	Tumour type (%)	
			Large	Small
AL	90	5.6 ± 1.7	87	13
25% ER	61	3.4 ± 0.6	77	23
40% ER	20	1.5 ± 0.5	33	66
p	0.007	0.05	< 0.0001	< 0.0001

* After Ruggeri et al. (56).
AL = *ad libitum*.

In a study of effects of different levels of energy restriction on DMBA-induced mammary tumourigenesis in rats (56), we examined the size of the tumours. We arbitrarily decided that any tumour weighing more than 100 mg was a "large" tumour. As can be seen from table 9, the ratio of large to small tumours was 6.7 in *ad libitum*–fed rats, fell to 3.3 in rats subjected to 25% energy restriction, and was

0.5 in rats whose energy intake was restricted by 40%. This observation suggests that the tumours had been implanted but were unable to grow. Thus there may be a competition between the tumour and host. In conditions of low energy availability the host wins out, but when there is excess of energy the tumour eventually triumphs.

The data show clearly that reduction of energy intake or increased energy output inhibits tumourigenesis (spontaneous, transplanted, or induced) in rodents. Since dietary fat supplies more calories than carbohydrate or protein it is immediately suspect, but as our studies show (17,19) energy restriction inhibits tumours even when the restricted animals ingest more fat than the freely fed controls. A modest reduction in energy intake may be a simple approach to reducing cancer risk in humans.

Interest in this area of research is borne out by the recent appearance of two books related to the effects of energy (caloric) restriction (see references 46 and 50).

REFERENCES

1 Watson AF, Mellanby E. Tar cancer in mice. II. The condition of the skin when modified by external treatment or diet, as a factor in influencing the cancerous reaction. *Br J Exp Pathol* 1930;11:311–322.

2 Baumann CA, Jacobi HP, Rusch HP. The effect of diet upon experimental tumor production. *Am J Hygiene* 1939;30:1–6.

3 Lavik PS, Baumann CA. Dietary fat and tumor formation. *Cancer Res* 1941;1:181–187.

4 Miller JA, Kline BE, Rusch HP, Baumann CA. The effect of certain lipids on the carcinogenicity of p-dimethylaminoazobenzene. *Cancer Res* 1944;4:756–761.

5 Kline BE, Nuller JA, Rusch HP, Baumann CA. Certain effects of dietary fats on the production of liver tumors in rats fed p-dimethylaminoazobenzene. *Cancer Res* 1946;6:5–7.

6 Gammal EB, Carroll KK, Plunkett ER. Effects of dietary fat on mammary carcinogenesis by 7,12-dimethylbenz(a) anthracene in rats. *Cancer Res* 1967;27:1737–1742.

7 Carroll KK, Khor H. Effect of level and type of dietary fat on incidence of mammary tumors induced in female Sprague-Dawley rats by 7,12-dimethylbenz(a) anthracene. *Lipids* 1971;6:415–420.

8 Ip C, Carter CA, Ip MM. Requirement of essential fatty acid for mammary tumorigenesis in the rat. *Cancer Res* 1985;45:1997–2001.

9 Tannenbaum A. Effects of varying caloric intake upon tumor incidence and tumor growth. *Ann NY Acad Sci* 1947;49:5–17.
10 Moreschi C. Beziehungen Zwischen Ernährung und Tumorwaschstum. *Z Immunitätsforsch* 1909;2:651–675.
11 Rous P. The influence of diet on transplanted and spontaneous tumors. *J Exp Med* 1914;3:150–167.
12 Lavik PS, Baumann CA. Further studies on the tumor-promoting action of fat. *Cancer Res* 1943;3:749–756.
13 Tannenbaum A. The dependence of the genesis of induced skin tumors on the caloric intake during different stages of carcinogenesis. *Cancer Res* 1944;4:683–687.
14 Tannenbaum A. The genesis and growth of tumors. II. Effects of caloric restriction per se. *Cancer Res* 1942;2:460–467.
15 Boutwell RK, Brush MK, Rusch HP. The stimulating effect of dietary fat on carcinogenesis. *Cancer Res* 1949;9:741–746.
16 Kritchevsky D. Calories and cancer. In: Carroll KK, ed. *Diet, nutrition, and health*. Montreal: McGill-Queen's University Press, 1990:250–255.
17 Kritchevsky D, Weber MM, Klurfeld DM. Dietary fat versus caloric content in initiation and promotion of 7,12-dimethylbenz(a)anthracene–induced mammary tumorigenesis in rats. *Cancer Res* 1984;44:3174–3177.
18 Klurfeld DM, Welch CB, Davis MJ, Kritchevsky D. Determination of degree of energy restriction necessary to reduce DMBA-induced mammary tumorigenesis in rats during the promotion phase. *J Nutr* 1989;119:286–291.
19 Klurfeld DM, Welch CB, Lloyd LM, Kritchevsky D. Inhibition of DMBA-induced mammary tumorigenesis by caloric restriction in rats fed high fat diets. *Int J Cancer* 1989;43:922–925.
20 Klurfeld DM, Lloyd LM, Buck CL, Davis MJ, Tulp ON, Kritchevsky D. Inhibition of mammary tumorigenesis in LA-N/cp (corpulent) rats. *Fed Proc* 1987;46:436.
21 Weindruch R, Walford RL. Dietary restriction in mice beginning at one year of age: effect on life span and spontaneous cancer incidence. *Science* 1982;215:1415–1418.
22 Kritchevsky D, Welch CB, Klurfeld DM. Response of mammary tumors to caloric restriction for different time periods during the promotion phase. *Nutr Cancer* 1989;12:259–269.
23 Rusch HP, Kline BE. The effect of exercise on the growth of a mouse tumor. *Cancer Res* 1944;4:116–118.
24 Klurfeld DM, Welch CB, Einhorn E, Kritchevsky D. Inhibition of colon tumor promotion by caloric restriction or exercise in rats. *FASEB J* 1988;2:A433.

25 Cohen LA, Chor K, Wang C-X. Influence of dietary fat, caloric restriction and voluntary exercise on N-nitrosomethylurea-induced mammary tumorigenesis in rats. *Cancer Res* 1988;48:4276–4283.

26 Hoffman FL. Cancer increase and overnutrition. Newark, NJ: Prudential Insurance Co, 1927.

27 Berg JW. Can nutrition explain the pattern of international epidemiology of hormone-dependent cancer? *Cancer Res* 1975;35:3345–3350.

28 Lew EA, Garfinkel L. Variations in mortality by weight in 750,000 men and women. *J Chronic Dis* 1979;32:563–576.

29 Garfinkel L. Overweight and cancer. *Ann Int Med* 1985;103:1034–1036.

30 Garabrant DH, Peters JM, Mack TM, Bernstein L. Job activity and colon cancer risk. *Am J Epidemiol* 1984;119:1005–1014.

31 Vena JE, Graham S, Zielezny M, Swanson MK, Barnes RE, Nolan J. Lifetime occupational exercise and colon cancer. *Am J Epidemiol* 1985;122:357–365.

32 Gerhardsson M, Floderus B, Norell SE. Physical activity and colon cancer risk. *Int J Epidemiol* 1988;17:743–746.

33 Sivertsen I, Dahlstrom AW. The relation of muscular activity to carcinoma. *Am J Cancer* 1921;6:365–377.

34 Jain M, Cook GM, Davis FG, Grace MG, Howe ER, Miller AB. A case-control study of diet and colorectal cancer. *Int J Cancer* 1980;26:757–768.

35 Bristol JB, Emmett PM, Heaton KW, Williamson RCN. Sugar, fat and the risk of colorectal cancer. *Br Med J* 1985;291:1467–1470.

36 Lyon JL, Mahoney AW, West DW, Gardner JW, Smith KR, Sorenson AW, Stanish W. Energy intake: its relation to colon cancer. *J Natl Cancer Inst* 1987;78:853–861.

37 Ruggeri BA. The effect of caloric restriction neoplasia and age-related degenerative processes. In: Alfin-Slater RB, Kritchevsky D, eds. *Human nutrition: a comprehensive treatise, cancer and nutrition*, vol 7. New York: Plenum Press, 1991:187–210.

38 Rao G, Xia E, Nadakuvukaren MJ, Richardson A. Effect of dietary restriction on the age-dependent changes in the expression of antioxidant enzymes in rat liver. *J Nutr* 1990;120:602–609.

39 Yu BP. Free radicals and modulation by dietary restriction. *Age and Nutrition* 1991;2:84–88.

40 Djuric Z, Lu MH, Lewis S, Luongo DA, Chen XW, Heilbrun LK, Reading BA, Duffy PH, Hart RW. Oxidative DNA damage in rats fed low fat, high fat or caloric-restricted diets. *Toxicol Appl Pharmacol* 1992;115:156–160.

41 Lipman JM, Turturro A, Hart RW. The influence of dietary restriction on DNA-repair in rodents: a preliminary study. *Mech Aging Dev* 1989;48:135–143.

42 Randerath E, Hart RW, Turturro A, Danna TF, Reddy R, Randerath K. Effects of aging and caloric restriction on I-compounds in liver, kidney, and white blood cell DNA of male brown Norway rats. *Mech Aging Dev* 1991;58:279–296.

43 Fernandes G, Khare A, Langamere S, Yu B, Sandberg L, Fredricks B. Effect of food restriction and aging on immune cell fatty acids, functions and oncogene expression in SPF Fischer 344 rats. *Fed Proc* 1987;46:567.

44 Nakamura KD, Duffy PH, Lu MS, Turturro A, Hart RW. The effect of dietary restriction on myc protooncogene expression in mice: a preliminary study. *Mech Aging Dev* 1989;48:199–205.

45 Himeno Y, Engelman RW, Good RA. Influence of caloric restriction on oncogene expression and DNA synthesis during liver regeneration. *Proc Natl Acad Sci USA* 1992;89:5497–5501.

46 Heydari A, Gutsmann A, You S, Takahashi R, Richardson A. Effect of dietary restriction on the genome functions of cells: alterations in the transcriptional apparatus of cells. In: Hart RW, Neumann DA, Robertson RT, eds. *Dietary restriction*. Washington: ILSI Press, 1995:213–228.

47 Boutwell RK, Brush MK, Rusch HP. Some physiological effects associated with chronic caloric restriction. *Am J Physiol* 1949;154:517–524.

48 Pashko LL, Schwartz AG. Reversal of food restriction–induced inhibition of mouse skin tumor promotion by adrenalectomy. *Carcinogenesis* 1992;13:1925–1928.

49 Pashko LL, Schwartz AG. Inhibition of 7,12-dimethylbenz(a) anthracene–induced lung tumorigenesis in A/J mice by food restriction is reversed by adrenalectomy. *Carcinogenesis* 1996;17:209–212.

50 Holson RR, Duffy PH, Ali SF, Scalzo FM. Aging, dietary restriction and glucocorticoids: a critical review of the glucocorticoid hypothesis. In: Fishbein L, ed. *Biological effects of dietary restriction*. Berlin: Springer Verlag, 1991:123–139.

51 Spindler SR, Grizzle JM, Walford RL, Mote PL. Aging and restriction of dietary calories increases insulin receptor mRNA and aging increases glucocorticoid receptor mRNA in the liver of female C3B10RF mice. *J Gerontol* 1991;46:B233–B237.

52 Cohen ND, Hilf R. Influence of insulin on growth and metabolism of 7,12-dimethylbenz(a) anthracene–induced mammary tumors. *Cancer Res* 1974;34:3245–3252.

53 Taub R, Roy A, Dieter R, Koontz J. Insulin as a growth factor in rat hepatoma cells. *J Biol Chem* 1987;262:10893–10897.

54 Ruggeri BA, Klurfeld DM, Kritchevsky D, Furlanetto RW. Caloric restriction and 7,12-dimethylbenz(a)-anthracene-induced mammary

tumor growth in rats: alterations in circulating insulin, insulin-like growth factors I and II, and epidermal growth factor. *Cancer Res* 1989;49:4130–4134.

55 Balage M, Manin M, Arnal M, Grizard J. Differential regulation of muscle and liver insulin receptor by energy restriction in growing rats. *Reproductive Nutr Dev* 1988;18:819–820.

56 Ruggeri RA, Klurfeld DM, Kritchevsky D. Biochemical alterations in 7,12-dimethylbenz(a)-anthracene-induced mammary tumors from rats subjected to caloric restriction. *Biochim Biophys Acta* 1987;929:239–246.

Priorities for
Nutrition Research
in Canada

HEATHER NIELSEN Representing
THE JOINT STEERING COMMITTEE RESPONSIBLE
FOR DEVELOPMENT OF A NATIONAL NUTRITION
PLAN FOR CANADA 1996

Nutrition for Health: An Agenda for Action

Nutritional well-being for all people in a peaceful, just, and environmentally safe world.

World Declaration on Nutrition

Dear Partners,

The health and well-being of individuals and the prosperity of the nation require a well nourished population. We all have a role to play in improving the nutritional health of Canadians.

Nutrition for Health: An Agenda for Action is the result of a multi-sectoral, Canada-wide process that gathered the collective wisdom of groups, organizations, and individuals. Communities and organizations can use this *Agenda for Action* to develop plans specific to their needs and capacities.

Implementation is up to all of us. The Joint Steering Committee recommends the establishment of a multisectoral network at the national level to provide leadership and co-ordination to this *Agenda for Action*.

Nutrition for Health: An Agenda for Action is focused on stimulating and accelerating action by all sectors towards achieving healthier people. Working together we can make a difference.

Joint Steering Committee
Spring 1996

1. Overview

The purpose of Nutrition for Health: An Agenda for Action *is to ensure integration of nutrition considerations into health, agriculture, education, social and economic policies and programs.*

WHY AN AGENDA FOR ACTION ...

Achieving "nutritional well-being for all people in a peaceful, just and environmentally safe world"* is an important goal and Canadians can make a significant contribution. Efforts to improve nutritional health require action by many sectors. *Nutrition for Health: An Agenda for Action* provides a model to address nutrition issues in communities across Canada. It includes a discussion of international issues and how foreign policy interconnects with domestic policy with regard to nutrition.

This document recognizes the following reasons to broaden support for nutrition.

- A well nourished population contributes to a healthier, more productive population, lower health care and social costs, and better quality of life.
- While the nutritional health of Canadians is good, it is not optimal.
- Eating patterns of many Canadians contribute to the high incidence of nutrition-related chronic diseases.
- Diet and activity patterns are second only to tobacco when considering non-genetic factors that contribute to mortality.
- Inequities in nutritional well-being exist, particularly for the socio-economically disadvantaged.
- Food choices are complex decisions which are influenced by a dynamic relationship between individual and environmental factors.

HOW IT WILL WORK ...

It is the intent of *Nutrition for Health: An Agenda for Action* to stimulate widespread action in mutually supportive directions, creating momentum and positive results for nutritional health.

---

* World Declaration on Nutrition

The action that communities undertake will be as unique as communities are unique. Local partners may differ, a community's needs and capacities will vary, but the sum of the actions will be significant.

Building on current knowledge and accomplishments, *Nutrition for Health: An Agenda for Action* encourages policy and program development that is coordinated, multisectoral, supports new and existing partnerships and promotes the efficient use of limited resources.

WHO IT IS FOR ...

Nutrition for Health: An Agenda for Action is targeted to community leaders and decision makers in a broad range of sectors. The policies and actions of governments, industry, non-government and voluntary organizations, affect the nutritional health of Canadians.

This *Agenda for Action* can be used by anyone committed to improving the nutritional health of the population. It has been specifically designed to facilitate nutrition planning at all levels. Its directional, rather than prescriptive nature, allows for application by many different players, in many different settings.

WHAT IT CONSISTS OF ...

It describes our current situation, builds on the Framework for Population Health, identifies priority areas for action, considers the implications of our international context, and includes indicators to monitor change in conditions related to nutritional health.

WHERE IT ALL BEGAN ...

Rome, 1992: At the International Conference on Nutrition, a joint venture of the World Health Organization (WHO) and the Food and Agriculture Organization (FAO), participating countries endorsed a *World Declaration on Nutrition* (Appendix 1) and made a commitment to develop national plans of action for nutrition.

With representation from diverse sectors across the country, Health Canada established a Joint Steering Committee (Appendix 2) to prepare a national nutrition plan. The Joint Steering Committee commissioned a series of studies (Appendix 3), drafted a plan, consulted stakeholders across Canada and then revised the plan. This document, *Nutrition for Health: An Agenda for Action*, is the result.

2. Current Situation

Nutrition-related conditions contribute to spiralling health care costs, lost economic productivity and decreased quality of life. The changing social, physical and health system environments can have a significant impact on nutritional health.

The Canadian people are changing. The population is aging, the elderly are staying in their homes longer, cultural diversity is increasing and the structure of the family is changing. Only 10% of families have a stay-at-home-spouse. Seventy percent of preschool children are in care arrangements while parents work or attend school. With growing time pressures, and less time to devote to food related activities, convenience foods and the food service sector play an increasingly important role in food choices and eating patterns.

The economic climate is suffering from new pressures. Accumulated debt, deficits, globalization, liberalizing trade, and the impact of technology are contributing to a fundamental restructuring of the economy. Domestic markets face increased competition. New export markets provide opportunity for wealth generation. At the same time, some people have become more vulnerable during this transition. Many Canadians have been affected by unemployment and reduced real income. Poverty among young families, lone seniors and socially isolated people is on the rise.

The social climate is undergoing change. For some, the primary influences on behaviour and life choices remain the traditional ones such as family, school, and religion, but for others, the media and peer groups are major sources of information and serve as role models for eating habits. Healthy food options must be provided in a variety of settings and the widespread promotion of healthy eating messages is needed.

Social programs are being re-evaluated as governments struggle with balancing budgets and reducing debt. Under review are traditional Canadian values such as universality, an income safety net, and the extent of social policy in general. The resulting shifts in social policies can have a significant impact on nutritional health.

Nutrition-related concerns do exist. In fact, nutrition problems contribute to spiralling health care costs, lost economic productivity and decreased quality of life. These problems are documented in the background papers outlined in Appendix 3.

Nutrition-related chronic diseases prevail. Cardiovascular disease, diabetes, osteoporosis and cancer result in premature death and

---

SELECTED NUTRITION-RELATED CONCERNS

- Cardiovascular disease accounts for 37% of all male deaths and 41% of all female deaths.
- Cancer accounts for 28% of all male deaths and 27% of all female deaths.
- Approximately 23% of Canadians are overweight.
- The prevalence of obesity in children has increased in the past decade from 14% to 24% among girls and from 18% to 26% among boys.
- Breastfeeding initiation and continuation varies widely across Canada, from an average of 75% initiation and only 30% continuation for 4–6 months.
- The rate of low birth weight in Canada is 5.7% while in certain subpopulations of the very poor living in the inner city, low birth weights are as high as 10%, rates comparable to those in developing countries.
- There are approximately 460 food banks helping 2,400,000 Canadians including 900,000 children.
- There are approximately 600 meal programs, with over 40,000 volunteers delivering meals to dependent seniors and shut-ins across the country.

---

disability for many people each year. The role of healthy eating and lifestyle in reducing the incidence of these multifactorial diseases is significant. Food choices of many Canadians result in inadequate amounts of some essential nutrients and excess amounts of fat and saturated fat.

Almost one quarter of Canadians are overweight. Physical inactivity combined with excess food energy intake, contribute to this problem. Obesity in children is increasing and appears to be related to inadequate exercise. Eating disorders remain a significant problem.

Disparities in nutritional well-being are evident. Health and nutritional problems are more common among vulnerable groups. There is evidence of micronutrient deficiency in some vulnerable groups, for example iron deficiency is seen in children within the aboriginal community.

Among those of lower socio-economic status, the incidence of low birth weights is higher and the rate of breastfeeding initiation is lower, than among the general population. Programs exist for groups such as high risk pregnant women, but they are not available to all who need them.

Some individuals see their access to foods threatened. The ability of certain vulnerable groups to obtain the food they need for their nutritional well-being without jeopardizing other basic needs, is of real concern. The use of food banks has risen dramatically and more food provision programs appear every day. Underlying causes of income insufficiency need effective solutions.

Health systems are being reformed, changing the way services are delivered, who delivers them and how resources are allocated. Health services are shifting from institutions to community-based delivery systems and the role of regional planning groups in decision making is expanding. Greater recognition is being given to the benefits of health promotion and disease prevention. Focused efforts to integrate nutrition services into existing and evolving health systems are necessary.

Nutrition research is lacking. Nutrition research includes a range of activities and methods – all integral to the understanding of nutrition problems and to the identification of solutions. Current priorities and existing research efforts are not aligned. Nutrition research is underfunded generally, and funding lies almost totally in biological sciences. The availability of nutrition expertise is threatened by insufficient funding of nutrition research. Monitoring the nutritional health of the population is essential, but is hampered by a lack of national data.

The food supply is being reshaped by many factors; new technologies in plant breeding, crop disease control, production, processing and novel ingredients; trade agreements that aim at a free flow of food between countries; and consumer demand for certain foods. Canada produces a safe, high quality food supply for domestic consumption and export, and imports many processed foods as well as out-of-season, tropical and non-traditional foods. Interest in the long term sustainability of the food supply is high. Issues related to sustainability of natural resources, including food, require cooperation between producers, food processors, retailers, governments and consumers.

The international context has always been important to Canada. It is becoming increasingly so. The rapid evolution of regional trading blocs and the liberalization of trade, the swift and relatively free flow of people across borders, Canada's significant immigration levels and the development of almost instantaneous communications capabilities have brought Canada closer to the rest of the world. Food and nutrition issues are no exception to this trend.

System wide reform is underway, resulting in policy and program redirection in many environments. Efforts to reduce nutrition problems will need to work within the climate of accelerated reform and must focus on innovative and collaborative solutions. The next section,

How Nutritional Health is Determined, discusses the Framework for
Population Health, a model that is both comprehensive and responsive to today's complex nutritional health issues.

3. How Nutritional Health is Determined

*Powerful economic and social forces, combined with individual practices and
capacities, influence what foods are available, and what foods are chosen.*

Canada has advanced understanding about the effect of people's
lifestyles and socio-economic circumstances on their health and
well-being. Reports such as the "Lalonde Report" (*A New Perspective
on the Health of Canadians,* 1974), *Achieving Health for All* (1986) and
the 1988 *Ottawa Charter on Health Promotion* have helped to create
this understanding.

A more recent report, *Strategies for Population Health, Investing in
the Health of Canadians* (1991),* builds on earlier work and positions
determinants of health within the Framework for Population Health.
This population health model has application to nutritional health.

Food choices, which play a direct role in nutritional health, significantly influence health status. Taking personal responsibility for
one's health is important, however food choices are not simply a
matter of personal choice. Economic and social forces, together with
factors related to the physical environment, influence what foods are
available and a person's individual capacity to make choices.

Actions by policy makers and community leaders must consider
all determinants of health and must be based on a foundation that
includes research, information and public policy.

INDIVIDUAL   FACTORS

Basic biology, genetic endowment, health status and individual
health practices impact on nutritional health. Nutrition programs
have long recognized the importance of knowledge, attitudes and
skills in developing positive health practices such as appropriate
food choice behaviour. The individual's capacity to adopt a healthy
pattern of eating is influenced by both the availability and understanding of information provided by sources such as *Canada's Food*

---

* Prepared by the Federal, Provincial and Territorial Advisory Committee on Population Health.

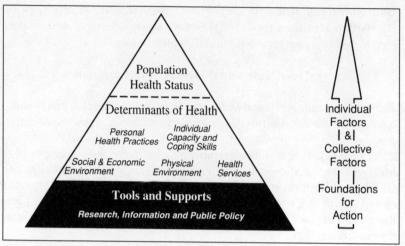

Framework for Population Health

Guide to Healthy Eating and food labels. Individual capacity involves more than knowledge about what to eat. It includes food preparation skills, time to prepare, and personal buying power, all of which are profoundly influenced by the following environmental factors.

COLLECTIVE FACTORS

Social and Economic Environment.   Economic conditions influence the ability of individuals to acquire a healthy diet. Unemployment and inadequate financial resources reduce individual capacity to meet daily need for food.

The social environment, with its diverse social mores, cultural values, support networks, traditions and practices, influences people's food choices. Settings vary – home, school, workplace, recreational site, restaurants – each affecting food choices. Advertising and the media are key sources of nutrition information.

Physical Environment.   Food is part of the physical environment. The type of food available in grocery stores, workplaces, schools and from the food service sector is a powerful influence on food choices. The composition of food can support the consumption of a diet consistent with nutrition guidelines and label information can assist consumers in making healthy food choices.

Not all consumers are in a position to choose their own food. Children at home, in day care and at school; individuals in hospitals and chronic care facilities; prison inmates; military personnel; individuals receiving meal services, such as Meals on Wheels; those in congregate dining programs, and others fed in institutional settings, are in environments where food is provided.

Health Services. Access to the full range of health, social and community services, including nutrition services, is essential. Appropriate nutrition services encompass healthy eating programs, public education, and access to individual care and counselling. Those with special nutrition needs or health conditions, such as pregnant women, breastfeeding mothers, the elderly, the sick and those with therapeutic nutrition needs, require access to care, counselling and education.

The collective and individual factors are intrinsically connected to the third component of the Framework for Population Health – the tools and supports that are the foundation for action.

FOUNDATIONS FOR ACTION

Research, information and public policy must form the foundations for action. Nutrition research encompasses a continuum of activity including research in basic biological sciences, epidemiology, clinical nutrition, determinants of food choices, dietary surveys, and the evaluation of programs, practices and policies. Information is essential for informed decision making at all levels from individual consumer decisions to organizational and public policy decisions. Public policy can help to create an environment that will promote health and nutritional well-being. Public policy must be based on informed decision making and research must provide relevant information to policy makers.

The Framework for Population Health provides an overview of the determinants of health and their interrelationships. The next section, *Strategic Directions*, builds on this population health model and describes a multilevel, multisectoral approach to improving the nutritional health of the population.

Canada does not exist in isolation. The world trade system increasingly affects domestic policy and programs. Internationally, Canada has a long tradition of assistance to developing countries. These linkages are discussed in section 5, *International Dimensions*.

4. Strategic Directions

- *Reinforce healthy eating practices*
- *Support nutritionally vulnerable populations*
- *Continue to enhance the availability of foods that support healthy eating*
- *Support nutrition research*

Nutritional health depends on several elements including comprehensive health and social policies, nutrition recommendations and guidelines, a safe food supply, and consumer interest in health and nutrition.

The four Strategic Directions arise from an analysis of the current situation in Canada. For each Direction, actions were considered to address the determinants identified in the Framework for Population Health, including individual factors, collective factors, and foundations for action. The selected actions are all high priority actions where resource allocation will have the greatest impact on health. All actions are interrelated, overlapping, and complementary.

Many communities across the country are already conducting health-enhancing activities. The intent of *Nutrition For Health: An Agenda for Action* is to build on these strengths, support activity already aligned with the Strategic Directions and stimulate new activity to achieve healthier people.

Nutrition issues are complex and involve many sectors. Intersectoral solutions are encouraged, with the formation of networks and coalitions being an essential component of successful action. The formation of a multisectoral co-ordinating network of interested partners will be an important first step. Sustained cooperation between sectors will require commitment, a willingness to align efforts, and the existence of facilitating structures. Involving people and their communities in comprehensive, multidisciplinary planning will yield positive health results.

REINFORCE HEALTHY EATING PRACTICES

National nutrition policies provide the foundation for healthy eating programs. *Nutrition Recommendations, Canada's Guidelines for Healthy Eating,* and *Canada's Food Guide to Healthy Eating* all contribute to our understanding of healthy eating practices.

Canadians need to improve their food choices and be more physically active in order to minimize the risk of nutrition-related chronic diseases. Eating patterns need more emphasis on bread, cereals, grains, fruit and vegetables, and adequate intakes of essential nutrients, and less emphasis on fat and saturated fat. Lack of physical activity, combined with excess food energy intakes, contributes to the continued prevalence of obesity.

Dietary change has been positive, but slow. Focused action to support healthy eating must occur in policies governing availability of nutrition services in health and community agencies, in programs enhancing consumer skills, and in services delivering care to individuals from birth to old age.

Healthy eating practices will be strengthened by the following: community-based services that include nutrition; schools that provide age-appropriate nutrition education; programs that emphasize practical skill development in reinforcing positive food choices; support for breastfeeding as the cultural norm; media and advertising which disseminate consistent, accurate messages; and food that is labelled to facilitate knowledgeable choice.

Key Actions:

1 Work to include and maintain nutrition services as part of comprehensive health services in both existing and evolving community-based settings.
2 Incorporate nutrition into curricula for children and youth and include quality daily physical education as part of all school programs.
3 Include nutrition in both the training and continuing education programs for health and other community service providers.
4 Improve usefulness of nutrition labelling, increase its availability, and broaden public education on its use.
5 Emphasize practical skill development (food selection, storage and preparations skills) in nutrition education programs for the public.
6 Work with the media to provide responsible public information on healthy eating and physical activity.
7 Protect and promote breastfeeding and improve access to community-based breastfeeding support groups.

SUPPORT NUTRITIONALLY VULNERABLE POPULATIONS

Vulnerability may result from several factors such as physical or mental disabilities, lack of education, acute and chronic illness, growth and aging. Poverty is frequently related to increased vulnerability and is often inter-related with other factors. Most at risk are those who are both physiologically vulnerable and socio-economically disadvantaged.

Nutritional vulnerability related to poverty is more prevalent within subgroups of the population including aboriginal people, seniors, refugees, high risk pregnant women, single mothers, low birth weight babies and children. The effects of poor nutrition prenatally and during infancy and childhood will be felt throughout the lifecycle. Data, however, are limited on the nutritional status of these vulnerable groups.

An increasing number of Canadians are turning to food banks in an attempt to meet their food needs. Food banks, originally seen as a temporary system of food relief, now provide charitable food support to growing numbers of Canadians. A variety of smaller scale, community food initiatives, such as collective kitchens, community gardens, food buying clubs, school-based breakfast and lunch clubs, have emerged to address the problem. The risk of chronically compromised food consumption is a serious public health concern.

Vulnerable groups require special support. Employment creation, income support and community-based food related policies and programs must be implemented to protect the nutritional health of vulnerable groups.

Key Actions:

1 Work with social policy decision makers to address the nutritional needs of vulnerable people.
2 Develop a data base to better define the vulnerable populations and to better understand their food and nutrition issues.
3 Monitor the cost of a nutritious food basket and use this information in the development of education programs and income support initiatives.
4 Strengthen the food and nutrition component of community programs and services for vulnerable groups, including acute and chronically ill people.
5 Provide broader and more consistent access to prenatal nutrition programs for vulnerable pregnant women.
6 Ensure that families have the supports they need to nourish their children adequately.
7 Ensure that nutrition is part of the continuing care programs in the community.

8 Support community meal programs to meet the nutritional needs of seniors or those who cannot leave home.

CONTINUE TO ENHANCE THE AVAILABILITY OF FOODS THAT SUPPORT HEALTHY EATING

Consumers value their access to quality foods. In Canada the food supply provides safe, nutritious food at both the retail and food service levels.

Policies that govern food production, pricing, composition, preparation, labelling, claims, and advertising influence the nutritional quality of the food supply. Food consumed away from home is making an increasingly important contribution to nutritional health. Small positive changes in the composition of food can have a significant impact on the nutrient content of the Canadian diet.

New technologies in food production and processing require ongoing evaluation. Public apprehension with respect to biotechnology in food production covers a range of issues including product safety, quality, and choice. Continued consumer participation in identifying their issues is fundamental.

Sustainability of all resources, including food, is essential to maintain a physical environment that supports health. In its broadest sense, sustainability refers to conserving or enhancing natural resources and the quality of the environment for future generations. This has special significance for indigenous food supplies which can be affected by environmental contamination as well as by physical changes to the land resulting from development activity.

Food imports and liberalized trade bring new challenges for policy makers and food inspection. Healthy eating patterns are supported by the continued review and evolution of policies which influence the sustainability, safety, availability and nutritional composition of food.

Key Actions:

1 Ensure that policies relating to food production, composition, addition of nutrients to foods, and marketing of food, promote increased availability of foods with compositional characteristics that support healthy eating.
2 Work with the food service sector to increase the availability of foods that support healthy eating.

3 Implement policies and incentives in publicly funded organizations (e.g. schools, hospitals, government agencies) to promote increased availability of foods that support healthy eating.
4 Maintain high standards of food safety through multisectoral cooperation to evolve food regulation, inspection, quality control and consumer safe food handling practices.
5 Engage in active dialogue with consumers about issues of food safety, food quality and new food technologies.
6 Support agriculture and food policies that are consistent with environmentally sustainable practices.

SUPPORT NUTRITION RESEARCH

Nutrition research covers a broad scope of activity. Biochemistry, molecular biology, clinical research, epidemiology and dietary surveys provide basic building blocks to better define the link between nutrition and chronic disease as well as essential nutrient requirements. Research on determinants of food choice and research to evaluate programs, practices and policies are equally important. Recognition of the value and importance of research across the continuum is essential.

There is inadequate total funding for nutrition research and an urgent need for long-term stable funding. Existing funds, while limited, are most often directed towards basic research. Program and practice-based research in clinical and population health settings needs strengthening. The availability of nutrition expertise is threatened by inadequate support for nutrition research.

Research efforts are not aligned with current nutrition priorities. Strengthening research to support nutrition priorities is vital.

Collaborative, multidisciplinary projects involving many sectors encourage combining of expertise and financial resources. Traditional scientific methods are being complemented with diverse methodologies such as qualitative research, program evaluation and case study discussions.

Improving the nutritional health of Canadians is dependent on our ability to monitor nutritional health and respond appropriately. A mechanism is needed to integrate and disseminate data to ensure it is available for practice, program and policy decisions.

Key Actions:

1 Establish research priorities that are aligned with the Strategic Directions and that consider the continuum of nutrition research activity.

2 Find effective mechanisms to expand access to research dollars from granting organizations for basic, clinical and applied research.
3 Access research funds from local, non-traditional sources (e.g. service clubs, industry).
4 Develop a data base on relevant indicators affecting nutritional health including nutritional status, food practices, social, economic, cultural and educational data.
5 Develop mechanisms to integrate and disseminate data to enable evidence-based program and policy decisions.

5. International Dimensions

Canada is part of the global community. Nutrition is integral to Canada's official development assistance, trade, and related knowledge and technologies.

The international context is increasingly important to nutrition at home and abroad. Canada is committed to a policy of strong international trade. To facilitate trade, Canada supports the international harmonization of regulations and the removal of trade barriers. In food trade the implications are important. By choice, and by necessity, Canada relies on importation for a substantial part of its food usage and on export of Canadian-produced food commodities to balance the trade picture. In a very real sense, Canada's food security depends upon the stability of world food trade. Canada has made a commitment to populations in developing countries and recently restated its commitment on making progress towards official development assistance as 0.7% GNP when the fiscal situation allows it. Featured in this commitment is Canada's involvement in health and nutrition worldwide.

Food, nutrition and health are priorities for Canadian Official Development Assistance (ODA). The United Nations currently estimates that approximately *eight hundred million* people in developing countries are malnourished. Many more suffer from micronutrient malnutrition. Malnutrition, even in mild to moderate cases, multiplies the number of child deaths caused by infections. Given the importance of well nourished populations for world peace and security, Canada is contributing resources to help alleviate this situation. Canada has identified six development program priorities, one of which is basic human needs, including nutrition.

Canada is collaborating with international organizations to promote breastfeeding, improve the nutrition of young children, and eliminate micronutrient malnutrition for all age groups in developing countries. Canada has taken a leadership role in the global program to eliminate iodine deficiency disorders and vitamin A deficiency. It is estimated that 2.8 million children under five suffer from clinical vitamin A deficiency (xerophthalmia). Another 251 million children live where vitamin A depletion is prevalent, putting them at increased risk of mortality and blindness. Approximately 1,570 million people live in regions where iodine deficiency diseases are common, 656 million exhibit goitre and 5.7 million overt cretinism. Children born in these situations are at risk of impaired brain development. There is room for Canada to expand its work in the control of these disorders and other forms of malnutrition.

Canada's development assistance is used in activities to alleviate poverty and improve food access. One focus is to increase incomes of the absolute poor, including landless labourers and subsistence farmers. Canada continues to play an important role in the international Expanded Programme of Immunization. There are three fundamental needs for improvement of young child nutrition: control of infection (including health care, immunization, water and sanitation), adequate care including feeding practices, and access to adequate food (quantity and nutritional quality). This thrust characterizes Canada's approach in the basic needs aspect of official development assistance. A recent Canadian target in this area is to commit 25% of its ODA to basic human needs.

Research can improve food security and nutrition. Over the last three decades, international research has helped stimulate the production of staple foods for many countries. This research has solved problems related to yields, pests, diseases, management as well as food storage and preservation. Through international collaboration in the collection, exchange and study of agricultural and wild plant materials, crop varieties with superior agronomic and nutritional characteristics have been developed. Higher yields have improved the incomes and diets of poor farm families and rural labourers, provided more affordable food and better nutrition for urban dwellers, and stimulated economic growth in many countries. With superior crop varieties made available world wide, the farm and food sectors of all countries benefit in terms of improved productivity, better disease resistance and more sustainable use of natural resources. International research centres also help preserve global biodiversity, the rich endowment of plant and animal species.

Food safety and quality benefit from global networks. Canadians consume a growing volume of imported foods. In order to ensure that foreign products meet the same high quality standards as Canadian products, the exporting countries must have appropriate food safety and quality programs. In addition, foods imported into Canada are monitored to ensure that they meet the standards Canada sets for our own producers and processors. International organizations such as the Food and Agriculture Organization (FAO) help developing countries establish their own food safety and quality programs through technical assistance. The FAO and the World Health Organization (WHO) have developed international food standards through the Codex Alimentarius Commission. Canadians have contributed to the development of these international standards. As developing countries put into place their own food safety and quality programs, international food standards are increasingly being used. In addition to ensuring food quality, this harmonization of standards facilitates international trade and access to global food markets.

6. Indicators of Change

Monitoring change is an important part of efforts to maintain and improve the nutritional health of the population. A system based on core indicators can provide valuable information.

Sixteen core indicators are included in *Nutrition for Health: An Agenda for Action*. Thirteen have a national focus and three relate to international issues. A rationale for the selection of each indicator, plus measurement specifications and data sources, are provided in a background paper (Appendix 3).

It is recognized that a limited number of indicators cannot capture the full breadth and depth of nutrition-related conditions, or replace a comprehensive nutrition monitoring system. However, a system based on core indicators can provide information in order to:

• monitor changes over time in nutrition-related conditions;
• provide a warning of need to consider planned actions; and
• maintain awareness of the state of nutrition among the various sectors involved in nutrition planning.

Key criteria for the selection of the core indicators include a recognition of their importance with regards to nutrition, the availability of data on an ongoing basis, and the feasability of data collection. In order to develop a workable nutrition indicator system, it was essential to make use of existing and readily available data. Certain

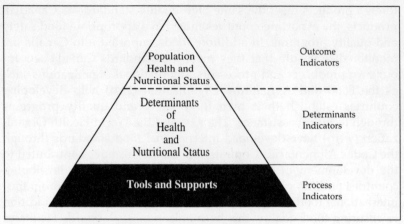

Model for the Selection of Nutrition-Related Indicators
Source: adapted from the "Framework for Population Health"

Core nutrition-related indicators

NATIONAL
Outcome Indicators:
potential years of life lost due to ischemic heart disease and stroke
prevalence of hypertension
incidence of certain site-specific cancers
incidence of low birth weight
prevalence of overweight and underweight
Determinant Indicators:
estimate intake of grains, fruits and vegetables
estimated intake of fat
level of recreational physical activity
initiation and duration of breastfeeding
nutrition awareness/attitudes
food bank use
cost of a "nutritious food basket" in relation to income
Process Indicator:
existence of a national multisectoral co-ordinating network

INTERNATIONAL
Outcome Indicators:
prevalence of iodine deficiency disorders worldwide
prevalence of vitamin A deficiency worldwide
Process Indicator:
Canada's total Official Development Assistance (ODA) as % of GNP and
proportion of ODA allotted to Basic Human Needs

indicators considered, therefore, were eliminated due to lack of data. The core indicators presented here will be reviewed and revised as dictated by need and the availability of data. In time, health promotion as well as health problem indicators will be more fully incorporated.

Data for the core nutrition indicators are available at the national level and for many of the indicators at the provincial and regional levels as well. In addition, data for many of the indicators are reported according to age groups, sex, and by proxy measures of socio-economic status.

The categories of core indicators are based on the Framework for Population Health. Core indicators include those that relate to outcomes, determinants and process.

The Framework for Population Health can be used for the development of national core indicators, and also provides a model for the collection of data according to the needs of different jurisdictions.

7. Action – A Shared Responsibility

Implementation, the next step, is the responsibility of all of us. The formation of networks of interested partners will allow for sharing of ideas and collaboration.

Implementation is the next step to *Nutrition for Health: An Agenda for Action* and is a shared responsibility. Individual commitment to improving nutritional health will be the stimulus for action. That action will be as unique as communities are unique. The flexible design and broad scope of this framework was intentional, in that it allows users to choose options best suited to their own needs and capacities.

The Joint Steering Committee believes that the formation of networks will be pivotal to implementation. Through networks, interested partners can share ideas, support one another, learn, collaborate and monitor progress. Joint Steering Committee members encourage users to establish networks appropriate for their own nutrition initiatives.

The cooperation of diverse sectors brought *Nutrition for Health* to this stage. That same cooperative spirit is needed to mobilize resources for the next phase. The establishment of a multisectoral network at the national level is recommended to provide leadership, coordination and ongoing support to the *Agenda for Action*.

Use *Nutrition for Health: An Agenda for Action* as a catalyst and support for:

- dialogue with decision makers and politicians;
- setting policy and advocating for policy change;
- discovering new channels of action;
- creating partnerships;
- gaining cooperation among agencies;
- establishing local goals and responsibilities;
- broadening support for nutrition;
- developing new products and services;
- expanding existing effective programs and services;
- setting priorities in programs, research, product development and resource allocation; and
- educating communities, community leaders, decision makers, media, clients, groups and agencies about the role of nutrition in health and their role in taking action.

Appendix 1   The *World Declaration on Nutrition* and *Global Plan of Action*: Highlights

Participating countries endorsed a *World Declaration on Nutrition* and a *Global Plan of Action for Nutrition*. The World Declaration on Nutrition affirms that "access to nutritionally adequate and safe food is a right of each individual." It further identifies nutrition as a precondition for the development of societies and a key objective of progress in human development. Asserting that nutritional well-being "must be at the centre of ... socio-economic development plans and strategies," the Declaration calls on countries to set measurable goals and timeframes for action on nutrition and food issues, with the overall goal of "nutritional well-being for all people in a peaceful, just and environmentally safe world." The *Global Plan for Action* sets out the following as universal objectives.

- Ensuring continued access by all people to sufficient supplies of safe foods for a nutritionally adequate diet
- Achieving and maintaining health and nutritional well-being of all people
- Achieving environmentally sound and socially sustainable development to contribute to improved nutrition and health
- Eliminating famines and famine deaths

To support achievement of these universal objectives, the Global Plan proposes nine theme areas for action, spanning the health, social, economic, environmental and foreign policy domains.

- Incorporating nutrition objectives, considerations and components into development policies and programmes
- Improving household food security
- Protecting consumers through improved food quality and safety
- Preventing and managing infectious diseases
- Promoting breastfeeding
- Caring for the socio-economically deprived and the nutritionally vulnerable
- Preventing and controlling specific micro-nutrient deficiencies
- Promoting appropriate diets and healthy lifestyles
- Assessing, analyzing and monitoring nutrition situations

Appendix 2 Members* of the Joint Steering Committee

Mr. E.M. Aiston (Chair)
Director General
International Affairs Directorate
Policy and Consultation Branch
Health Canada

Mrs. Iowne Anderson
Aboriginal Community
Representative
Ohsweken, Ontario

Ms. Carolyn Barber
Nutrition Coordinator
Department of Public Health
City of Toronto

Ms. Susan Beaubier
Nutrition Specialist
Indian and Northern Health
Services Directorate
Medical Services Branch
Health Canada

Dr. Micheline Beaudry
Professeure
Département de nutrition
humaine et de consommation
Faculté des sciences de
l'agriculture et de l'alimentation
Université Laval

Ms. Helen Brown
Senior Nutrition Consultant
Public Health Branch
Ontario Ministry of Health

Ms. Mary Bush
Nutrition Programs Officer
Systems for Health Directorate
Health Promotion and Programs
Branch
Health Canada

---

* Position at the time of involvement with the Joint Steering Committee (JSC). The work spanned the period of 1993 to 1996; some members moved to new positions and were not able to continue their involvement with the JSC.

Ms. Anne Carrow
Director, Nutrition
Health Promotion and Disease
Prevention
British Columbia Ministry of
Health

Ms. Carmen Connolly
Chief, Nutrition Programs Unit
Health Promotion Directorate
Health Programs and Services
Branch
Health Canada

Mrs. Mary Jane Green
Senior Advisor
International Affairs Directorate
Policy and Consultation Branch
Health Canada

Ms. Suzanne Hendricks
President
National Institute of Nutrition

Mr. H. Philip Hepworth
Director, Program Information
and Training
Cost Shared Programs Directorate
Social Development, Education
and Employment Group
Human Resources Development
Canada

Mr. Wardie Leppan
Executive Director
World Food Day Association of
Canada

Dr. Guy Nantel
Senior Scientific Advisor
Health Affairs Division
International Affairs Directorate
Health Canada

Mrs. Heather Nielsen
Nutrition Programs Officer
Systems for Health Directorate
Health Promotion and Programs
Branch
Health Canada

Dr. Sonya Rabeneck
Senior Nutrition Specialist
Multilateral Programs Branch
Canadian International
Development Agency

Mrs. Lina Robichon-Hunt
Technical Advisor – Nutrition
Food Programs
Centre for Food and Animal
Research
Agriculture and Agri-Food
Canada

Ms. Marsha Sharp
Chief Executive Officer
The Canadian Dietetic
Association

Ms. Christina Zehaluk
Nutritionist
Food Directorate
Health Protection Branch
Health Canada

The Joint Steering Committee would like to acknowledge the contribution of Barbara Davis, Lavada Pinder and Norman Tape in the development of *Nutrition for Health: An Agenda for Action*.

Appendix 3   Background Working Documents

In developing *Nutrition for Health: An Agenda for Action*, the following documents were commissioned:

- *Country Paper Canada–Supplement*, an updated and expanded version of the country paper submitted by Canada's delegation to the International Congress on Nutrition (ICN), that provides information and data on nutrition issues and activities in Canada.
- *Environmental Scan*, commissioned to elicit insights and views from leaders in industry, health, social services and economics on how to position nutrition as an integral element of a health strategy for Canada.
- *Nutrition in Action Survey*, a survey of activities in the area of nutrition and food, that assessed progress in key sectors on implementation of the 106 Action Towards Healthy Eating recommendations and action on the ICN theme areas.
- *Summary of the Regional Think Tank Sessions*, a series of "Think Tank" sessions held in Vancouver, Toronto, Halifax and Montreal, and drawing upon expertise from governments, the academic community, industry and non-governmental organizations, developed proposals for objectives, strategies and actions.
- *Food Quality and Safety Programs in Canada*, review of federal food regulatory programs, assessment/management of foodborne risk, new initiatives and emerging issues in food quality and education on safe food handling.
- *Review of National Programs*, review of Canadian programs relative to three ICN Themes; monitoring, preventing micronutrient diseases and preventing and managing infectious diseases.
- *A Report on the Use of Indicators in "Nutrition for Health: An Agenda for Action"*, identifies and describes key issues relating to the use of indicators, proposes core indicators and discusses rationale, measurement issues and sources of data.
- *The Consultation Summary Report*, a consolidation of the results of the nation-wide consultation process.

Nutrition for Health: An Agenda for Action and the above background working papers are available through Internet at: *http://www.hwc.ca* or by contacting a member of the Joint Steering Committee.

Index

Trust for Mutual Under-
standing, 36
Tubers, 147
Tumour: burden, 260;
growth, 258, 260; host
composition, 265; inci-
dence, 258–9; initia-
tion, 259; metastasis,
194; multiplicity, 258,
260; promotion, 259.
See also Cancer
Tumourigenesis, 258–62,
265
Tumours: chemically
induced, 258–60, 263;
colon, 217, 260;
induced by heterocy-
clic amines, 216; mam-
mary, 259–60, 262, 264;
skin, 258–9, 262; spon-
taneous, 259–60; trans-
planted, 259–60
Turkey, 68, 85
Twins, 104–5, 170

Ulcers, decubitus, 206
Underfeeding, effect on
cancer, 258–60
Undernutrition, 201
Underweight, 203, 290
UNICEF Regional Moni-
toring Study, 33
United States Agency for
International Develop-
ment (USAID), 33
United States Depart-
ment of Agriculture
(USDA), 6
United States Environ-
mental Protection
Agency's Environmen-
tal Committee, 38
University of California,
San Francisco, 26, 29
University of California's
Cardiovascular
Research Institute, 30
University: of Massachu-
setts, 36; of Pittsburgh,
36; of Wisconsin, 258
Urbanization, 105
Uremia, 120–1, 124

Uric acid, 51
Urinary: bladder, 216,
221; calcium excretion,
171–2; levels of MeIQx,
221; nitrate, 232–3;
potassium, 109, 113
Urine, 220, 229
Uterus, 262
Utrecht University, 7

Valsalva manœuvre, 110
Vascular resistance, 106,
110; peripheral, 107,
112; smooth muscle,
106–7
Vasoactive peptides,
endothelial derived,
106
Vasoconstrictor endothe-
lin, 106
Vasodilator, bradykinin,
107; insulin, 106
Vegetable: consumption,
45; hydrogenated, 51–
2, 54; intake, 12; liq-
uid, 65–6; oil, 70, 72–5,
85; protein, 60, 78
Vegetables, 84, 186, 196,
201; and breast cancer,
241; complex carbohy-
drate and micronutri-
ents, 8; consumption,
41, 43–4, 46, 59, 78, 81,
83, 85, 185, 192, 205,
231, 283; determinant
indicators, 290; in Med-
iterranean diet, 72; recipes, 86; source of fibre,
88, 147; source of
omega-3 fatty acids,
73; and stomach can-
cer, 228–9
Vegetarians, 173
Vein grafts, intimal
hyperplasia, 75
Ventricle, 108
Ventricular hypertrophy,
107–8, 112–13
Vertebrae, 168
Vertebral fracture, 202
Very low density lipopro-
tein (VLDL), 87, 245;

cholesterol, 93; effect
of dietary cholesterol,
62; effect of low-fat,
low cholesterol diet,
89; effect of omega-3
fatty acids, 51, 74–5;
levels, 92–3; overpro-
duction, 61, 79; produc-
tion, 81, 247; synthesis,
79–80, 88, 94. *See also*
Lipoprotein(s)
Vitamin A: deficiency,
288; effect of alcohol,
177; in foods, 201, 241;
function, 8; intake,
181, 200, 202, 204–5,
208; metabolism, 8; rec-
ommendation for
older adults, 207; trans-
port, 8. *See also* Retinal
Vitamin B_6, 205, 207–8
Vitamin B_{12}, 181, 202,
204–5, 207–8
Vitamin C: antioxidant
effects, 182–3; and car-
diovascular disease,
11; deficiency, 104, 205;
in foods, 186, 201, 241;
intake, 14, 181, 187,
200, 202, 204–5; recom-
mendation for older
adults, 207; require-
ment, 81
Vitamin D, 4; and cal-
cium absorption, 171;
intake, 202, 205, 208;
and osteoporosis, 167,
170–1, 202; recommen-
dation for older
adults, 207; sources,
174, 201
Vitamin E, 196; antioxi-
dant, 60, 78, 182–3;
effects of alcohol, 180,
182–3; intake, 180, 208;
recommendations for
older adults, 207;
requirement, 81
Vitamin K, 172, 205
Vitamins, 178; antioxi-
dant, 78; deficiency,
and drug use, 205;